NEUROSCIENCE RESEARCH PROGRESS

SHORT-TERM MEMORY

NEW RESEARCH

NEUROSCIENCE RESEARCH PROGRESS

Additional books in this series can be found on Nova's website under the Series tab.

Additional e-books in this series can be found on Nova's website under the e-book tab.

NEUROSCIENCE RESEARCH PROGRESS

SHORT-TERM MEMORY

NEW RESEARCH

GARIFALLIA KALIVAS
AND
SAPPHO F. PETRALIA
EDITORS

Nova Science Publishers, Inc.
New York

Library of Congress Cataloging-in-Publication Data

Short-term memory : new research / editors, Garifallia Kalivas and Sappho F. Petralia.
p. ; cm.
Includes bibliographical references and index.
ISBN 978-1-62100-860-6 (hardcover)
I. Kalivas, Garifallia. II. Petralia, Sappho F.
[DNLM: 1. Memory, Short-Term--physiology. WL 337]

612.823312--dc23

2011039652

Published by Nova Science Publishers, Inc. † New York

CONTENTS

PREFACE

The capacity for holding a small amount of information in mind in an active, readily available state for a short period of time is known as short-term memory. The duration of short-term memory (when rehearsal or active maintenance is prevented) is believed to be in the order of seconds. This book presents research in the shared object representation in visual short-term memory and visual attention; neuron-astroglial communication in short-term memory; visual short-term memory and the bilateral field advantage; working memory and language processing and reading acquisition; an in vitro model for analyzing the conversion of short-term to long-term memory and Cav2.1-mediated NMDA receptor signaling in short-term memory.

Chapter 1 - Although it is generally accepted that short-term memory and working memory deficits are prevalent among children with developmental dyslexia and attention-deficit/hyperactivity disorder (ADHD), the nature of the deficit remains under debate despite decades of research on the topic. Therefore, this chapter will review the literature on the topic, addressing several key issues. What are the disparities in the literature and some of the pertinent findings which underlie them? What are potential sources of these discrepancies? What role do comorbid diagnoses play in these findings? What are some potential neurobiological substrates that may underlie the short-term memory and working memory deficits in developmental dyslexia and ADHD? Finally, given the disparities in the research, what should be the authors' future directions on the topic?

Chapter 2 - For several decades the stated Holy Grail of chemical, biological and biophysical research into neocortical information processing has been to reduce such neocortical phenomena into specific bottom-up molecular and smaller-scale processes. Over the past three decades, with regard to short-term memory (**STM**) and long-term memory (**LTM**) phenomena, which themselves are likely components of other phenomena like attention and consciousness, a statistical mechanics of neocortical interactions (**SMNI**) approach has yielded specific details of **STM** capacity, duration and stability not present in molecular approaches, but it is clear that most molecular approaches consider it inevitable that their reductionist approaches at molecular and possibly even quantum scales will yet prove to be causal explanations of such phenomena. The **SMNI** approach is a bottom-up aggregation from synaptic scales to columnar and regional scales of neocortex, and has been merged with larger non-invasive **EEG** scales with other colleagues – all at scales much coarser than molecular scales. As with many Crusades for some truths, other truths can be trampled. It is proposed that an **SMNI** vector potential (**SMNI-VP**) constructed from magnetic fields induced by neuronal electrical firings, at thresholds of collective minicolumnar activity with laminar specification, can give rise to causal top-down mechanisms that effect molecular excitatory and inhibitory processes in **STM** and **LTM**. A specific example might be causal influences on momentum **p** of Ca^{2+} ions by the **SMNI-VP A**, as calculated by the canonical momentum **q**, $\mathbf{q} = \mathbf{p} - e\mathbf{A}$, where e is the electron coulomb charge, which may be applied either classically or quantum-mechanically. Such a smoking gun for top-down effects awaits forensic in vivo experimental verification, requiring appreciating the necessity and due diligence of including true multiple-scale interactions across orders of magnitude in the complex neocortical environment.

Chapter 3 - Visual short-term memory (VSTM) mediates the storage of visual information over a period of several seconds. Its relationship to visual attention has been the focus of much research. In this chapter the authors describe research investigating whether VSTM and visual attention share the same means of representing objects. First, the authors review the evidence and theories in the literature that relate visual attention and VSTM. From this review, the authors propose that VSTM and visual attention share the same object representations. Second, the authors describe new research investigating whether a process facilitating the perception of objects as being continuous over changes in space and time depend on both visual attention and VSTM. The tasks required participants to maintain the continuity of object representations as the display changed. The results suggested that periodically sampling visual information and matching it to representations in VSTM preserve object continuity. These experimental results support the claim that a critical link between VSTM and visual attention may be a shared means of representing objects.

Chapter 4 - It is thought that there is a very close structure-function relationship in cerebral neocortex and present neurobiological concepts regarding short-term and long-term memory are based on synaptic neurotransmission and plasticity. However, the diversity and complexity of neurocortical connections, circuits, maps and their relationships with superior cognitive functions are not fully understood requiring a re-evaluation of the classical approach. It is proposed that cerebral neocortex is organized fundamentally in two functionally complementary and closely interrelated three-dimensional structures formed by the neuronal and the astroglial networks, which in addition to chemical and electrical signals may communicate with each other through magnetic fields and electromagnetic waves. If ultra-weak electromagnetic waves (bio-photons) generated as cellular by-products of reactive oxygen species and reactive nitrogen species could play a biological function in information processing and short-term memory it must be under the driving of neuron-astroglial interactions. There is evidence that changes of bio-photonic activity is related to consciousness and other neuro-cognitive functions, suggesting that bio-photons may play some role in the function of the nervous system. Moreover, the discovery that human brain has magnetite nano-particles has opened new possibilities about the role of these nano-crystals in information processing and memory at quantum level. Neuro-electrophysiological data have shown a close correlation between external magnetic pulses and neural activity, which have been explained based on mechanical, chemical and specific spin-electronic mechanisms. This chapter reviews recent discoveries concerning the ability of neuronal cells to perceive and process electro-magnetic information, and put forward the possible role of bio-photons generated as consequence of neuronal and astroglial metabolisms in short-term memory. A final discussion concerns relationship between the bio-photonic activity and bio-electro-magnetic activity in the neocortex. The authors' present concept suggests that in the human cerebral cortex there is an electro-magnetic interplay between neurons and astrocytes that allows the generation of innumerable bio-phonic-mediated nano-holograms, which are based on magnetite-compounds associated to neuronal and astroglial membranes. In the present chapter the authors put forward that bio-photons generated by neuronal and astroglial metabolism may produce holographic pictures explaining retrieval of short-term and long-term memories as well as other neuro-cognitive representations such as dreams produced during sleep. The authors' hypothesis proposes that interactions between bio-electric, bio-magnetic and bio-photonic activities in neurons and astrocytes in the human neocortex may play important roles in cognitive functions, providing new perspectives for better understand complex functions of the central nervous system such as short-term memory.

Chapter 5 - Past research has demonstrated superior visual processing when the information is distributed across the left and right visual fields rather than within the same single hemifield. This effect is known as the *bilateral field advantage* (BFA). Recent studies have recently begun to investigate whether a BFA also arises in visual short-term memory (VSTM), with a direct effect on its storage capacity. In other words, the question is whether it is possible to remember more visual objects when they are distributed between the two hemifields than when they are all located within a single one.

The goal of this chapter is to provide a synthesis of the current data regarding the possible existence of a BFA in VSTM. Those data reveal that a BFA can be found in spatial short-term memory, namely when the task requires holding spatial information. However, no BFA has been found in object short-term memory (i.e., when the task is to hold detailed visual properties of the objects), unless attentional selective processes are dominantly engaged in the task, suggesting that the BFA is a general feature of selective attention.

Chapter 6 - Short-term working memory provides a basis for performance of current behavioral and cognitive tasks. It is based on repeated circulation of impulses in a circuit of neurons in the cortical and subcortical structures through which the perception of this information, its analysis and storage is carried out. Disruption of short-term working memory (and in particular of its spatial form) is observed in ageing and, to a greater extent, in Alzheimer's disease patients. Prenatal stress also leads to disruption of short-term memory in later life and according to authors' data one of the reasons of short-term memory deficit after prenatal hypoxia lies in a decrease in the number of synaptopodin-positive labile spines and the levels of activity and expression of a metallopeptidase neprilysin (NEP) which is involved in metabolism of some neuropeptides and, in particular, in amyloid β peptide degradation. As such, the authors postulate that there is a link between the decrease of the amyloid-degrading enzymes activity, in particular of NEP and a reduced number of labile interneuronal contacts which might be one of the reasons of short-term working memory decline caused by early development pathology, normal ageing or neurodegenerative deceases. This decline can be compensated by up-regulation of NEP expression and activity.

Chapter 7 - In the present chapter the author proposes an extension of the interactive model of short-term memory proposed by R. Martin and Lesch (1996), and R. Martin, Lesch, and Bartha (1999) – which was developed to capture word-level processing – so that it can capture, in addition, sentence-level information. The author will illustrate the extended model's explanatory power with data from a Greek-speaking agrammatic patient on four previously reported tasks: sentence repetition task, sentence grammaticality judgment task, sentence-picture matching task, sentence completion task.

Chapter 8 - Previous research has shown that the process of reading acquisition in Arabic by beginning readers is more challenging and might be slower than in other languages. Furthermore, recent study showed that reading in Arabic is slower than reading in other languages, even among skilled native Arabic speakers. This chapter summerize the role of short-term memory, represented by Working Memory (WM) measures in developmental reading problems, considering: 1) The unique contribution of WM to reading in language that has a unique and complex structure, Arabic; 2) Domain-general or -specific explanations of decoding and reading difficulties. Specifically, the chapter tries to explain whether a supra-lexical factor (working memory), affects meta-lingual performance, which is critical for the development of reading skill in Arabic language readers; and whether this effect differs with age, from 1st through 12th grade of school. Based on recent published studies, short-term memory was found to be involved in and affect phonemic manipulations at all grade levels: the longer the manipulated stimulus, the poorer the performance. The implications of these findings in addition to other aspects of the related issue are discussed.

Chapter 9 - Short-term memory is instantaneously established by modifying the synaptic transmission efficiency of existing synapses.

Long-Term Potentiation (LTP) of the rodent hippocampus is a cellular model most often used to investigate this instantaneous synaptic modification, as it has been shown that intense activity in an input pathway leads to an immediate enhancement in synaptic transmission efficiency.

Although such instantaneous synaptic modification is assumed to lead to structural changes that ensure life-long memory, how this conversion occurs is poorly understood. While morphological changes observed in the late phase of LTP are expected to offer some insight on the matter, the longevity of these changes is unknown. Using stable cultures of rodent hippocampal slices, the authors recently found that repeated, but not single, inductions of LTP lead to a distinct, slow developing and long lasting enhancement of synaptic strength coupled with the formation of new synapses, a phenomenon the authors name RISE (Repetitive LTP-Induced Synaptic Enhancement).

In this article, the authors describe fundamental properties of this novel synaptic plasticity phenomenon and propose an *in vitro* model for analyzing its cellular mechanisms that underlie the conversion of short- to long-term memory.

Chapter 10 - The Cav2.1 channel is highly expressed in the nervous system and regulates the presynaptic modulation of the glutamate release machinery. N-methyl-D-aspartate (NMDA)-receptor signaling mediates short-term memory. Because Cav2.1 and NMDA receptors are present at a variety of synapses, the use of systemic injections makes it difficult to evaluate the behavioral performance. In this regard, studies using microinfusions into specific neural regions are a useful tool to understand the relevant neuronal circuits. The antiepileptic drug levetiracetam has been reported to inhibit presynaptic Cav2.1 functions, reducing glutamate release. Rolling Nagoya mice carrying a mutation in the $\alpha1$ subunit of the Cav2.1 (Cav2.1$\alpha1$) demonstrate severe ataxia from about 2 weeks of age. Heterozygous rolling Nagoya (rol/+) mice show normal spontaneous alternations in behavior in the Y-maze test, a measure of short-term spatial memory. In this chapter, the authors have shown that a dose of levetiracetam injected into the hippocampus did not affect the controls but decreased the spontaneous alternation in rol/+ mice. The results suggest that the Cav2.1$\alpha1$ mutation, through a decrease in the Ca^{2+} influx, lowers the threshold for learning impairment and that Cav2.1-mediated NMDA receptor signaling in the hippocampus is involved in short-term spatial memory. The combination of the sub-threshold pharmacological and genetic approach presented here is easily performed and can be used to study functional signaling pathways in neuronal circuits.

In: Short-Term Memory: New Research
Editors: Garifallia Kalivas and Sappho F. Petralia
ISBN: 978-1-62100-860-6

Chapter 1

WORKING MEMORY FUNCTIONING IN DEVELOPMENTAL DYSLEXIA AND ADHD

Michelle Y. Kibby
Southern Illinois University-Carbondale, Department of Psychology
and Center for Integrated Research in Cognitive & Neural Sciences, IL, US

ABSTRACT

Although it is generally accepted that short-term memory and working memory deficits are prevalent among children with developmental dyslexia and attention-deficit/hyperactivity disorder (ADHD), the nature of the deficit remains under debate despite decades of research on the topic. Therefore, this chapter will review the literature on the topic, addressing several key issues. What are the disparities in the literature and some of the pertinent findings which underlie them? What are potential sources of these discrepancies? What role do comorbid diagnoses play in these findings? What are some potential neurobiological substrates that may underlie the short-term memory and working memory deficits in developmental dyslexia and ADHD? Finally, given the disparities in the research, what should be our future directions on the topic?

INTRODUCTION

Often the term 'short-term memory' (STM) is used to represent short-term storage of information when distracters are not present. It is believed to be a limited capacity system. This chapter will include STM via its focus on working memory in developmental dyslexia and ADHD. Working memory (WM) goes beyond STM by including both short-term storage and mental operations on the information stored, similar to RAM on a computer. When a task requires the active use of strategies to encode material, adds distracters, or adds concurrent tasks to the encoding or delay interval, many argue that the task goes from measuring STM to measuring WM. Working memory is used during mental arithmetic, problem-solving, fluid reasoning, and purposeful learning, among other tasks. Because Baddeley's model of WM is one of the most commonly used models in the developmental dyslexia literature and is often used in the ADHD literature, it will be the one used in this chapter.

Baddeley (1986) originally defined working memory as being comprised of three components, the central executive (CE) and two slave systems: the phonological loop (PL) and the visuospatial sketchpad (VSS). The phonological loop is the short-term storage buffer for verbal/auditory material, and the visuospatial sketchpad is the short-term storage buffer for visual and spatial material. The PL can hold as much material as an individual can say in 2 seconds. It is comprised of the phonological store (the storage buffer) and the subvocal rehearsal mechanism (the rehearsal mechanism used to maintain the memory trace in the store). The phonological store is assessed through the phonological similarity effect. The phonological similarity effect is when rhyming words are harder to recall than non-rhyming words, presumably because the store utilizes phonological codes, and rhyming words require discrimination amongst similar codes. Thus, if the store is functioning properly, individuals should perform worse when lists rhyme as compared to when they do not. The subvocal rehearsal mechanism is assessed through the word length effect. This effect is when lists of short words are easier to recall than lists of long words. Since long words take longer to say, they can be lost easier to decay during rehearsal compared to short words. Thus, when the subvocal rehearsal mechanism is working effectively, individuals should perform worse on lists containing long words than on lists containing short words. It should be noted that subvocal rehearsal mechanism as proposed by Baddeley is under some dispute, but given its common use in the literature, it will be used in the chapter. The visuospatial sketchpad likely has at least two subcomponents as well: one for static pictures and geometric patterns/figures and another for spatial material using grids, tones, movements, etc. (Logie, 1995). The nature of these two subcomponents is debated, but they have been shown to be separable in research (Abdullaev and Bechtereva, 1993; Della Sala, Gray, Baddeley, Allamano, and Wilson, 1999; Logie and Pearson, 1997).

Under most debate in this model is the central executive: what it is and what it does. Baddeley suggested that it is a multi-component attentional control system which is involved with focused attention when ignoring distractions, divided attention including dual task synchronization, attention switching such as flexibly switching attention from one task to another, and monitoring and updating information held in WM (Baddeley, 1986, 1996, 2002). It is believed to be domain general, involved with mental manipulation of both verbal and visual material.

Accordingly, the phonological loop and visuospatial sketchpad can be thought of as separate short-term memory systems, whereas the central executive is what brings the model from merely assessing STM to assessing WM. Recently Baddeley introduced a fourth component to his model, the episodic buffer (Baddeley, 1986, 2000). Because research in developmental dyslexia and ADHD does not focus on this newer component much, it will not be addressed in this chapter.

As a segue to the discussion on the topic, it is important to discuss what constitutes developmental dyslexia and ADHD. There is a great deal of debate on what should constitute the diagnosis of developmental dyslexia, although many agree it to be a biologically-based disorder of reading. There are two main definitions used in the field: the IQ-achievement discrepancy model, commonly referred to as 'dyslexia', and the poor reader definition, commonly referred to as 'poor readers'. Various other terms are used to label the disorder as well, such as 'reading disability' and 'reading disorder', along with 'developmental dyslexia', and one needs to read the Methods section carefully to see which operational definition is being used. I will use the term 'dyslexia' when referring to the discrepancy definition, 'poor reader' when referring to the poor reader definition, and 'reading disorder' (RD) or developmental dyslexia when lumping them together into one group.

At the source of this debate is the argument over what constitutes developmental dyslexia. Some believe it to be a genetically-based, specific disorder in reading despite average intellect, adequate sensory/motor functioning, and adequate education. Proponents of this definition are the World Federation of Neurology (1968) and the Orton Dyslexia Society (1994). Many of the researchers in this camp adhere to the IQ-achievement discrepancy definition in some form. Others believe that IQ is irrelevant to the definition of RD, as long as the child is not mentally retarded, and all that matters for the definition is below average reading ability. Linda Siegel (Siegel, 1988) is one of the forerunners of this approach. Researchers in this camp believe that since phonological processing is a core deficit in RD, and both dyslexia and poor reader groups have poor phonological processing, an IQ-achievement discrepancy is irrelevant to the definition. Moreover, an IQ-achievement discrepancy often disqualifies poor readers with below average IQ who are greatly in need of services.

Also of interest is the type of reading deficit required for a diagnosis of developmental dyslexia. This chapter will focus on children with deficits in basic reading, regardless of whether having dyslexia or being a poor reader. Basic reading includes word identification, decoding of words and non-words, and reading rate (often called reading fluency). The chapter will not focus on reading comprehension, as different, but overlapping, skills contribute to reading comprehension as compared to basic reading. Many believe developmental dyslexia to be a disorder of basic reading (Orton Dyslexia Society, 1994), whereas poor reading comprehension, when not due to a deficit in basic reading, is a separate disorder (see Vukovic and Siegel, 2006).

There is relatively less controversy over the definition of Attention-Deficit/Hyperactivity Disorder (ADHD), as most researchers use the DSM to diagnose it. The DSM-IV discusses three subtypes, two of which are ADHD Predominately Inattentive type (ADHD-PI) and ADHD Combined type (ADHD-C). ADHD-PI requires at least 6 symptoms of inattention, such as distractibility, forgetfulness, and daydreaming, symptoms commonly related to poor sustained attention. ADHD-C requires at least 6 symptoms of inattention and 6 symptoms of hyperactivity/impulsivity for diagnosis. Most individuals with ADHD who are school-aged or older do not have the Hyperactive/Impulsive type (see Mash and Wolfe, 2010), and it is questionable whether it should be a separate subtype at all (Mash and Wolfe); therefore, this subtype will not be addressed in the chapter.

Why focus on developmental dyslexia and ADHD together in one chapter? Simply put, it is their comorbidity. Developmental dyslexia occurs in approximately 20-40% of children with ADHD, and ADHD occurs in approximately 15-40% of children with RD (Shaywitz, Fletcher, and Shaywitz, 1995; Semrud-Clikeman et al., 1992; Willcutt and Pennington, 2000). Both disorders are heterogeneous in their causes, even beyond definitional issues, with some of the contributors overlapping between the two disorders and some of them differing. To better illustrate this point, some individuals with RD have reduced processing speed (Shanahan et al., 2006), poor executive functioning (de Jonge and de Jonge, 1996; de Jong, 1998; Meltzer, 1991; Nigg, Hinshaw, Carte, and Treuting, 1998; Reiter, Tucha, and Lange, 2005; Willcutt et al., 2001), poor orthographic functioning (Berninger and Abbott, 1994;

Olson, Forsberg, Wise, and Rack, 1994) and/or slow retrieval of phonemes from long-term memory (Bowers, Sunseth, and Golden, 1999; Sunseth and Bowers, 2002). Most children with RD have poor phonological processing, which is why it is believed to be a core deficit in RD (Brady, 1991; Gottardo, Stanovich, and Siegel, 1996; Swank, 1994; Wagner, Torgesen, and Rashotte, 1994). Nonetheless, some children with RD have additional deficits, and a minority has intact phonological processing. Despite differing contributors, they still meet criteria for the disorder according to the RD definition used. The disorder of ADHD also is quite heterogeneous in its etiologies. Although a majority of these children have deficits in at least one aspect of executive functioning, some do not (see Nigg, Willcutt, Doyle, and Sonuga-Barke, 2005). Some have slow processing speed (Shanahan et al., 2006). Nonetheless, most do not have problems with phonological processing unless they have comorbid RD (Purvis and Tannock, 2000; Shaywitz, et al., 1995; Willcutt et al., 2001). Given the two disorders' comorbidity, it is important to control for one disorder when studying the other; otherwise, one is unable to know if the findings are driven by the disorder of interest or a comorbid one.

DEVELOPMENTAL DYSLEXIA

Most researchers have found children with developmental dyslexia to be impaired on measures of verbal STM, irrespective of the RD definition used. This is true regardless of whether tasks include serial ordered recall of words, digits, or nonwords (see Alloway and Gathercole, 2006; Baddeley, 1986; Jorm, 1983; Mann, Cowin, and Schoenheimer, 1989; McDougall, 1994; Snowling, 1991; Wagner and Torgesen, 1987). These types of measures encourage phonetic coding of material (Henry, 2001; Swank, 1994). In contrast, the literature on visual STM and the central executive is more varied in its findings.

Phonological Loop

Overview. As just noted, many researchers find children with developmental dyslexia to have impaired verbal short-term memory. What is under debate is why. Some suggest that it is due to children with RD having faulty phonological codes which leads to the phonological store being highly defective to abolished (Mann, Liberman, and Shankweiler, 1980; Shankweiler, Liberman, Mark, Fowler, and Fischer, 1979). These researchers failed to find the phonological similarity effect in RD. However, some have found the phonological similarity effect to be intact in RD when floor effects are controlled (Hall, Wilson, Humphreys, Tinzmann, and Bowyer, 1983; Johnston, 1982), which suggests the store is intact. Others state that the source of the verbal STM deficit lies outside of the phonological store, perhaps due to slow articulation rate in RD since the phonological loop can hold as much as one can articulate in 2 seconds (McDougall, 1994; McDougall, Hulme, Ellis, and Monk, 1994). Some researchers suggest the deficit is due to poor subvocal rehearsal (Bauer, 1977; Done and Miles, 1978), but others have found the word length effect to be intact in RD (Baddeley, 1986; McDougall and Donohoe, 2002; McDougall, et al., 1994). Still others suggest that the STM deficit is related to poor central executive functioning in RD (de Jong,

1998; Isaki and Plante, 1997; Siegel, 1994; Swanson and Ashbaker, 2000). Given the controversy in the literature, this issue was of particular interest to me.

Study 1. In a carefully designed study[1] (Kibby, Marks, Morgan, and Long, 2004), we assessed working memory in dyslexia according to Baddeley's model (1986). Participants included 20 typically developing controls and 20 children with dyslexia, ages 9-13 years. The groups were equated on IQ, gender, socio-economic status (SES), and history of ADHD. They also were comparable in arithmetic and articulation rate. Neither group had a history of neurological disorder or psychiatric disorder other than ADHD.

The phonological loop was assessed through a word list task. The lists were comprised of 3, 5, or 7 words that were not easily clustered semantically. The lists either rhymed or did not rhyme to assess the phonological store via the phonological similarity effect, and they were comprised of either one or three syllable words to assess the subvocal rehearsal mechanism via the word length effect. All lists were to be repeated in serial order. This resulted in a 2 (group membership) X 3 (list length) X 2 (phonemic similarity) X 2 (word length) X 3 (level of central executive load) design. The word lists were equated for age of acquisition, concreteness and word frequency in English. The central executive was assessed through dual-task performance, with participants having to perform a concurrent motor task of moderate or high load during list presentation on two thirds of the trials (1/3 of the trials for each type of load). A third of the trials only required learning of the lists (no central executive load). The visuospatial sketchpad was assessed through learning a series of spatial positions as discussed in the visuospatial section on developmental dyslexia. All within-subject conditions were counter-balanced.

Analysis revealed all main effects were significant and in the expected direction. There were two significant interactions: between group membership, phonemic similarity and central executive load and between group membership, phonemic similarity and word length. In terms of the former interaction, children with dyslexia did not show a phonological similarity effect at any level of central executive load. Controls had a significant phonological similarity effect under moderate load and no central executive load conditions, but they did not show a phonological similarity effect under high central executive load, hitting a floor in performance. In terms of the central executive, although both groups performed better under no central executive load than under dual-task conditions, children with dyslexia did not perform differentially worse on the lists with increasing central executive load. If the central executive were impaired, one would expect an additional decrease in performance with increasing central executive load as compared to controls. Because the central executive was found to be intact in the visual condition as well, and it may be domain-general, these findings suggest that it is intact in dyslexia. Hence, the deficits in verbal STM memory are not likely due to central executive dysfunction in dyslexia.

Analysis of the group X phonemic similarity X word length interaction revealed an intact word length effect for both groups. In contrast to controls, the dyslexia group showed a significant phonological similarity effect for short words but not long words. The control group showed a significant phonological similarity effect for short and long words. These results suggest the subvocal rehearsal mechanism is intact in dyslexia, consistent with the findings of Baddeley (1986). In contrast, the phonological store appears to function with

[1] Please refer to the Kibby, Marks et al., 2004 article for a more thorough description of the study and additional information.

reduced effectiveness, as it was intact for words with less of a phonological load (short words), but it was impaired for words with more of a phonological load (long words). This result helps to rectify earlier findings of an abolished phonological store in RD due to lack of a phonological similarity effect (Mann et al., 1980; Shankweiler, et al., 1979) with later findings suggesting the phonological similarity effect, and thus the store, is intact in developmental dyslexia (Hall et al., 1983; Holligan and Johnston, 1988; Johnston, 1982).

When analyzing predictors of verbal short-term memory performance in the children with dyslexia under the no central executive load condition, articulation rate, verbal IQ and word identification were not significant predictors, but a measure highly sensitive to phonological processing was, pseudoword decoding. This lead to my interest in whether the verbal STM deficit could be accounted for by simply poor phonological awareness which leads to defective input/encoding of material, or if it was due to a defective phonological store itself, or a combination of the two.

Study 2. In a subsequent study[2] (Kibby, 2009b), I tested four possible contributors to the verbal STM deficit in developmental dyslexia: slow articulation rate (Baddeley. 1986; McDougall et al., 2004), an impaired phonological store (Kibby, Marks, et al., 2004; Mann, et al., 1980; Shankweiler, et al., 1979), poor phonological awareness which affects phonological coding into verbal STM (Kibby, Marks, et al., 2004; Mark, Shankweiler, Liberman, and Fowler, 1977; Torgesen, 1985; Wagner, et al., 1994), and fewer/poorer quality long-term memory (LTM) representations of items for STM to use (McDougall and Donohoe, 2002; Roodenrys and Stokes, 2001). The central executive was not examined as it has been shown to be intact in dyslexia when the definition focuses on basic reading and deficits in short-term storage are controlled (Kibby and Cohen, 2008; Kibby, Marks, et al., 2004; Roodenrys, Koloski, and Grainger, 2001). Baddeley's (1986) model of the phonological loop was used, including the phonological similarity effect and the word length effect, to study the phonological store and subvocal rehearsal mechanism, respectively.

Participants included 18 children with dyslexia and 18 typically developing controls, without a history of ADHD, other psychiatric disorder or neurological disorder. Participants were between 9 and 14 years of age. Groups were equated for nonverbal intelligence, age, grade, socio-economic status, and gender. They differed in Verbal IQ so Verbal IQ was used as a covariate in the analyses, as above average Verbal IQ in the controls would contribute to the verbal STM differences found. When Verbal IQ was statistically controlled, groups were comparable in articulation rate but differed in phoneme deletion, a measure of phonological awareness requiring segmenting and blending of phonemes (taken from McDougall et al., 2004), with the dyslexia group performing worse. Despite this, articulation rate also was used as a covariate in the analyses because my goal was to see if groups differed in verbal STM even when articulation rate and Verbal IQ were statistically controlled.

There were 2 blocks in this experiment: one assessing the phonological store and the other assessing the subvocal rehearsal mechanism. Items in a given list were either highly frequent words (early age of acquisition), less frequent words (late age of acquisition), or presumably novel items (pronounceable nonwords) for both blocks. Thus, the phonological store block utilized a 2 (group membership) X 3 (item frequency) X 2 (similarity: rhyming or not) design, and the subvocal rehearsal block utilized a 2 (group membership) X 3 (frequency) X 2 (length: one or three syllables) design. Lists did not rhyme in the subvocal

[2] Please refer to the Kibby, 2009b article for a more thorough description of the study and additional information.

rehearsal block, and the phonological store block utilized all one syllable stimuli. Participants were instructed to recall the lists in serial order.

In the subvocal rehearsal block, significant main effects were found for group and length, and there were group X length and group X frequency interactions. Articulation rate was a significant covariate; Verbal IQ was not. In terms of the word length interaction, both groups had significant length effects, but the control group's was larger. This difference in word length effect likely was related to range effects, as the dyslexia group recalled fewer items than controls in general. Moreover, as the word length effect in dyslexia may be influenced by the amount of phonological processing required (Kibby, Marks, et al., 2004), phoneme deletion was added as a covariate in the analysis. When this was done, the group X length interaction was no longer significant, but the length X phonological awareness interaction was. These findings suggest that the subvocal rehearsal mechanism is intact in dyslexia, similar to what has been found by others (Baddeley, 1986; Kibby, Marks, et al., 2004; McDougall and Donohoe, 2002; McDougall, et al., 1994). Hence, it likely is not the source of the verbal STM deficit in dyslexia. In terms of the group X frequency interaction, groups were quite comparable on frequent words, but controls performed better on the low frequency words and nonwords.

For the phonological store block, MANCOVA revealed a significant main effect for group, and articulation rate was a significant covariate. The three-way interaction also was significant: group X frequency X similarity. Similar to the subvocal rehearsal block, group differences in performance increased as items became less frequent. The dyslexia group did not display a significant phonological similarity effect at any level of item frequency. Controls displayed the typical phonological similarity effect for frequent items, but a reversed similarity effect for low frequency items and a non-significant effect for nonwords. This suggests that the store is impaired in dyslexia even when controlling for articulation rate and verbal intellect, consistent with prior work in this area (Kibby, Marks, et al., 2004; Rack, Snowling, and Olson, 1992; Roodenrys, et al., 2001; Swanson and Ashbaker, 2000; Swanson and Howell, 2001). A discussion of control findings will follow shortly.

Prior research has suggested two primary sources contribute to verbal STM for words in general: articulation rate and long-term memory (LTM) representations (Hulme, Maughan, and Brown, 1991; Roodenrys, Hulme, and Brown, 1993). I found that for both blocks of the verbal STM task, children with dyslexia performed worse on low frequency words but quite similarly to controls on high frequency words, even when a measure of phonological awareness was controlled along with Verbal IQ and articulation rate. As the words used for the frequent condition had a young age of acquisition, it is quite likely that the children with dyslexia knew them and had good LTM representations for them. In contrast, they likely did not have good LTM representations for the low frequency/high age of acquisition words due to weaknesses in semantic/lexical knowledge as they had lower verbal intellect than controls and likely had less exposure to the words via more limited exposure to grade level and higher text (Cunningham and Stanovich, 1993; McDougall and Donohoe, 2002; Stadler, 1993; Torgesen, 1985).

Going beyond the work of Hulme and colleagues I believe that verbal STM is multi-faceted, with contributors to it varying with the type of material being utilized. Thus, articulation rate and LTM representations are two probable contributors to verbal STM, but there are likely others as well such as effectiveness of the phonological store itself and phonological awareness which affects encoding. The entire sample was used to test this assertion given small sample size. Phoneme deletion, articulation rate, Verbal IQ and word identification were entered into regression equations to assess how well they predicted verbal STM for the various types of material. When using Stepwise linear regression, performance on low frequency words was predicted by articulation rate and Verbal IQ, but verbal STM for high frequency words was predicted by articulation rate alone. Given that all participants likely knew the high frequency words, it is not surprising that Verbal IQ did not enter the high frequency word equation. Nonword STM performance was predicted by phoneme deletion and articulation rate. Word identification ability did not enter into any equation.

The findings, when taken together, suggest all four beliefs on the source of the verbal STM deficit in RD are correct. Articulation rate was a significant covariate in both MANCOVA equations, and it was related to all types of material studied in the regression equations. Thus, slow articulation rate likely contributes to reduced verbal STM performance when it is present in a given individual. Some children with RD have slow articulation rate in general (McDougall et al., 2004; Roodenrys and Stokes, 2001), and some had slow articulation rate in this sample, as the dyslexia group had a longer mean articulation rate than controls, just not significantly so. In the regression equations phonological awareness predicted STM for nonwords, which are encoded phonetically. Children with dyslexia had reduced phonological awareness in this study, and typically do in general, so poor phonological awareness likely contributes to the verbal STM deficit in RD. This may be especially true for novel items, given the additional decrement in performance in dyslexia as compared to controls during the nonword condition. Nonetheless, the deficit in verbal STM in dyslexia likely goes beyond this, as reduced verbal STM was found when phonological awareness was controlled. Based on the phonological store block and prior research in this area (Kibby, Marks, et al., 2004; Mann, et al., 1980; Rack, et al., 1992; Roodenrys, et al., 2001; Swanson and Ashbaker, 2000; Swanson and Howell, 2001), the phonological store appears to function less effectively in RD, even when articulation rate, Verbal IQ, and phonological awareness are controlled. Finally, children with dyslexia performed worse than controls on low frequency words, likely related to fewer/worse quality LTM representations for them as noted above. Overall, these findings suggest that the phonological store and phonological awareness are impaired in RD, affecting verbal STM for items that are coded phonetically. In contrast, verbal STM for familiar words is intact, and the deficit in STM for less common words may be the result of fewer/poorer quality LTM representations for these words. When slow articulation rate is present, it affects verbal STM for all types of verbal material.

As reported earlier, controls' performance on the phonological store block varied, demonstrating the expected phonological similarity effect for familiar words, a reversed similarity effect for less common words, and a non-significant effect for nonwords. When asked about what strategy they used for less common words, they stated that they would say words that rhymed for items on the phonetically similar lists. This strategy was not available for the phonetically dissimilar lists. This report is consistent with behavioral observations and suggests that they were using a phonetic coding/retrieval strategy for these lists. In contrast, children with dyslexia did not have a reversed phonological similarity effect for the less common words. Instead, they continued to try to provide words on the list. Neither group had a significant phonological similarity effect in the nonword condition, but both groups showed a slight reversed similarity effect. Neither group could use a semantic/lexical strategy here.

Baddeley's model proposes a unitary verbal store which utilizes phonological codes. According to Hulme and colleagues (1991), LTM contributions aid retrieval of the words when partially decayed in the phonological store. Much of the research cited thus far utilizes this approach. Nonetheless, the work of Martin and colleagues (Martin and Romani, 1994; Martin, Shelton, and Yaffee, 1994) suggests there are at least two verbal short-term storage mechanisms: one for semantically coded material and one for phonetically coded material. The neuroimaging literature is consistent with this, with the pars triangularis being the potential site of the subvocal rehearsal mechanism, the supramarginal gyrus being the potential site of the phonological store, and multiple areas being involved with short-term storage of items by their meaning including the temporal lobes and prefrontal regions (Baddeley, 1998; Cabeza and Nyberg, 2000; Fiez et al., 1996; Jonides et al., 1998; Kibby et al., 2004; Smith and Jonides, 1997).

Commensurate with the notion of two verbal STM systems, I consistently have found children with dyslexia to be impaired in phonological STM but comparable to controls for semantically coded material, even when using different samples and different measures (Kibby, 2009a, 2009b; Kibby and Cohen, 2008). Others also have found dyslexia to be intact for stories/passages and familiar word lists that can be coded semantically (Lee and Obrzut, 1994; McDougall and Donohoe, 2002) but impaired on material that is coded/stored phonetically (Swank, 1994; Wagner et al., 1994). Taking my 2004 and 2009 studies together, children with dyslexia are better able to successfully use their phonological store when items/lists are less challenging phonetically (Kibby, Marks, et al., 2004; Kibby, 2009a,b). They are more likely to opt for another strategy, such as semantic coding/storage, when words/lists have more of a phonological load. Prior research suggests children with dyslexia prefer coding/storing items by their meaning rather than phonetically (Waterman and Lewandowski, 1993).

While it is interesting to note that the verbal STM deficit in RD is likely multifaceted in nature, another important issue is whether verbal STM contributes to reading performance. Some argue that verbal STM is related to reading performance but does not contribute substantially to it. Rather, both verbal STM and reading ability are affected by phonological awareness, which is frequently deficient in RD (Rapala and Brady, 1990; Wadsworth, DeFries, Fulker, and Olson, 1995). In contrast, others suggest that verbal STM is an important contributor to reading performance even when controlling phonological awareness (Cormier and Dea, 1997; Gathercole, Willis, and Baddeley, 1991; Hansen and Bowey, 1994; Tractenberg, 2002). In the present chapter I used hierarchical regression to determine how well verbal IQ, phoneme deletion, and verbal STM predicted basic reading performance, with the variables being entered in this order. Verbal IQ and phonological awareness were significant predictors of word identification. In contrast, phonological awareness and verbal STM were predictive of pseudoword decoding. Thus, verbal STM may play less of a role in identifying words, but it is related to the decoding of novel items, helping to reconcile the two camps of research in this area.

In my follow-up study assessing the 2004 and 2009 samples on clinical measures, similar results were found (Kibby, 2009a). The study included material coded semantically from the 2004 sample (Wide Range Assessment of Memory and Learning [WRAML], STM for stories) and the 2009 sample (California Verbal Learning Test, Children's Version [CVLT-C], STM free recall of a word list containing items that are easily clustered semantically). The study also included material coded phonetically (WRAML number/letter span from the 2004 sample). Material coded semantically was not related to basic reading ability, but material coded phonetically was. Number/letter span was moderately related to word recognition and highly correlated with pseudoword decoding. In a separate sample (Kibby and Cohen, 2008), a different measure of phonological STM (Children's Memory Scale [CMS] Numbers Forward) was related to word identification to a small degree, explaining 4% of the variance when verbal IQ and phonological awareness were controlled, but it was not significant when a measure of verbal working memory was entered into the equation (Sequences).

How phonological STM contributes to basic reading ability is unclear, but some suggest it may play a role in decoding by providing a buffer where words are held while sound segmentation and blending take place (Baddeley, 1986; Snowling, 1991; Wagner and Torgesen, 1987). Thus, phonological STM may be involved with word identification only when decoding is required. Reading unknown words encourages use of a decoding approach. Reading phonetically-regular words may facilitate use of a decoding strategy as well. Therefore, presence of a significant correlation between phonological STM and word identification may depend upon the percentage of unknown and phonetically regular words in the word identification list, as well as the type of STM task used and power. In contrast to word identification, phonological STM is more consistently related to pseudoword identification because it requires decoding of all items. Hence, phonological STM's relationship with word identification is variable, possibly depending upon the amount of decoding required, whereas the relationship between phonological STM and decoding is more consistent. This proposition helps to explain the variable findings in the literature on verbal STM in basic reading. Clearly further research in this area is indicated.

Visuospatial Sketchpad

There is some controversy over the presence of visual STM deficits in developmental dyslexia. While some researchers have found visual or visual-spatial STM deficits in RD, many have not when the possibility for verbal coding was controlled (for reviews see Jorm, 1983; Mann, Cowin, and Schoenheimer, 1989; McDougall, 1994; Snowling, 1991; Torgesen, 1985). Nonetheless, a study using spatial positions with limited possibility for verbal coding showed a visual-spatial STM deficit in RD (Morrison, Giordani, and Nagy, 1977). Kaplan and colleagues (Kaplan, Dewey, Crawford, and Fisher, 1998) also found deficits in visual STM for spatial positions in RD. Moreover, when studying the central executive and visual-spatial sketchpad in poor readers, Swanson and colleagues found poor memory for position as well as poor memory for words, especially when central executive demands were high, displaying a domain-general deficit in working memory (Swanson, Ashbaker, and Lee, 1996; Swanson and Howell, 2001). Thus, it was important to me to examine this issue while controlling potential central executive deficits.

In the 2004 study described previously (Kibby, Marks et al., 2004)[1], the visual-spatial sketchpad was assessed in a separate block from the phonological loop, using Baddeley's (1986) model. This block included the same 40 participants as the phonological loop block. All participants had to learn and recall a series of spatial positions, being 3, 5, or 7 items long. The positions were presented one at a time on a 4 X 4 grid, and participants were asked to retrieve the positions by pointing to them in order after a 3 second delay interval. Identical to the phonological loop block, the central executive was assessed through dual-task performance, with participants having to perform a concurrent motor task of moderate or high difficulty during list presentation on two thirds of the trials (1/3 of the trials for each type of load). A third of the trials only required learning of the lists (no central executive load). This resulted in a 2 (group membership) X 3 (list length) X 3 (amount of central executive load) design.

Results indicated significant main effects for the within subject variables: list length and central executive load. In contrast, the group membership main effect was highly non-significant. This suggests that the visual-spatial sketchpad and central executive are intact in dyslexia. Furthermore, my later research found visual-spatial STM to be intact in dyslexia when using different measures and samples. More specifically, in a clinic sample of dyslexia, ADHD, comorbid dyslexia/ADHD and controls, children with dyslexia were found to be intact on visual and spatial STM as compared to those without dyslexia; there was no interaction between dyslexia and ADHD diagnosis (Kibby and Cohen, 2008). The measures used included CMS Picture Locations and Dot Locations (visual-spatial) and Faces (visual, non-spatial). Moreover, in a university laboratory setting using the 2004 sample (Kibby, Marks, et al., 2004), children with dyslexia were found to be intact on the visual measures from the WRAML which include both visual/non-spatial and visual-spatial measures of STM (Kibby, 2009a). Hence, the visual-spatial sketchpad likely is intact in RD when the dyslexia definition is used and the presence of ADHD is controlled (Jeffries and Everatt, 2004; Jorm, 1983; McDougall, et al., 1994; also see the reviews on STM mentioned earlier). The former is important because poor readers, who are more likely to have below average IQ, may be more likely to have broad ranging deficits in cognition that extend beyond phonological processing. The latter is important because children with ADHD have been shown to have deficits in visual-spatial STM, which will be discussed more thoroughly in the ADHD section.

Central Executive

In the 1980s it was more commonly believed that executive dysfunction may be a robust contributor to developmental dyslexia. For example, several researchers found poor strategy usage, poor self-monitoring and self-regulation during cognitive tasks, and difficulty coordinating and integrating information to solve a problem (Brown and Palincsar, 1989; Short and Ryan, 1984; Swanson, 1989; Swanson, Cochran, and Ewers, 1989; for a review see Meltzer, 1991). As a result, some believed RD to be caused by a deficit in the ability to coordinate the multiple processes involved with reading rather than a deficit in a basic component such as phonological and/or orthographic processing (see Meltzer, 1991). Although some currently believe that at least a portion of children with RD have executive dysfunction (Altemeier, Abbott, and Berninger, 2008; Asbjørnsen, Helland, Obrzut, and Boliek, 2003; de Jong et al., 2009; Willcutt, et al., 2001), the focus on executive functioning largely fell by the wayside in the 90s when the focus on phonological processing became prominent.

Nonetheless, executive functioning has remained of interest to working memory researchers studying RD. Here the controversy focused on whether the WM deficit is in the phonological loop component and/or the central executive component. Central executive functioning is one aspect of executive functioning in general. As discussed in the phonological loop section, several researchers believe that the phonological loop is affected in

RD, along with phonological awareness, and both phonological awareness and phonological STM are believed to be separable but inter-related aspects of phonological processing, a core deficit in RD (Wagner et al., 1994). In contrast, other researchers believe there is a domain general deficit in WM in RD affecting WM for all types of material, with the source of the deficit being poor central executive functioning (de Jong, 1998; Swanson et al., 1996; Swanson and Howell, 2001; Swanson and Sachse-Lee, 2001). Hence, the working memory literature reflects the overall debate in the literature over whether the deficits in RD are primarily phonological or executive in nature, or a combination of the two.

In terms of the central executive in particular, the literature on developmental dyslexia has been disparate. Various researchers have found the central executive to be affected in RD (de Jong, 1998; Swanson and Howell, 2001; Swanson and Sachse-Lee; 2001; Willcutt et al., 2001). A primary researcher on the central executive in RD is Swanson. He has indicated that poor central executive functioning is a common deficit in reading disabilities (Swanson, 2006; Swanson, et al., 1996) and that children with learning disabilities have difficulty coordinating the multiple skills involved with reading (Swanson, 1989). This notion is consistent with what was suggested by Meltzer (1991), as noted above. Swanson (2006) suggested that the deficits in the central executive in RD are related to difficulty with controlled attention processing (allocating attention appropriately in dual task situations, suppressing conflicting/irrelevant information, updating information held in WM). He has frequently found deficits in central executive functioning using various tasks in poor readers. For example, Swanson and colleagues have found central executive deficits when using verbal and visual material during complex span tasks, updating tasks, tasks involving distracters, and concurrent task performance (see Swanson, 2006). As a result, he has stated that there is a domain-general central executive deficit, as well as a deficit in the phonological loop, in poor readers (Swanson et al., 1996; Swanson, 2006). Nevertheless, others have found the central executive to be intact in RD when deficits in the slave systems, the phonological loop and visuospatial sketchpad, are controlled (Kibby et al., 2004, Kibby and Cohen, 2008; Roodenrys et al., 2001).

What appear to be key issues here is the definition of RD used, whether phonological loop deficits are controlled when assessing the central executive in verbal WM, how well comorbid diagnoses are controlled, and whether there are reading comprehension problems along with problems in basic reading. More specifically, the work by Kibby and colleagues (2004, 2008) used a dyslexia definition of RD, which tends to result in specific deficits in phonological processing at a group level (see Bishop and Snowling, 2004). Thus, when using this definition, problems in the central executive may be less common, whereas deficits in the phonological loop are frequent. In contrast, the work by Swanson and colleagues often used a poor reader definition. Poor readers are more likely to have deficits that extend beyond poor phonological processing to include various other cognitive and linguistic skills related to the lower IQ in this group (Bishop and Snowling). Hence, this group may be more likely to have central executive dysfunction along with executive dysfunction in general.

In some studies on RD, verbal WM deficits may be found because the effects of the phonological loop and phonological awareness deficits are not controlled. Thus, while it may look like children with dyslexia have verbal WM deficits that are due to the central executive, it may be that the WM deficits are due to a faulty phonological store and/or poor phonological processing/coding. In terms of comorbid diagnoses, both dyslexia and poor readers are comorbid with ADHD, and some children with ADHD have central executive deficits

(Barkley, 1997; Korkman and Pesonen, 1994; Mariani and Barkley, 1997; Shue and Douglas, 1992.bio-ph]). Therefore, if a study does not control for the presence of ADHD, central executive deficits may be found related to the ADHD rather than RD specifically. Finally, Swanson and Berninger (1995) noted that poor phonological loop functioning is more related to deficits in word identification, whereas poor central executive functioning is more related to deficits in reading comprehension. Given that dyslexia often is associated with a specific deficit in phonological processing and basic reading without additional reading comprehension problems, it follows that the phonological loop would be the aspect of WM affected in this group. Poor readers often have deficits in reading comprehension, along with their word identification problems, related to the non-phonological linguistic deficits found in this group (see Bishop and Snowling, 2004). Thus, it follows that deficits in both the phonological loop and central executive would be common in this group.

Although the central executive does not appear to be impaired in pure dyslexia (those meeting the dyslexia definition with no ADHD or receptive/expressive language impairment), its functioning does appear to be related to academic achievement in general. For example, several studies have found central executive functioning to be related to reading comprehension (Perfetti, 1985; Swanson and Ashbaker, 2000; Stone and Brady, 1995), and some studies have found it be related to word recognition (Kibby and Cohen, 2008; Swanson and Ashbaker, 2000). In 1992 Walczyk and Raska demonstrated that WM is important for maintaining access to information while reading, allowing for better comprehension. Maintaining access to the information read may aid word recognition as well, particularly for less familiar words where the context may aid recognition of the word. Research also has illustrated that WM may be involved with math skills (Denckla, 1996; Hulme and Roodenrys, 1995; Wilson and Swanson, 2001). More specifically, WM may be important for solving mathematical application problems (Swanson and Sachse-Lee, 2001) and for solving calculations that require problem decomposition, retrieval of math facts, and/or problem-solving (Geary, 2004).

Confounding Factors

Many of the factors leading to the conflicting findings on WM in RD have been described above: the definition of RD used (poor reader versus dyslexia), the types of tasks/methods used to assess STM/WM, and whether or not comorbid diagnoses such as ADHD and receptive/expressive language impairment were controlled. Nonetheless, a key factor that I have not addressed yet is the varying operational definitions of RD used within the field in terms of dyslexia and poor readers. For example, some use a set discrepancy (such as a 20 point discrepancy) between IQ and basic reading ability whereas others use a regression formula that takes into account properties of the normal curve when defining dyslexia. Even those using a set discrepancy vary in the amount of points required for a discrepancy (e.g. 1 standard deviation vs. 1.5 or 2 standard deviations), reflecting the States' heterogeneity in the definition. The regression formulas used also vary, although Shaywitzs' and colleagues' definition is commonly utilized (Shaywitz, Shaywitz, Fletcher, and Escobar, 1990). Moreover, authors differ in whether they use WISC/WAIS Full-Scale IQ, Verbal IQ/Verbal Comprehension Index, Performance IQ/Perceptual Reasoning Index, or some other measure of intelligence. For both types of definition, discrepancy and poor reader, the measures of basic reading used differ across studies. Some include reading rate, whereas others focus on word identification and/or phonological decoding without including reading rate. In terms of the poor reader definition, some researchers require poor readers to read at least 1 standard deviation below the mean, whereas others require reading to be at least 1.5 standard deviations below the mean. This issue is important because the more severe the reading deficit must be to make a diagnosis, the more likely deficits beyond phonological processing will occur.

Attention-Deficit/Hyperactivity Disorder

The literature on Attention-Deficit/Hyperactivity Disorder (ADHD) is even more disparate than the literature on developmental dyslexia, as the literature on RD at least shows deficits in phonological STM and the phonological loop consistently. For example, some research suggests that the central executive is impaired in ADHD, but the phonological loop and visuospatial sketchpad are spared. Others find at least one of the slave systems to be affected, and some find the central executive to be intact. These issues and the corresponding research will be elaborated upon next.

Phonological Loop

Some children with ADHD have various subtle, language weaknesses (Camarata and Gibson, 1999; Carte, Nigg, and Hinshaw, 1996; McInnes, Humphries, Hogg-Johnson, and Tannock, 2003; Purvis and Tannock, 1997). Furthermore, specific language impairment is found in 30-60% of children with ADHD (D'Incau, 2000; Riccio and Hynd, 1993). Nonetheless, phonological processing is typically spared in ADHD (Purvis and Tannock, 2000; Shaywitz et al., 1995; Willcutt et al., 2001). Hence, an interesting dichotomy is found between developmental dyslexia and ADHD, in which aspects of linguistic functioning are affected in some individuals with ADHD with better preserved phonological processing in comparison, and phonological processing is the primary linguistic deficit in RD with other aspects of language functioning being better preserved in comparison.

Corresponding with the spared phonological processing in ADHD at the group level, verbal STM and the phonological loop frequently are shown to be intact in ADHD (Karatekin, 2005; Korkman and Pesonen, 1994; McInnes et al., 2003; Rucklidge and Tannock, 2002; Willcutt et al., 2001; see Roodenrys, 2006). Nonetheless, some researchers have found verbal STM deficits in this population (Pallas, 2003; Quinlin and Brown, 2003; Stevens, Quittner, Zuckerman, and Moore, 2002). Perhaps the verbal STM deficits are related to the comorbid language problems present in some individuals with ADHD, if these individuals are included in the sample. This may be more likely the case when items are coded semantically given their non-phonological linguistic deficits. Alternatively, the verbal STM deficit could be related to inattention which is a common deficit in ADHD. Attention problems may affect their performance on some phonetic memory measures due to these measures being particularly sensitive to inattention. The latter notion will be elaborated upon subsequently.

In our 2008 study using the Children's Memory Scale, Kibby and Cohen assessed children with ADHD, dyslexia, comorbid dyslexia/ADHD, and controls. When assessing children with ADHD, we found them to be intact on most aspects of verbal STM assessed: Stories, Word Pairs (a verbal paired associate learning task), Word Lists (a selective reminding task), and Numbers Backward (backwards digit span), demonstrating good semantic and phonological STM in general. Nonetheless, they performed worse than controls on Numbers Forward (forward digit span). Simple span tasks typically are considered to be measures of the phonological loop, as is the case with Numbers Forward. However, if the phonological loop were impaired in ADHD, Word Lists should have been affected too, because Word Lists is a list learning task using semantically unrelated words. This type of list encourages phonetic coding in general, and Word Lists was found to be related to phonetic coding rather than semantic coding in our study. Moreover, children with dyslexia, who showed a phonological loop deficit, were deficient on all phonological STM tasks, including Words Lists and Numbers Forward. What was hypothesized in this study is that Numbers Forward is sensitive to fluctuations in attention because the items are only presented once and must be repeated in serial order to be correct. In contrast, Word Lists utilizes a long list and does not need to be recalled in serial order. Thus, even though a word or two is missed, a sufficient number of items may be focused upon to achieve an average score. As children with ADHD often have fluctuations in attention, these fluctuations may have differentially affected their Numbers Forward score. Consistent with this notion, children with ADHD performed significantly better on Numbers Backward than Numbers Forward. Numbers Backward is often perceived to be harder than Numbers Forward and, thus, may better drive focused attention, even though both tasks require sufficient span to perform well. Taken together, our findings suggest verbal STM is intact in ADHD, consistent with the bulk of the literature on ADHD, and their phonological loop functions adequately at the group level when they are focused upon the task at hand and do not have comorbid RD or receptive/expressive language deficits.

Visuospatial Sketchpad

Similar to verbal STM, some researchers have shown visual STM to be intact in ADHD (French, Zentall, and Bennett, 2001; Karatekin, 2004; see Alloway and Gathercole, 2006), whereas others have found visual STM deficits in ADHD (Kirk, 2001; Martinussen, Hayden, Hogg-Johnson, and Tannock, 2005; Martinussen and Tannock, 2006; McInnes et al., 2003; Roodenrys, 2006). Given that the visuospatial sketchpad has separable subcomponents for visual/non-spatial and spatial material, what may be of key importance to this topic is the type of material utilized.

In the study by Kibby and Cohen (2008) mentioned above it was found that visual STM performance in children with ADHD was related to the type of material utilized. Although their STM for visual/non-spatial material was intact (CMS Faces Immediate memory), their STM for visual-spatial material was reduced (CMS Picture Locations and Dot Locations). This finding is consistent with prior research which suggests that spatial STM is affected in ADHD (Aman, Roberts, and Pennington, 1998; Bedard, Martinussen, Ickowicz, and Tannock, 2004; Martinussen et al., 2005; McInnes et al., 2003; Sonuga-Barke, Sereant, Nigg, and Willcutt, 2008). It also is consistent with Kempton's and colleagues' 1999 findings which suggest that visual memory (pattern recognition) is intact in ADHD but spatial STM is impaired. Moreover, children with ADHD have been shown to have inadequate spatial processing at the group level and atypical parietal lobe functioning and structure, which is consistent with our findings (Aman et al., 1998; Farmer, 2003; Fillipek et al., 1997; Kim, Lee, Shin, Cho, and Lee, 2002; Lane, 2004; Silk et al., 2005; Vance et al., 2007). Therefore, it appears that the spatial aspect of the visuospatial sketchpad is deficient in ADHD at the group level.

Of interest to this topic is the effect that stimulant medication has on the visual-spatial STM deficit in ADHD. Kibby and Cohen (2008) found children with ADHD tested on stimulant medication performed better on STM for Dot Locations than children with ADHD tested off it. This study could not assess who was medication naïve versus just tested off medication, however. Prior literature has found similar results, as children with ADHD performed better on spatial STM tasks when on methylphenidate compared to when they were off it (Barnett et al., 2001; Bedard, Jain, Hogg-Johnson, and Tannock, 2007; Bedard, et al., 2004; Mehta, Goodyer, and Sahakian, 2004). Also of interest is that the medication effect was specific to Dot Locations in our study; performance on the other STM measures did not differ between ADHD on and off medication. This specificity also was demonstrated by Bedard and colleagues (2007) who found methylphenidate improved spatial STM performance but not verbal STM performance in ADHD.

Central Executive

Children with ADHD frequently present with executive dysfunction (see Barkley, 1997; Korkman and Pesonen, 1994; Pennington and Ozonoff, 1996), likely due to poor frontal-striatal functioning (Casey, Castellanos, Giedd, and Marsh, 1997; Castellanos, 1997). Although executive functioning may be spared in ~20% of children with ADHD (see Nigg, Willcutt, Doyle and Sonuga-Barke, 2005), a large body of research suggests that they often have impairment in at least one aspect of executive functioning including self-regulation, response inhibition, shifting of mental set, WM, vigilance, problem solving, organization, and/or nonverbal and verbal fluency (Barkley, 1997; Berlin, Bohlin, Nyberg, and Janols, 2004; Miller and Castellanos, 1998; Korkman and Pesonen, 1994; Nigg, 2006; Pennington and Ozonoff, 1996; Reader, Harris, Schuerholz, and Denckla, 1994; Shallice et al., 2002). The specific type of executive deficit(s) a child has likely varies across children with ADHD. Nonetheless, their deficits in executive functioning often include poor sustained effort on effortful tasks and poor strategy usage (Ackerman, Anhalt, Dykman, and Holcomb, 1986; Douglas and Benezra, 1990; Shallice et al., 2002). This deficit in strategy usage may affect WM performance, as Cornoldi, Barbieri, Gaiani, and Zocchi (1999) found that children with ADHD performed comparably to controls on a WM task when they were taught to use a strategy. Similar to other aspects of WM, the research on the central executive in ADHD is disparate, with some researchers finding it is affected (Barkley, 1997; Douglas and Benezra; 1990; Karatekin, 2004; Martinussen and Tannock, 2006; Muir-Broaddus, Rosenstein, Medina, and Soderberg, 2002; Shallice et al., 2002; Willcutt, Doyle, Nigg, Faraone, and Pennington, 2005) and others finding it to be spared, especially when tasks utilize verbal material (Kerns, McInerney, and Wilde, 2001; Kibby and Cohen, 2008; Kuntsi, Oosterlaan, and Stevenson, 2001; Pallas, 2003; Rucklidge and Tannock, 2002; Willcutt et al., 2001).

In the study by Kibby and Cohen (2008) we found children with ADHD, as well as children with dyslexia, have intact central executive (CE) functioning when controlling focused attention/short-term storage. More specifically, children with ADHD performed worse than controls on a measure of verbal WM, Sequences. Nonetheless, when the effects of reduced focused attention/short-term storage were controlled by subtracting the Numbers Forward score from the Sequences score, children with ADHD performed comparably to controls. This was true for the RD group as well. Moreover, children with ADHD performed better on Numbers Backward than Numbers Forward as previously stated. These findings suggest the CE is intact in ADHD and that verbal WM deficits, when found, are related to focused attention and/or linguistic deficits. This proposition is consistent with the literature suggesting verbal WM is intact in many individuals with ADHD (Kerns et al., 2001; Kibby and Cohen, 2008; Kuntsi et al., 2001; Pallas, 2003; Rucklidge and Tannock, 2002; Sonuga-Barke et al., 2008; Willcutt et al., 2001). It should be noted, however, that the tasks used to measure CE functioning in this study were verbal in nature; we did not have a nonverbal measure of CE functioning.

A key issue here is the nature of the central executive. Both verbal and visual WM should be equally affected by CE deficits if the CE is domain-general. Because verbal WM frequently is found to be intact in ADHD while visual-spatial WM frequently is found to be impaired (see Sonuga-Barke et al., 2008), visual-spatial short-term storage deficits must be driving the WM deficits in ADHD if the CE is domain-general. STM deficits causing the WM deficits in ADHD is a possibility given that the phonological loop often is intact and the visuospatial sketchpad often is impaired in individuals with ADHD based upon the bulk of the literature reviewed. Taken together, if the CE is domain-general, the CE likely is intact in ADHD at the group level. If the CE is not domain-general as proposed by Baddeley (1986, 2000), then CE deficits could be present in one modality and not in another, which would help to explain why deficits in visual-spatial WM are more commonly found in ADHD than deficits in verbal WM, even when short-term storage deficits are controlled. The notion of an at least partially domain-specific CE is consistent with research on the CE in the general population (Fastame, Mammarella, Carretti, and Meneghetti, 2008), and it is consistent with the research on ADHD (Martinussen et al., 2005).

Recent research by Cornoldi and Vecchi (2003) suggests that the CE is not always domain-general, and WM functions somewhat differently than what was proposed by Baddeley (1986, 2000). Cornoldi and Vecchi believe WM operates in two continuous dimensions: horizontal, reflecting domain, and vertical, reflecting level of active processing. The horizontal dimension is material specific and includes several modalities such as visual, spatial, phonological and semantic, corresponding with Baddeley's slave systems (Fastane et al., 2008). The vertical dimension reflects the level of executive control required to complete a task. This dimension is similar to Baddeley's notion of the CE, but it is continuous in nature from very passive (simple span) to very active. For passive tasks low on the vertical dimension, there is a great deal of modality specificity, consistent with Baddeley's notion of the slave systems. For tasks midway on the dimension, the CE is at least partially domain-specific. For tasks at the top of the vertical dimension, the CE is domain-general. Hence, the CE may be at least partially modality specific, although not as much so as STM.

When using this model, the meta-analytic findings by Martinussen and colleagues (2005) on ADHD make more sense. They found spatial STM was more affected than verbal STM, as would be expected based upon the literature I reviewed. However, they also found visual-spatial CE was more impaired than verbal CE. Furthermore, the CE was slightly more impaired than the store for visual material but comparable to, to less impaired than, the store for verbal material. The differences in CE effect sizes across modalities and the differences in STM and CE effect sizes within modality are more readily explained by Cornoldi and Vecchi's model (2003) than Baddeley's (1986) domain-general model. Correspondingly, spatial STM and spatial CE effect sizes were large, whereas verbal STM and verbal CE effect sizes were moderate. The moderate verbal CE effect size helps to explain why researchers vary in being able to find verbal WM deficits in ADHD, since such deficits would take more power to find. Second, similar to the verbal STM deficit, the verbal CE deficit also may be related to the comorbid language weaknesses present in some individuals with ADHD, making the verbal CE deficit more difficult to find in a given sample as some children with ADHD would not have language deficits. More work is needed to determine this. Third, it may take the right type of task to find CE deficits in ADHD, as the CE deficits found in ADHD may be specific to task rather than global. This third supposition will be elaborated upon next. Of course, all three possibilities could be correct.

Findings of task-specific deficits in central executive functioning in ADHD are consistent with the model proposed by Cornoldi and Vecchi (2003). For example, initially Willcutt and colleagues found children with ADHD scored comparably to controls on all verbal WM measures administered (Willcutt et al., 2001). Willcutt, Pennington, Olson, Chabildas, and Hulslander (2005) found similar results; however, the ADHD group performed worse on one of the various verbal WM measures administered, Counting Span; visual WM was not assessed in either study. Roodenrys and colleagues (2001) also found task specific deficits in CE functioning in ADHD, with deficits being found on the more challenging verbal tasks. In a recent review, Roodenrys (2006) noted verbal WM is frequently found to be intact in ADHD, and CE deficits are only found on specific tasks. In contrast, spatial STM and spatial WM functioning are frequently found to be impaired. When analyzing types of tasks, Roodenrys found tasks requiring updating, planning/strategy, switching of attention, and generating novel/random sequences are affected in ADHD. It could be argued that these are challenging tasks and higher on the vertical domain of Cornoldi and Vecchi's model.

Also of importance to the examination of WM functioning in ADHD is the subtype used in the study. Many of the studies cited combined the ADHD subtypes into one group of children with ADHD. However, other studies focused on only one subtype or compared WM deficits across subtypes. For example, Barkley typically studies ADHD-Combined type (ADHD-C) and states that both verbal and visual WM are deficient in this population (1997, 2000). Other researchers also have found reduced verbal and visual WM in this subtype (Kunin-Batson, 2002; Tripp, Ryan, and Peace, 2002). When comparing ADHD-Predominantly Inattentive type (ADHD-PI) to ADHD-C, Klorman and colleagues (1999) only found executive deficits in ADHD-C. Moreover, Lane (2004) found ADHD-C performed worse than ADHD-PI on measures of WM despite the two groups being comparable in sustained attention. In contrast, other researchers have shown children with ADHD-PI perform comparably to children with ADHD-C but worse than controls on cognitive executive functioning measures including WM; the two subtypes differ only on measures of behavioral inhibition systematically (Chhabildas, Pennington, and Willcutt, 2001; Houghton et al., 1999; Nigg, Blaskey, Huang-Pollock, and Rappley, 2002).

In a preliminary study we found children with ADHD-PI and ADHD-C performed comparably to each other on the various traditional neuropsychological measures of executive functioning administered, including WM (Molnar and Kibby, unpublished data). These measures of cognitive executive functioning were administered in the laboratory. When using a behavioral questionnaire on executive functioning in daily life, children with ADHD-C had worse scores than children with ADHD-PI, dyslexia and controls on response inhibition. In contrast, the two subtypes were comparable to each other but worse than dyslexia and controls on working memory and other cognitive executive functioning scales. Thus, our findings are consistent with other research which suggests that ADHD-PI and ADHD-C are comparable on cognitive executive measures including WM, but differ in behavioral/response inhibition (Chhabildas et al., 2001; Houghton et al., 1999; Nigg et al., 2002).

Along with the type of deficits potentially varying between ADHD-PI and ADHD-C, the source of the WM deficit may differ between ADHD-PI and ADHD-C as well. Some researchers believe the two subtypes are actually separate disorders, with ADHD-PI having problems with under-arousal, daydreaming and processing speed which affect WM, and ADHD-C having problems with response inhibition which affects WM (see Diamond, 2005). Thus, with this explanation, the types of WM deficits may differ between subtypes, as was found by Farmer (2003). Nonetheless, there is debate over the nature of ADHD as other researchers believe the two subtypes are truly subtypes of the same disorder. They suggest cognitive deficits such as inattention, slow processing speed, and poor WM are associated with the inattention dimension of ADHD, whereas behavioral inhibition is associated with the hyperactive/impulsive dimension of ADHD (Chhabildas et al., 2001; Houghton et al., 1999; Nigg et al., 2002). Hence, both subtypes would have problems consistent with the inattention dimension, and ADHD-C would have additional problems consistent with the hyperactive/impulsive dimension. Therefore, both subtypes should have similar problems with WM for similar reasons according to this explanation, although children with ADHD-C may have worse deficits than ADHD-PI given the additional deficits in behavioral inhibition. Some research is consistent with this supposition (Klorman et al., 1999; Lane, 2004; Martinussen and Tannock, 2006; Sarkari, 2003; Molnar and Kibby, unpublished data). Clearly more research is indicated in this area.

Confounding Factors

Older research often used the DSM-III or III-R to diagnose ADHD, whereas more recent research typically utilizes the DSM-IV. The DSM-III recognized Attention Deficit Disorder with and without Hyperactivity, allowing for inattention to be sufficient for diagnosis; the DSM-III-R only recognized ADHD, with children having to have a combination of inattention, hyperactivity and impulsivity symptoms to meet criteria; and the DSM-IV recognizes ADHD Predominately Inattentive type, ADHD Hyperactive/Impulsive type, and ADHD Combined type, with the symptoms needed for diagnosis varying with subtype. Thus, the version of the DSM used will affect the composition of the sample.

Despite many researchers using the DSM to define ADHD, researchers differ somewhat in their operational definitions of ADHD. Some researches use questionnaires to define ADHD along with, or instead of, the DSM, whereas others rely solely on the DSM. Researchers also differ on which score should be used as the cut-off on the questionnaires when used. More specifically, some require children to be 1, 1.5, or 2 standard deviations above the mean in inattention and/or hyperactive/impulsive behaviors on a questionnaire to define ADHD. Moreover, the questionnaires used to define ADHD vary across studies. Furthermore, there is a debate over who is the best informant, the parent or the teacher, when scores are discordant on the questionnaires and, thus, which informant should be used or both.

Also of concern is that researchers differ in whether they lump the subtypes together into one group of children with ADHD broadly defined, whether they focus on only one subtype of ADHD, or whether they break down ADHD by subtypes in their study, as noted above. Furthermore, some researchers do not focus on categorical subtypes, but instead use inattention and hyperactivity as continuous dimensions of behavior as noted earlier. Since the subtype/dimension assessed may affect the findings on WM, this inconsistency in which subtype(s)/dimension(s) is studied may contribute to the variability in findings on WM in ADHD.

An additional issue of importance is whether the effects of medication were controlled when studying WM. As noted earlier, we found visual STM to be affected in children with ADHD off medication; performance was better for children on stimulant medication (Kibby and Cohen, 2008). Moreover, when comparing children with ADHD on and off medication, several studies have found children with ADHD to perform better on visual STM and/or CE tasks when on medication (Barnett et al., 2001; Bedard et al., 2007; Bedard et al., 2004; Kunin-Batson, 2002; Mehta et al., 2004), as noted earlier, Thus, the variability in findings on WM in ADHD could be related to whether the sample was allowed to be on medication or not during the study. This may be particularly true for tasks measuring visual storage and CE functioning (Bedard et al., 2007; Kibby and Cohen, 2008; Kunin-Batson, 2002).

Similar to RD, another factor that can affect WM performance in ADHD is the presence of comorbid disorders. Some studies assess and control for comorbid disorders that affect WM performance such as RD and language impairment, whereas other studies do not. For those studies that do not control for comorbid disorders, it is difficult to determine which WM deficits are due to the comorbid disorder, and to what extent, and which are due to ADHD.

Comorbid Attention-Deficit/Hyperactivity Disorder and Developmental Dyslexia

Research on comorbid RD/ADHD is slowly emerging. Thus far it shows that children with comorbid RD/ADHD have deficits consistent with both disorders. For example, researchers have demonstrated that children with RD have poor phonological processing and phonological loop functioning whereas children with ADHD have poor inhibitory control but generally intact phonological loop functioning; those with comorbid dyslexia/ADHD have problems consistent with both disorders (Korkman and Pesonen, 1994; Klorman et al., 1999; Rucklidge andTannock, 2002; Willcutt et al., 2001, Willcutt, Pennington et al.,, 2005). When examining verbal WM, Roodenrys and colleagues (2001) found that the comorbid RD/ADHD group had problems on phonological loop measures (word span and digit span) consistent with the RD group, but they also had poor central executive functioning on measures requiring mental manipulation and generation whereas the RD group did not. This study did not have an ADHD-only group.

In our study on ADHD and RD discussed above (Kibby and Cohen, 2008), we found no interaction when using a 2 X 2 MANOVA comparing those with and without ADHD and those with and without dyslexia. Thus, the RD/ADHD group presented with the visual-spatial STM deficits consistent with the ADHD group and the verbal STM deficits consistent with the RD group. None of the groups presented with verbal CE deficits. The RD/ADHD group had the lowest mean on Numbers Forward and Sequences, but their scores were not significantly different from the RD and ADHD groups. Furthermore, the RD/ADHD group did not present with additional WM deficits extending beyond those of RD-only or ADHD-only based on our MANOVA results.

Taken together, our results are consistent with the "common etiology hypothesis" of RD/ADHD proposed by Willcutt and colleagues (2001). According to this hypothesis, ADHD and RD share a common etiology given their comorbidity, along with having deficits specific to the given disorder. They proposed slow processing speed to be the shared cause (Willcutt et al., 2001; Willcutt, Pennington et al., 2005; Shanahan et al., 2006). The common cause should contribute to most cases of each disorder, along with comorbid RD/ADHD. Thus, those with RD/ADHD should have a deficit in the shared etiology(s), along with the deficits specific to each disorder. Our data is consistent with this hypothesis as children with RD/ADHD had the phonological STM/phonological loop deficits consistent with RD and the visual-spatial STM/visuospatial sketchpad deficits consistent with ADHD. They also had reduced forward digit span, consistent with both disorders. Thus, reduced verbal span may be a common etiology for the two disorders, although the reason why span is reduced may differ between RD and ADHD.

Neurobiology of Working Memory in Developmental Dyslexia and ADHD

When looking at the general population it appears that multiple areas of the brain are involved with working memory. In terms of verbal WM, the pars triangularis appears to be part of the network responsible for the subvocal rehearsal mechanism; the supramarginal gyrus likely is a site for the phonological store; and multiple areas of the brain are involved with short-term storage of items by their meaning, including the temporal lobes and prefrontal regions (Baddeley, 1998; Cabeza and Nyberg, 2000; Fiez et al., 1996; Jonides et al., 1998; Kibby, Kroese et al., 2004; Smith and Jonides, 1997), as noted earlier. In terms of visual-spatial STM; the ventrolateral prefrontal cortex and ventral stream may be involved with the visual/non-spatial subcomponent, and the dorsolateral prefrontal cortex and dorsal stream, including superior parietal cortex, may be involved with the spatial component (see Wang and Zhang, 2008; Wendelken, 2008). The frontal-striatal network has been shown to be involved with the CE (Chein and Fiez, 2001; Jonides et al., 1997; Nyberg et al., 2002; Vassileva, 2003).

In terms of the pars triangularis, size of the pars triangularis is correlated with phonological awareness, rapid automatic naming, and verbal STM in general (Eckert et al., 2003; Kibby, Kroese, Krebbs, Hill, and Hynd, 2009). Moreover, the pars triangularis has been shown to be smaller in dyslexia than controls when using manual tracing techniques (Eckert et al., 2003, Kibby, Johnson et al., unpublished data), although inconsistently so (Kibby,

Kroese et al., 2009), and the inferior frontal region, which includes the pars triangularis, differs in size between RD and controls when using voxel-based morphometry (VBM; Brown et al., 2001). When using functional neuroimaging, hypoactivation of the right frontotemporal region was found in RD during a memory task for tones (Rumsey et al., 1994). However, research on left inferior frontal activation is disparate, with some studies demonstrating similar activation to controls (Chiron et al., 1999; Paulesu et al., 1996; Rumsey et al., 1997), some demonstrating overactivation related to its use in compensating for left posterior dysfunction (Pugh et al., 2000; Shaywitz et al., 1998), and others demonstrating hypoactivation during phonological tasks (Georgiewa et al. 1999). Thus, the functioning of the pars triangularis in dyslexia is likely task dependent. Taking a network rather than a localization approach, the network involved with the subvocal rehearsal mechanism likely is intact in dyslexia given the literature reviewed earlier, but other networks to which the pars contributes may be affected in RD (such as those involved with other aspects of STM and/or with phonological awareness).

When examining ADHD, we found children with ADHD had smaller right pars triangularis size than those without ADHD (Kibby, Kroese et al., 2009). This finding is consistent with other neuroimaging literature implicating inferior frontal involvement in ADHD (Filipek et al., 1997; Sowell et al., 2003; Swanson et al., 1998). In a preliminary study, we measured both the pars triangularis and the pars opercularis (Kibby, Johnson, et al., unpublished data). The main effects for dyslexia and ADHD were significant. However, the interaction between dyslexia and ADHD was not significant, similar to the cognitive literature. At the univariate level those with and without dyslexia differed in pars triangularis volume, as did those with and without ADHD, being a possible source of shared etiology. No group differences were found for the pars opercularis, and none of the interaction terms were significant. Pearson correlations using the total sample found pars opercularis volume and pars triangularis volume were correlated with verbal WM functioning. Thus, this study suggests possible involvement of the bilateral inferior frontal region in short-term maintenance of material consistent with previous research on WM in controls (D'Esposito and Postle, 2002) as well as RD (Eckert et al., 2003; Kibby, Kroese et al., 2009)

A dissociation between RD and ADHD is found when examining regions other than the inferior frontal region, with the posterior perisylvian region being affected in RD (Brown et al., 2001; Eliez et al., 2000; Pugh et al., 2000; Shaywitz et al., 1998) and the frontal-striatal and frontal-parietal circuits being affected in ADHD (Casey et al., 1997; Castellanos, 1997; Semrud-Clikeman et al., 2000). Consistent with this, the supramarginal gyrus is often atypical in size in RD (Leonard et al., 2001; Leonard et al., 1993; Kibby, LaMacchia et al., unpublished data), and it may be involved with the phonological store based on functional and structural MRI studies (Jonides et al., 1998; Kibby, Kroese et al., 2004; Smith and Jonides, 1997). Thus, this site may be contributing to the deficits in the phonological loop in RD given the atypical structure in this region and the hypoactivation in the left inferior parietal area, which includes the supramarginal gyrus, during functional neuroimaging studies (Pugh et al., 2000; Shaywitz et al., 1998).

In terms of the frontal-parietal circuit, children with ADHD have been shown to have atypical size/activation in frontal and parietal regions (Castellanos, Giedd, Marsh, and Hamburger, 1996; Durston, van Belle, and de Zeeuw, 2011; Fillipek et al., 1997; Mostofsky, Cooper, Kates, Denckla, and Kaufmann, 2002; Silk et al., 2005; Vaidya and Stollstorff, 2008; Zametkin et al., 1993). Furthermore, the atypical parietal structure/activation may be related to the visual-spatial STM deficits in ADHD and their atypical visual-spatial processing in general (Aman et al., 1998; Farmer, 2003; Vance et al., 2007). In terms of the CE, the frontal-striatal system may be more active in ADHD than controls when engaged in an n-back task (Vassileva, 2003), suggesting greater resources are required by individuals with ADHD to complete the task.

CONCLUSION

Based upon the literature reviewed, both children with developmental dyslexia and children with ADHD present with deficits in WM functioning. Whereas children with dyslexia frequently present with deficits in the phonological loop and phonological STM, children with ADHD frequently present with deficits in the visuospatial sketchpad and spatial STM. They also occasionally present with deficits in forward digit span, likely due to fluctuations in attention. The bulk of the literature suggests the central executive is intact in RD when deficits in short-term storage are controlled, the dyslexia definition is used, the reading deficit is specific to basic reading, and the presence of comorbid ADHD and language impairment is controlled. In contrast to RD, the CE may be deficient in ADHD for tasks involving greater executive control, with visual CE being more affected than verbal CE. Children with comorbid RD/ADHD present with deficits associated with both disorders. When looking at the findings in total, forward digit span may be impaired in both RD and ADHD, being a potential source of shared etiology between the two disorders, although the sources of this deficit may differ between groups.

In terms of the neurobiological bases of the STM/WM deficits in RD and ADHD, the literature is inconclusive. Nonetheless, certain trends can be found across the studies currently available. The supramarginal gyrus is atypical in RD at the group level, and this may be related to their poor phonological store functioning. The parietal lobes, part of the frontal-parietal circuit, are atypical in ADHD at the group level which may be related to their deficits in visual-spatial STM/CE. The frontal-striatal circuit also has been shown to be atypical in ADHD and may be related to the CE deficits found in this group. Both RD and ADHD occasionally have atypical structure in the lateral inferior frontal region at the group level, which may be a potential source of shared etiology between the two disorders. Structure of this region is related to short-term maintenance of material.

As noted throughout this literature review, RD and ADHD are heterogeneous disorders in etiology that are defined by behavioral description, which likely contributes to the variability in findings across studies. Other sources of the variability in findings are differing operational definitions of RD and ADHD, variability in the measures used to make diagnoses, variability in the tasks used to assess STM/WM, small sample sizes which affect the ability to generalize to the respective populations, insufficient control of store deficits when assessing CE functioning, and lack of control for common comorbidities such as language impairment and ADHD when assessing RD, and RD and language impairment when assessing ADHD. As all of these factors likely contribute to the heterogeneity in findings on STM/WM in RD and ADHD, it is important for researchers to address these issues when investigating STM/WM in the future.

Therefore, future research on STM/WM in RD and ADHD should focus on correcting the common sources of variability in the findings to date. This will not be an easy task, however, as there is not a consensus on the best definition of RD and ADHD, on the best tasks to use to assess RD and ADHD, or on the best tasks to use to measure STM/WM. Furthermore, it will require a thorough battery of tests to assess for common comorbid disorders. It also will require more time and resources or collaborative effort to derive larger sample sizes. Nonetheless, doing this will greatly facilitate advances in our knowledge of STM/WM functioning in RD and ADHD.

Acknowledgment

The writing of this chapter was supported by a grant from the National Institutes of Health (NIH), National Institute of Child Health and Human Development (NICHD: R15 HD065627). Many of the studies discussed from my lab were at least partially supported by a grant from NIH/NICHD (R03 HD048752). The content of this chapter is the sole responsibility of the author and does not necessarily represent the views of NIH or NICHD.

References

Abdullaev, Y. G., and Bechtereva, N. P. (1993). Neuronal correlate of the higher-order semantic code in human prefrontal cortex in language tasks. *Int. J. Psychophysiol.,* 14(3), 167-177.

Ackerman, P. T., Anhalt, J. M., Dykman, R. A., and Holcomb, P. J. (1986). Effortful processing deficits in children with reading and/or attention disorders. *Brain and Cognition,* 5(1), 22-40. doi: 10.1016/0278-2626(86)90060-6

Alloway, T. P., and Gathercole, S. E. (2006). *Working memory and neurodevelopmental disorders*. New York: Psychology Press.

Altemeier, L. E., Abbott, R. D., and Berninger, V. W. (2008). Executive functions for reading and writing in typical literacy development and dyslexia. *Journal of Clinical and Experimental Neuropsychology,* 30(5), 588-606. doi: 10.1080/13803390701562818

Aman, C. J., Roberts, R. J., Jr., and Pennington, B. F. (1998). A neuropsychological examination of the underlying deficit in attention deficit hyperactivity disorder: Frontal lobe versus right parietal lobe theories. *Developmental Psychology,* 34(5), *956-969.*

Asbjørnsen, A. E., Helland, T., Obrzut, J. E., and Boliek, C. A. (2003). The Role of Dichotic Listening Performance and Tasks of Executive Functions in Reading Impairment: A Discriminant Function Analysis. *Child Neuropsychology,* 9(4), 277-288.

Baddeley, A. (1998). Recent developments in working memory. *Current Opinion in Neurobiology* 8(2), 234-238. doi: 10.1016/s0959-4388(98)80145-1

Baddeley, A. D. (1986). *Working Memory*. Oxford: Oxford University Press.

Baddeley, A. D. (1996). Exploring the central executive. *The Quarterly Journal of Experimental Psychology A: Human Experimental Psychology,* 49A(1), 5-28.

Baddeley, A. D. (2000). The episodic buffer: A new component of working memory? *Trends in Cognitive Sciences,* 4(11), 417-423.

Baddeley, A. D. (2002). Is working memory still working? *European Psychologist,* 7(2), 85-97.

Barkley, R. A. (1997). Attention-deficit/hyperactivity disorder, self-regulation, and time: Toward a more comprehensive theory. *Journal of Developmental and Behavioral Pediatrics,* 18(4), 271-279.

Barkley, R. A. (2000). Genetics of childhood disorders: XVII. ADHD, Part 1: The executive functions and ADHD. *Journal of the American Academy of Child and Adolescent Psychiatry* 39(8), 1064-1068.

Barnett, R., Maruff, P., Vance, A., Luk, E. S. L., Costin, J., Wood, C., and Pantelis, C. (2001). Abnormal execution function in attention deficit hyperactivity disorder: The effect of stimulant medication and age on spatial working memory. *Psychological Medicine,* 31(6), 1107-1115.

Bauer, R. H. (1977). Memory processes in children with learning disabilities: Evidence for deficient rehearsal. *Journal of Experimental Child Psychology,* 24(3), 415-430. doi: 10.1016/0022-0965(77)90088-1

Bedard, A. C., Jain, U., Hogg-Johnson, S., and Tannock, R. (2007). Effects of methylphenidate on working memory components: Influence of measurement. *Journal of Child Psychology and Psychiatry,* 48(9), 872-880.

Bedard, A. C., Martinussen, R., Ickowicz, A., and Tannock, R. (2004). Methylphenidate improves visual-spatial memory in children with attention-deficit/hyperactivity disorder. *Journal of the American Academy of Child and Adolescent Psychiatry,* 43(3), 260-268.

Berlin, L., Bohlin, G., Nyberg, L., and Janols, L. O. (2004). How well do measures of inhibition and other executive functions discriminate between children with ADHD and controls? *Child Neuropsychology,* 10(1), 1-13.

Berninger, V. W., and Abbott, R. D. (1994). Multiple orthographic and phonological codes in literacy acquisition: An evolving research program. In V. W. Berninger (Ed.), *The varieties of orthographic knowledge, 1: Theoretical and developmental issues.* (pp. 277-319). New York: Kluwer Academic/Plenum Publishers.

Bishop, D. V. M., and Snowling, M. J. (2004). Developmental Dyslexia and Specific Language Impairment: Same or Different? *Psychological Bulletin,* 130(6), 858-886. doi: 10.1037/0033-2909.130.6.858

Brady, S. A. (1991). The role of working memory in reading disability. In S. A. Brady and D. P. Shankweiler (Eds.), *Phonological processes in literacy: A tribute to Isabelle Y Liberman.* (pp. 129-151). Hillsdale, N. J.: Lawrence Erlbaum Associates, Inc.

Bowers, P. G., Sunseth, K., and Golden, J. (1999). The route between rapid naming and reading progress. *Scientific Studies of Reading,* 3(1), 31-53. doi: 10.1207/s1532799xssr0301_2

Brown, A. L., and Palincsar, A. S. (1989). Guided, cooperative learning and individual knowledge acquisition. In L. B. Resnick (Ed.), *Knowing, learning, and instruction: Essays in honor of Robert Glaser.* (pp. 393-451). Hillsdale, NJ: Lawrence Erlbaum Associates, Inc.

Brown, W., Eliez, S., Menon, V., Rumsey, J., White, C., and Reiss, A. (2001). Preliminary evidence of widespread morphological variations of the brain in dyslexia. *Neurology,* 56(6), 781-783.

Cabeza, R., and Nyberg, L. (2000). Neural bases of learning and memory: Functional neuroimaging evidence. *Curr. Opin. Neurol.,* 13(4), 415-421.

Camarata, S. M., and Gibson, T. (1999). Pragmatic language deficits in attention-deficit hyperactivity disorder (ADHD). *Mental Retardation and Developmental Disabilities Research Reviews,* 5(3), 207-214. doi: 10.1002/(sici)1098-2779(1999)5:3<207::aid-mrdd7>3.0.co;2-o

Carte, E. T., Nigg, J. T., and Hinshaw, S. P. (1996). Neuropsychological functioning, motor speed, and language processing in boys with and without ADHD. *Journal of Abnormal Child Psychology,* 24(4), 481-498. doi: 10.1007/bf01441570

Casey, B. J., Castellanos, F. X., Giedd, J. N., and Marsh, W. L. (1997). Implication of right frontostriatal circuitry in response inhibition and attention-deficit/hyperactivity disorder. *Journal of the American Academy of Child and Adolescent Psychiatry,* 36(3), 374-383.

Castellanos, F. (1997). Toward a pathophysiology of attention-deficit/hyperactivity disorder. *Clinical Pediatrics,* 36(7), 381-393.

Castellanos, F. X., Giedd, J. N., Marsh, W. L., and Hamburger, S. D. (1996). Quantitative brain magnetic resonance imaging in attention-deficit hyperactivity disorder. *Archives of General Psychiatry,* 53(7), 607-616.

Chein, J. M., and Fiez, J. A. (2001). Dissociation of verbal working memory system components using a delayed serial recall task. *Cereb. Cortex,* 11(11), 1003-1014.

Chhabildas, N., Pennington, B. F., and Willcutt, E. G. (2001). A comparison of the neuropsychological profiles of the DSM-IV subtypes of ADHD. *Journal of Abnormal Child Psychology,* 29(6), 529-540. doi: 10.1023/a:1012281226028

Chiron, C., Pinton, F., Masure, M. C., Duvelleroy-Hommet, C., Leon, F., and Billard, C. (1999). Hemispheric specialization using SPECT and stimulation tasks in children with dysphasia and dystrophia. *Dev. Med. Child Neurol.,* 41(8), 512-520.

Cormier, P., and Dea, S. (1997). Distinctive patterns of relationship of phonological awareness and working memory with reading development. *Reading and Writing,* 9(3), 193-206.

Cornoldi, C., Barbieri, A., Gaiani, C., and Zocchi, S. (1999). Strategic memory deficits in attention deficit disorder with hyperactivity participants: The role of executive processes. *Developmental Neuropsychology,* 15(1), 53-71.

Cornoldi, C., and Vecchi, T. (2003). *Visuo-spatial working memory and individual differences. Essays in cognitive psychology.* Hove: Psychology Press.

Cunningham, A. E., and Stanovich, K. E. (1993). Children's literacy environments and early word recognition subskills. *Reading and Writing,* 5(2), 193-204. doi: 10.1007/bf01027484

D'Esposito, M., and Postle, B. R. (2002). The neural basis of working memory storage, rehearsal, and control processes: Evidence from patient and functional magnetic resonance imaging studies. In L. R. Squire and D. L. Schacter (Eds.), *Neuropsychology of memory* (3rd ed.). (pp. 215-224). New York: Guilford Press.

D'Incau, B. J. (2000). Comorbidity of language disorder with attention-deficit/hyperactivity disorder in a sample of early elementary children: A preliminary investigation. *Dissertation Abstracts International: Section B: The Sciences and Engineering,* 61(1-B), pp. 561.

De Jong, C. G. W., Van De Voorde, S., Roeyers, H., Raymaekers, R., Oosterlaan, J., and Sergeant, J. A. (2009). How distinctive are ADHD and RD? Results of a double dissociation study. *Journal of Abnormal Child Psychology,* 37(7), 1007-1017. doi: 10.1007/s10802-009-9328-y

De Jong, P. F. (1998). Working memory deficits of reading disabled children. *Journal of Experimental Child Psychology,* 70(2), 75-96.

De Jonge, P., and de Jonge, P. F. (1996). Working memory, intelligence and reading ability in children. *Personality and Individual Differences, 21*(6), 1007-1020. doi: 10.1016/s0191-8869(96)00161-4

Della Sala, S., Gray, C., Baddeley, A. D., Allamano, N., and Wilson, L. (1999). Pattern span: a tool for unwelding visuospatial memory. *Neuropsychologia*, 37(10), 1189-1199. doi: 10.1016/s0028-3932(98)00159-6

Denckla, M. B. (1996). Biological correlates of learning and attention: What is relevant to learning disability and attention-deficit hyperactivity disorder? *Journal of Developmental and Behavioral Pediatrics,* 17(2), 114-119.

Diamond, A. (2005). Attention-deficit disorder (attention-deficit/hyperactivity disorder without hyperactivity): A neurobiologically and behaviorally distinct disorder from attention-deficit/hyperactivity disorder (with hyperactivity). *Development and Psychopathology,* 17(3), 807-825.

Done, D. J., and Miles, T. R. (1978). Learning, memory and reading disabilities. In M. M. Gruneberg, P. E. Morris and R. N. Sykes (Eds.), *Practical aspects of memory*. London: Academic Press.

Douglas, V. I., and Benezra, E. (1990). Supraspan verbal memory in attention deficit disorder with hyperactivity normal and reading-disabled boys. *Journal of Abnormal Child Psychology,* 18(6), 617-638. doi: 10.1007/bf01342751

Durston, S., van Belle, J., and de Zeeuw, P. (2011). Differentiating Frontostriatal and Fronto-Cerebellar Circuits in Attention-Deficit/Hyperactivity Disorder. *Biological Psychiatry,* 69(12), 1178-1184. doi: 10.1016/j.biopsych.2010.07.037

Eckert, M. A., Leonard, C. M., Richards, T. L., Aylward, E. H., Thomson, J., and Berninger, V. W. (2003). Anatomical correlates of dyslexia: Frontal and cerebellar findings. *Brain,* 126(2), 482-494.

Eliez, S., Rumsey, J. M., Giedd, J. N., Schmitt, J., Patwardhan, A. J., and Reiss, A. L. (2000). Morphological alteration of temporal lobe gray matter in dyslexia: An MRI study. *Journal of Child Psychology and Psychiatry,* 41(5), 637-644.

Farmer, L. J. (2003). A comparison between children with inattentive and combined subtypes of ADHD using neuropsychological and neuroanatomical measures. *Dissertation Abstracts International: Section B: The Sciences and Engineering,* 63(11-B), pp. 5549.

Fastame, M. C., Mammarella, I. C., Carretti, B., and Meneghetti, C. (2008). The continuous architecture of working memory: Evidence from Learning Disabilities and Genetic Syndromes. In N. B. Johansen (Ed.), *New Research on Short-Term Memory* (pp. 283-310). New York: Nova Science Publishers.

Fiez, J. A., Raife, E. A., Balota, D. A., Schwarz, J. P., Raichle, M. E., and Petersen, S. E. (1996). A positron emission tomography study of the short-term maintenance of verbal information. *The Journal of Neuroscience,* 16(2), 808-22;

Filipek, P. A., Semrud-Clikemann, M., Steingard, R., Renshaw, P., Kennedy, D., and Biederman, J. (1997). Volumetric MRI analysis comparing subjects having attention-deficit hyperactivity disorder with normal controls. *Neurology,* 48(3), 589-601.

French, B. F., Zentall, S. S., and Bennett, D. (2001). Short-term memory of children with and without characteristics of attention deficit hyperactivity disorder. *Learning and Individual Differences,* 13(3), 205-225.

Gathercole, S. E., Willis, C., and Baddeley, A. D. (1991). Differentiating phonological memory and awareness of rhyme: Reading and vocabulary development in children. *British Journal of Psychology, 82*(3), 387-406.

Geary, D. C. (2004). Mathematics and Learning Disabilities. *Journal of Learning Disabilities,* 37(1), 4-15.

Georgiewa, P., Rzanny, R., Hopf, J. M., Knab, R., Glauche, V., Kaiser, W. A., and Blanz, B. (1999). fMRI during word processing in dyslexic and normal reading children. *Neuroreport,* 10(16), 3459-3465.

Gottardo, A., Stanovich, K. E., and Siegel, L. S. (1996). The relationships between phonological sensitivity, syntactic processing, and verbal working memory in the reading performance of third-grade children. *Journal of Experimental Child Psychology,* 63(3), 563-582.

Hall, J. W., Wilson, K. P., Humphreys, M. S., Tinzmann, M. B., and Bowyer, P. M. (1983). Phonemic-similarity effects in good vs. poor readers. *Memory and Cognition,* 11(5), 520-527.

Hansen, J., and Bowey, J. A. (1994). Phonological analysis skills, verbal working memory, and reading ability in second-grade children. *Child Development,* 65(3), 938-950.

Henry, L. A. (2001). How does the severity of a learning disability affect working memory performance? *Memory,* 9(4-6), 233-247. doi: 10.1080/09658210042000085

Holligan, C., and Johnston, R. S. (1988). The use of phonological information by good and poor readers in memory and reading tasks. *Memory and Cognition,* 16(6), 522-532.

Houghton, S., Douglas, G., West, J., Whiting, K., Wall, M., Langsford, S., Carroll, A. (1999). Differential patterns of executive function in children with attention-deficit hyperactivity disorder according to gender and subtype. *Journal of Child Neurology,* 14(12), 801-805. doi: 10.1177/088307389901401206

Hulme, C., Maughan, S., and Brown, G. D. (1991). Memory for familiar and unfamiliar words: Evidence for a long-term memory contribution to short-term memory span. *Journal of Memory and Language,* 30(6), 685-701. doi: 10.1016/0749-596x(91)90032-f

Hulme, C., and Roodenrys, S. (1995). Verbal working memory development and its disorders. *Journal of Child Psychology and Psychiatry,* 36(3), 373-398.

Isaki, E., and Plante, E. (1997). Short-term and working memory differences in language/learning disabled and normal adults. *Journal of Communication Disorders,* 30(6), 427-437.

Jeffries, S., and Everatt, J. (2004). Working memory: Its role in dyslexia and other specific learning difficulties. *Dyslexia,* 10(3), 196-214.

Johnston, R. S. (1982). Phonological coding in dyslexic readers. *Br. J. Psychol.,* 73(Pt 4), 455-460.

Jonides, J., Schumacher, E. H., Smith, E. E., Koeppe, R. A., Awh, E., Reuter-Lorenz, P. A.,Willis, C. R. (1998). The role of parietal cortex in verbal working memory. *J. Neurosci.,* 18(13), 5026-5034.

Jonides, J., Schumacher, E. H., Smith, E. E., Lauber, E. J., et al. (1997). Verbal working memory load affects regional brain activation as measured by PET. *Journal of Cognitive Neuroscience,* 9(4), 462-475.

Jorm, A. F. (1983). Specific reading retardation and working memory: A review. *British Journal of Psychology,* 74(3), 311-342.

Kaplan, B. J., Dewey, D., Crawford, S. G., and Fisher, G. C. (1998). Deficits in long-term memory are not characteristic of ADHD. *Journal of Clinical and Experimental Neuropsychology,* 20(4), 518-528.

Karatekin, C. (2004). A test of the integrity of the components of Baddeley's model of working memory in attention-deficit/hyperactivity disorder (ADHD). *Journal of Child Psychology and Psychiatry, 45*(5), 912-926.

Kerns, K. A., McInerney, R. J., and Wilde, N. J. (2001). Time reproduction, working memory, and behavioral inhibition in children with ADHD. *Child Neuropsychology*, 7(1), 21-31.

Kibby, M. Y. (2009a). Memory Functioning in Developmental Dyslexia: An Analysis Using Two Clinical Memory Measures. *Archives of Clinical Neuropsychology*, 14(6), 525-546. doi: 10.1080/09297040701821752

Kibby, M. Y. (2009b). There are multiple contributors to the verbal short-term memory deficit in children with developmental reading disabilities. *Child Neuropsychology,* 15(5), 485-506. doi: 10.1080/09297040902748218

Kibby, M. Y., and Cohen, M. J. (2008). Memory functioning in children with reading disabilities and/or attention deficit/ hyperactivity disorder: A clinical investigation of their working memory and long-term memory functioning. *Child Neuropsychology,* 14(6), 525-546. doi: 10.1080/09297040701821752

Kibby, M. Y., Kroese, J., Morgan, A., Hiemenz, J., Cohen, M., and Hynd, G. (2004). The relationship between perisylvian morphology and verbal short-term memory functioning in children with neurodevelopmental disorders. *Brain and Language, 89(1),* 122-135. doi: DOI 10.1016/S0093-934X(03)00310-9

Kibby, M. Y., Marks, W., Morgan, S., and Long, C. J. (2004). Specific Impairment in Developmental Reading Disabilities: A Working Memory Approach. *Journal of Learning Disabilities,* 37(4), 349-363. doi: 10.1177/00222194040370040601

Kim, B.-N., Lee, J.-S., Shin, M.-S., Cho, S.-C., and Lee, D.-S. (2002). Regional cerebral perfusion abnormalities in attention deficit/hyperactivity disorder: Statistical parametric mapping analysis. *European Archives of Psychiatry and Clinical Neuroscience,* 252(5), 219-225.

Kirk, K. S. (2001). Relations between measures of attention and memory in the assessment of children with attentional difficulties. *Dissertation Abstracts International: Section B: The Sciences and Engineering,* 62(1-B), pp. 553.

Klorman, R., Hazel-Fernandez, L. A., Shaywitz, S. E., Fletcher, J. M., Marchione, K. E., Holahan, J. M., Shaywitz, B. A. (1999). Executive functioning deficits in attention-deficit/hyperactivity disorder are independent of oppositional defiant or reading disorder. *Journal of the American Academy of Child and Adolescent Psychiatry,* 38(9), 1148-1155.

Korkman, M., and Pesonen, A. E. (1994). A comparison of neuropsychological test profiles of children with attention deficit-hyperactivity disorder and/or learning disorder. *Journal of Learning Disabilities,* 27(6), 383-392.

Kunin-Batson, A. S. (2002). The effects of methylphenidate on neuropsychological functioning in children with attention deficit hyperactivity disorder. *Dissertation Abstracts International: Section B: The Sciences and Engineering*, 62(11-B), pp. 5380.

Kuntsi, J., Oosterlaan, J., and Stevenson, J. (2001). Psychological mechanisms in hyperactivity: I Response inhibition deficit, working memory impairment, delay aversion, or something else? *Journal of Child Psychology and Psychiatry,* 42(2), 199-210.

Lane, B. A. (2004). The differential neuropsychological/cognitive profiles of ADHD subtypes: A meta-analysis. *Dissertation Abstracts International: Section B: The Sciences and Engineering,* 64(11-B), pp. 5590.

Lee, C. P., and Obrzut, J. E. (1994). Taxonomic clustering and frequency associations as features of semantic memory development in children with learning disabilities. *Journal of Learning Disabilities,* 27(7), 454-462.

Leonard, C. M., Eckert, M. A., Lombardino, L. J., Oakland, T., Kranzler, J., Mohr, C. M., Freeman, A. (2001). Anatomical risk factors for phonological dyslexia. *Cerebral Cortex, 11*(2), 148-157.

Leonard, C. M., Voeller, K. K. S., Lombardino, L. J., Morris, M. K., Hynd, G. W., Alexander, A. W., Staab, E. V. (1993). Anomalous cerebral structure in dyslexia revealed with magnetic resonance imaging. *Archives of Neurology,* 50(5), 461-469.

Logie, R. H. (1995). *Visuo-spatial working memory*. Hillsdale, NJ: Lawrence Erlbaum Associates, Inc.

Logie, R. H., and Pearson, D. G. (1997). The Inner Eye and the Inner Scribe of Visuo-spatial Working Memory: Evidence from Developmental Fractionation. *European Journal of Cognitive Psychology,* 9(3), 241-257. doi: 10.1080/095414497382806

Mann, V. A., Cowin, E., and Schoenheimer, J. (1989). Phonological processing, language comprehension, and reading ability. *Journal of Learning Disabilities*, 22(2), 76-89.

Mann, V. A., Liberman, I. Y., and Shankweiler, D. (1980). Children's memory for sentences and word strings in relation to reading ability. *Memory and Cognition,* 8(4), 329-335.

Mariani, M. A., and Barkley, R. A. (1997). Neuropsychological and academic functioning in preschool boys with attention deficit hyperactivity disorder. *Developmental Neuropsychology,* 13(1), 111-129.

Mark, L. S., Shankweiler, D., Liberman, I. Y., and Fowler, C. A. (1977). Phonetic recoding and reading difficulty in beginning readers. *Memory and Cognition*, 5(6), 623-629.

Martin, R. C., and Romani, C. (1994). Verbal working memory and sentence comprehension: A multiple-components view. *Neuropsychology,* 8(4), 506-523.

Martin, R. C., Shelton, J. R., and Yaffee, L. S. (1994). Language processing and working memory: Neuropsychological evidence for separate phonological and semantic capacities. *Journal of Memory and Language,* 33(1), 83-111.

Martinussen, R., Hayden, J., Hogg-Johnson, S., and Tannock, R. (2005). A Meta-Analysis of Working Memory Impairments in Children With Attention-Deficit/Hyperactivity Disorder. *Journal of the American Academy of Child and Adolescent Psychiatry*, 44(4), 377-384.

Martinussen, R., and Tannock, R. (2006). Working Memory Impairments in Children with Attention-Deficit Hyperactivity Disorder With and Without Comorbid Language Learning Disorders. *Journal of Clinical and Experimental Neuropsychology,* 28(7), 1073-1094.

Mash, E. J., and Wolfe, D. A. (2010). *Abnormal Child Psychology* (4th ed.). Belmont, C. A.: Wadsworth.

McDougall, S. (1994). Short-term memory, speech rate and phonological awareness as predictors of learning to read. In C. Hulme and M. Snowling (Eds.), *Reading Development and Dyslexia* (pp. 31-44). London: Whurr Publishers, Ltd.

McDougall, S., and Donohoe, R. (2002). Reading ability and memory span: Long-term memory contributions to span for good and poor readers. *Reading and Writing,* 15(3-4), 359-387.

McDougall, S., Hulme, C., Ellis, A., and Monk, A. (1994). Learning to read: the role of short-term memory and phonological skills. *J. Exp. Child Psychol.,* 58(1), 112-133.

McInnes, A., Humphries, T., Hogg-Johnson, S., and Tannock, R. (2003). Listening comprehension and working memory are impaired in attention-deficit hyperactivity disorder irrespective of language impairment. *Journal of Abnormal Child Psychology,* 31(4), 427-443.

Mehta, M. A., Goodyer, I. M., and Sahakian, B. J. (2004). Methylphenidate improves working memory and set-shifting in AD/HD: Relationships to baseline memory capacity. *Journal of Child Psychology and Psychiatry,* 45(2), 293-305.

Meltzer, L. (1991). Problem-solving strategies and academic performance in learning disabled students: Do subtypes exist? In L. V. Feagans, E.J. Short and L. J. Meltzer (Eds.), *Subtypes of learning disabilities: Theoretical perspectives and research.* (pp. 163-188). Hillsdale, N. J.: Lawrence Erlbaum Associates.

Miller, K. J., and Castellanos, F. X. (1998). Attention deficit/hyperactivity disorders. *Pediatrics In Review / American Academy Of Pediatrics,* 19(11), 373-384.

Morrison, F. J., Giordani, B., and Nagy, J. (1977). Reading disability: an information-processing analysis. *Science,* 196(4285), 77-79.

Mostofsky, S. H., Cooper, K. L., Kates, W. R., Denckla, M. B., and Kaufmann, W. E. (2002). Smaller prefrontal and premotor volumes in boys with attention-deficit/hyperactivity disorder. *Biological Psychiatry,* 52(8), 785-794.

Muir-Broaddus, J. E., Rosenstein, L. D., Medina, D. E., and Soderberg, C. (2002). Neuropsychological test performance of children with ADHD relative to test norms and parent behavioral ratings. *Archives of Clinical Neuropsychology,* 17(7), 671-689.

Nigg, J. T. (2006). *What causes ADHD?: Understanding what goes wrong and why*. New York: Guilford Press.

Nigg, J. T., Blaskey, L. G., Huang-Pollock, C. L., and Rappley, M. D. (2002). Neuropsychological executive functions and DSM-IV ADHD subtypes. *Journal of the American Academy of Child and Adolescent Psychiatry,* 41(1), 59-66. doi: 10.1097/00004583-200201000-00012

Nigg, J. T., Hinshaw, S. P., Carte, E. T., and Treuting, J. J. (1998). Neuropsychological correlates of childhood attention-deficit/hyperactivity disorder: Explainable by comorbid disruptive behavior or reading problems? *Journal of Abnormal Psychology,* 107(3), 468-480. doi: 10.1037/0021-843x.107.3.468

Nigg, J. T., Willcutt, E. G., Doyle, A. E., and Sonuga-Barke, E. J. S. (2005). Causal Heterogeneity in Attention-Deficit/Hyperactivity Disorder: Do We Need Neuropsychologically Impaired Subtypes?. *Biological Psychiatry,* 57(11), 1224-1230. doi: 10.1016/j.biopsych.2004.08.025

Nyberg, L., Forkstam, C., Petersson, K. M., Cabeza, R., and Ingvar, M. (2002). Brain imaging of human memory systems: between-systems similarities and within-system differences. *Cognitive Brain Research*, 13(2), 281.

Olson, R. K., Forsberg, H., and Wise, B. (1994). Genes, environment, and the development of orthographic skills. In V. W. Berninger (Ed.), *The varieties of orthographic knowledge,*

1: Theoretical and developmental issues. (pp. 27-71). New York: Kluwer Academic/Plenum Publishers.

Pallas, D. M. (2003). A comparison of children with and without ADHD on verbal short-term and working memory tasks. *Dissertation Abstracts International: Section B: The Sciences and Engineering,* 63(7-B), pp. 3482.

Paulesu, E., Frith, U., Snowling, M., Gallagher, A., Morton, J., Frackowiak, R. S., and Frith, C. D. (1996). Is developmental dyslexia a disconnection syndrome? Evidence from PET scanning. *Brain,* 119(Pt 1), 143-157.

Pennington, B. F., and Ozonoff, S. (1996). Executive functions and developmental psychopathology. *Journal of Child Psychology and Psychiatry,* 37(1), 51-87.

Perfetti, C. A. (1985). *Reading ability*. New York: Oxford University Press.

Pugh, K. R., Mencl, W., Jenner, A. R., Katz, L., Frost, S. J., Lee, J. R., Shaywitz, B. A. (2000). Functional neuroimaging studies of reading and reading disability (developmental dyslexia). *Mental Retardation and Developmental Disabilities Research Reviews,* 6(3), 207-213.

Purvis, K. L., and Tannock, R. (1997). Language abilities in children with attention deficit hyperactivity disorder, reading disabilities, and normal controls. *Journal of Abnormal Child Psychology,* 25(2), 133-144. doi: 10.1023/a:1025731529006

Purvis, K. L., and Tannock, R. (2000). Phonological processing, not inhibitory control, differentiates ADHD and reading disability. *Journal of the American Academy of Child and Adolescent Psychiatry,* 39(4), 485-494.

Quinlan, D. M., and Brown, T. E. (2003). Assessment of short-term verbal memory impairments in adolescents and adults with ADHD. *Journal of Attention Disorders,* 6(4), 143-152.

Rack, J. P., Snowling, M. J., and Olson, R. K. (1992). The Nonword Reading Deficit in Developmental Dyslexia - a Review. *Reading Research Quarterly,* 27(1), 28-53.

Rapala, M. M., and Brady, S. (1990). Reading ability and short-term memory: The role of phonological processing. *Reading and Writing,* 2(1), 1-25.

Reader, M. J., Harris, E. L., Schuerholz, L. J., and Denckla, M. B. (1994). Attention deficit hyperactivity disorder and executive dysfunction. *Developmental Neuropsychology,* 10(4), 493-512.

Reiter, A., Tucha, O., and Lange, K. W. (2005). Executive functions in children with dyslexia. *Dyslexia,* 11(2), 116-131. doi: 10.1002/dys.289

Riccio, C. A., and Hynd, G. W. (1993). Developmental language disorders in children: Relationship with learning disability and Attention Deficit Hyperactivity Disorder. *School Psychology Review,* 22(4), 696-709.

Roodenrys, S. (2006). *Working memory function in attention deficit hyperactivity disorder.* New York: Psychology Press.

Roodenrys, S., Hulme, C., and Brown, G. (1993). The development of short-term memory span: Separable effects of speech rate and long-term memory. *Journal of Experimental Child Psychology,* 56(3), 431-442. doi: 10.1006/jecp.1993.1043

Roodenrys, S., Koloski, N., and Grainger, J. (2001). Working memory function in attention deficit hyperactivity disordered and reading disabled children. *British Journal of Developmental Psychology,* 19(3), 325-337.

Roodenrys, S., and Stokes, J. (2001). Serial recall and nonword repetition in reading disabled children. *Reading and Writing,* 14(5-6), 379-394.

Rucklidge, J. J., and Tannock, R. (2002). Neuropsychological profiles of adolescents with ADHD: Effects of reading difficulties and gender. *Journal of Child Psychology and Psychiatry and Allied Disciplines,* 43(8), 988-1003.

Rumsey, J. M., Andreason, P., Zametkin, A. J., King, A., Hamburger S.D., Aquino T. ... Cohen R.M. (1994). Right frontotemporal activation by tonal memory in dyslexia, an O-1-5 PET study. *Biological Psychiatry,* 36(3), *171-180.*

Rumsey, J. M., Nace, K., Donohue, B., Wise, D., Maisog, J. M., and Andreason, P. (1997). A positron emission tomographic study of impaired word recognition and phonological processing in dyslexic men. *Archives of Neurology,* 54(5), 562-573.

Sarkari, S. (2003). Do verbal working memory and reconstitution differentiate children with AD/HD. hyperactive-impulsive/combined type from children with ad/hd - predominantly inattentive type and controls? *Dissertation Abstracts International: Section B: The Sciences and Engineering,* 63(7-B), pp. 3483.

Semrud-Clikeman, M., Biederman, J., Sprich-Buckminster, S., Lehman, B. K., Faraone SV, and Norman D, (1992). Comorbidity between ADDH and learning disability: A review and report in a clinically referred sample. *Journal of the American Academy of Child and Adolescent Psychiatry,* 31(3), 439-448.

Semrud-Clikeman, M., Steingard, R. J., Filipek, P., Biederman, J., Bekken, K., and Renshaw, P. F. (2000). Using MRI to examine brain-behavior relationships in males with attention deficit disorder with hyperactivity. *Journal of the American Academy of Child and Adolescent Psychiatry,* 39(4), 477-484.

Shallice, T., Marzocchi, G. M., Coser, S., Del Savio, M., Meuter, R. F., and Rumiati, R. I. (2002). Executive function profile of children with attention deficit hyperactivity disorder. *Developmental Neuropsychology,* 21(1), 43-71.

Shanahan, M. A., Pennington, B. F., Yerys, B. E., Scott, A., Boada, R., Willcutt, E. G., DeFries, J. C. (2006). Processing Speed Deficits in Attention Deficit/Hyperactivity Disorder and Reading Disability. *Journal of Abnormal Child Psycholog,* 34(5), 585-602. doi: 10.1007/s10802-006-9037-8

Shankweiler, D., Liberman, I. Y., Mark, L. S., Fowler, C. A., and Fischer, F. W. (1979). The speech code and learning to read. *Journal of Experimental Psychology: Human Learning and Memory,* 5(6), 531-545. doi: 10.1037/0278-7393.5.6.531

Shaywitz, B. A., Fletcher, J. M., Holahan, J. M., Shneider, A. E., Marchione, K. E., Stuebing, K. K., Shaywitz, S. E. (1995). Interrelationships between reading disability and attention-deficit/hyperactivity disorder. *Child Neuropsychology,* 1(3), 170-186.

Shaywitz, B. A., Fletcher, J. M., and Shaywitz, S. E. (1995). Defining and classifying learning disabilities and attention-deficit/hyperactivity disorder. *Journal of Child Neurology,* 10(Suppl 1), S50-S57.

Shaywitz, S. E., Shaywitz, B. A., Fletcher, J. M., and Escobar, M. D. (1990). Prevalence of reading disability in boys and girls: Results of the Connecticut Longitudinal Study. *Journal of the American Medical Association, 264*(8), 998-1002.

Shaywitz, S. E., Shaywitz, B. A., Pugh, K. R., Fulbright, R. K., Constable, R. T., Mencl, W. E., Gore, J. C. (1998). Functional disruption in the organization of the brain for reading in dyslexia. *Proc. Natl.Acad. Sci. U S A,* 95(5), 2636-2641.

Short, E. J., and Ryan, E. B. (1984). Metacognitive differences between skilled and less skilled readers: Remediating deficits through story grammar and attribution training. *Journal of Educational Psychology,* 76(2), 225-235. doi: 10.1037/0022-0663.76.2.225

Shue, K. L., and Douglas, V. I. (1992). Attention deficit hyperactivity disorder and the frontal lobe syndrome. *Brain and Cognition,* 20(1), 104-124.

Siegel, L. S. (1988). Evidence that IQ scores are irrelevant to the definition and analysis of reading disability. *Can. J. Psychol.,* 42(2), 201-215.

Siegel, L. S. (1994). Working memory and reading: A life-span perspective. *International Journal of Behavioral Development Special Issue: The development of working memory,* 17(1), 109-124.

Silk, T., Vance, A., Rinehart, N., Egan, G., O'Boyle, M., Bradshaw, J., and Cunnington, R. (2005). Fronto-parietal activation in attention-deficit hyperactivity disorder, combined type: Functional magnetic resonance imaging study. *British Journal of Psychiatry,* 187(3), 282-283.

Smith, E. E., and Jonides, J. (1997). Working memory: A view from neuroimaging. *Cognitive Psychology,* 33(1), 5-42.

Snowling, M. J. (1991). Developmental Reading Disorders. *Journal of Child Psychology and Psychiatry and Allied Disciplines,* 32(1), 49-77. doi: 10.1111/1469-7610.ep11651178

Sonuga-Barke, E. J. S., Sergeant, J. A., Nigg, J., and Willcutt, E. (2008). Executive dysfunction and delay aversion in attention deficit hyperactivity disorder: Nosologic and diagnostic implications. *Child and Adolescent Psychiatric Clinics of North America,* 17(2), 367-384. doi: 10.1016/j.chc.2007.11.008

Sowell, E. R., Thompson, P. M., Welcome, S. E., Henkenius, A. L., Toga, A. W., and Peterson, B. S. (2003). Cortical abnormalities in children and adolescents with attention-deficit hyperactivity disorder. *Lancet,* 362(9397), 1699-1707.

Stadler, M. A. (1993). Implicit serial learning: Questions inspired by Hebb (1961). *Memory and Cognition,* 21(6), 819.

Stevens, J., Quittner, A. L., Zuckerman, J. B., and Moore, S. (2002). Behavioral inhibition, self-regulation of motivation, and working memory in children with attention deficit hyperactivity disorder. *Developmental Neuropsychology,* 21(2), 117-140.

Stone, B., and Brady, S. (1995). Evidence for Phonological Processing Deficits in Less-Skilled Readers. *Annals of Dyslexia,* 45, 51-78.

Sunseth, K., and Bowers, P. G. (2002). Rapid naming and phonemic awareness: Contributions to reading, spelling, and orthographic knowledge. *Scientific Studies of Reading*, 6(4), 401-429. doi: 10.1207/s1532799xssr0604_05

Swank, L. K. (1994). Phonological coding abilities: Identification of impairments related to phonologically based reading problems. *Topics in Language Disorders, 14*(2), 56-71.

Swanson, H. L. (1989). Verbal coding deficits in learning-disabled readers: A multiple stage model. *Educational Psychology Review,* 1(3*),* 235-277.

Swanson, H. L. (2006). Working memory and reading disabilities: Both phonological and executive processing deficits are important. In T. P. Alloway and S. E. Gathercole (Eds.), *Working memory and neurodevelopmental disorders.* (pp. 59-88). New York: Psychology Press.

Swanson, H. L., and Ashbaker, M. H. (2000). Working memory, short-term memory, speech rate, word recognition and reading comprehension in learning disabled readers: Does the executive system have a role? *Intelligence,* 28(1), 1-30.

Swanson, H. L., Ashbaker, M. H., and Lee, C. (1996). Learning-disabled readers' working memory as a function of processing demands. *J. Exp. Child. Psychol.*, 61(3), 242-275.

Swanson, H. L., and Berninger, V. (1995). The role of working memory in skilled and less skilled readers' comprehension. *Intelligence,* 21(1), 83-108.

Swanson, H. L., Cochran, K. F., and Ewers, C. A. (1989). Working memory in skilled and less skilled readers. *Journal of Abnormal Child Psychology,* 17(2), 145-156.

Swanson, H. L., and Howell, M. (2001). Working memory, short-term memory, and speech rate as predictors of children's reading performance at different ages. *Journal of Educational Psychology,* 93(4), 720-734.

Swanson, H. L., and Sachse-Lee, C. (2001). A subgroup analysis of working memory in children with reading disabilities: Domain-general or domain-specific deficiency? *Journal of Learning Disabilities Special Issue,* 34(3), 249-263.

Swanson, J., Castellanos, F., Murias, M., LaHoste, G., and Kennedy, J. (1998). Cognitive neuroscience of attention deficit hyperactivity disorder and hyperkinetic disorder. *Current Opinion in Neurobiology*, 8(2), 263-271.

Torgesen, J. K. (1985). Memory processes in reading disabled children. *Journal of Learning Disabilities,* 18(6), 350-357. doi: 10.1177/002221948501800608

Tractenberg, R. E. (2002). Exploring hypotheses about phonological awareness, memory, and reading achievement. *Journal of Learning Disabilities, 35*(5), 407-424.

Tripp, G., Ryan, J., and Peace, K. (2002). Neuropsychological functioning in children with DSM-IV combined type attention deficit hyperactivity disorder. *Australian and New Zealand Journal of Psychiatry,* 36(6), 771-779.

Vaidya, C. J., and Stollstorff, M. (2008). Cognitive neuroscience of Attention Deficit Hyperactivity Disorder: Current status and working hypotheses. *Developmental Disabilities Research Reviews,* 14(4), 261-267. doi: 10.1002/ddrr.40

Vance, A., Silk, T. J., Casey, M., Rinehart, N. J., Bradshaw, J. L., Bellgrove, M. A., and Cunnington, R. (2007). Right parietal dysfunction in children with attention deficit hyperactivity disorder, combined type: A functional MRI study, *Molecular Psychiatry,* 12(9), 826-832.

Vassileva, J. L. (2003). A functional magnetic resonance imaging study of verbal working memory in adults with attention deficit hyperactivity disorder. *Dissertation Abstracts International: Section B: The Sciences and Engineering,* 63(8-B), pp. 3973.

Vukovic, R. K., and Siegel, L. (2006). The role of working memory in specific reading comprehension difficulties. In T. P. Alloway and S. E. Gathercole (Eds.), *Working memory and neurodevelopmental disorders.* (pp. 89-112). New York: Psychology Press.

Wadsworth, S. J., DeFries, J. C., Fulker, D. W., and Olson, R. K. (1995). Reading performance and verbal short-term memory: A twin study of reciprocal causation. *Intelligence,* 20(2), 145-167. doi: 10.1016/0160-2896(95)90030-6

Wagner, R. K., and Torgesen, J. K. (1987). The nature of phonological processing and its causal role in the acquisition of reading skills. *Psychological Bulletin,* 101(2), 192-212. doi: 10.1037/0033-2909.101.2.192

Wagner, R. K., Torgesen, J. K., and Rashotte, C. A. (1994). Development of reading-related phonological processing abilities: New evidence of bidirectional causality from a latent variable longitudinal study. *Developmental Psychology,* 30(1), 73-87. doi: 10.1037/0012-1649.30.1.73

Walczyk, J. J., and Raska, L. J. (1992). The relation between low- and high-level reading skills in children. *Contemporary Educational Psychology,* 17(1), 38-46.

Wang, Y., and Zhang, X. (2008). Event-related potentials and working memory. In N. B. Johansen (Ed.), *New Resarch on Short-Term Memory* (pp. 437-455). New York, NY: Nova Science Pubishers.

Waterman, B., and Lewandowski, L. (1993). Phonologic and semantic processing in reading-disabled and nondisabled males at two age levels. *Journal of Experimental Child Psychology*, 55(1), 87-103. doi: 10.1006/jecp.1993.1004

Wendelken, C. (2008). Maintaining organized information: Modeling and fMRI investigation of working memory processes in prefrontal and parietal cortices. In N. B. Johansen (Ed.), *New Research on Short-Term Memory* (pp. 485-491). New York: NY: Nova Science Publishers.

Willcutt, E. G., Doyle, A. E., Nigg, J. T., Faraone, S. V., and Pennington, B. F. (2005). Validity of the Executive Function Theory of Attention-Deficit/Hyperactivity Disorder: A Meta-Analytic Review. *Biological Psychiatry,* 57(11), 1336-1346. doi: 10.1016/j.biopsych.2005.02.006

Willcutt, E. G., and Pennington, B. F. (2000). Comorbidity of reading disability and attention-deficit/hyperactivity disorder: Differences by gender and subtype. *Journal of Learning Disabilities Vol.* 33(2), 179-191.

Willcutt, E. G., Pennington, B. F., Boada, R., Ogline, J. S., Tunick, R. A., Chhabildas, N. A., and Olson, R. K. (2001). A comparison of the cognitive deficits in reading disability and attention-deficit/hyperactivity disorder. *Journal of Abnormal Psychology:,* 110(1), 157-172.

Willcutt, E. G., Pennington, B. F., Olson, R. K., Chhabildas, N., and Hulslander, J. (2005). Neuropsychological Analyses of Comorbidity Between Reading Disability and Attention Deficit Hyperactivity Disorder: In Search of the Common Deficit. *Developmental Neuropsychology,* 27(1), 35-78.

Wilson, K. M., and Swanson, H. L. (2001). Are mathematics disabilities due to a domain-general or a domain-specific working memory deficit? *Journal of Learning Disabilities,* 34(3), 237-248.

Zametkin, A. J., Liebenauer, L. L., Fitzgerald, G. A., King, A. C., Minkunas, D. V., Herscovitch, P., Cohen, R. M. (1993). Brain metabolism in teenagers with attention-deficit hyperactivity disorder. *Archives of General Psychiatry,* 50(5), 333-340.

In: Short-Term Memory: New Research
Editors: Garifallia Kalivas and Sappho F. Petralia
ISBN: 978-1-62100-860-6

Chapter 2

COLUMNAR EEG MAGNETIC INFLUENCES ON MOLECULAR DEVELOPMENT OF SHORT-TERM MEMORY

Lester Ingber*
Lester Ingber Research, US

Abstract

For several decades the stated Holy Grail of chemical, biological and biophysical research into neocortical information processing has been to reduce such neocortical phenomena into specific bottom-up molecular and smaller-scale processes. Over the past three decades, with regard to short-term memory (STM) and long-term memory (LTM) phenomena, which themselves are likely components of other phenomena like attention and consciousness, a statistical mechanics of neocortical interactions (SMNI) approach has yielded specific details of STM capacity, duration and stability not present in molecular approaches, but it is clear that most molecular approaches consider it inevitable that their reductionist approaches at molecular and possibly even quantum scales will yet prove to be causal explanations of such phenomena. The SMNI approach is a bottom-up aggregation from synaptic scales to columnar and regional scales of neocortex, and has been merged with larger non-invasive EEG scales with other colleagues – all at scales much coarser than molecular scales. As with many Crusades for some truths, other truths can be trampled. It is proposed that an SMNI vector potential (SMNI-VP) constructed from magnetic fields induced by neuronal electrical firings, at thresholds of collective minicolumnar activity with laminar specification, can give rise to causal top-down mechanisms that effect molecular excitatory and inhibitory processes in STM and LTM. A specific example might be causal influences on momentum $\mathbf{p}$ of Ca^{2+} ions by the SMNI-VP $\mathbf{A}$, as calculated by the canonical momentum $\mathbf{q}$, $\mathbf{q} = \mathbf{p} - e\mathbf{A}$, where e is the electron coulomb charge, which may be applied either classically or quantum-mechanically. Such a smoking gun for top-down effects awaits forensic in vivo experimental verification, requiring appreciating the necessity and due diligence of including true multiple-scale interactions across orders of magnitude in the complex neocortical environment.

*E-mail address: ingber@alumni.caltech.edu

PACS 05.10.Gg, 87.50.yg, 87.19.-j

AMS Subject Classification: 82Dxx, 92Cxx, 60Gxx

Keywords: short-term memory, astrocytes, neocortical dynamics, vector potential

1. Introduction and Rational

The phenomenon of short-term memory (STM) has many aspects and observed as well as conjectured mechanisms. The approach here is to take one approach based on a statistical mechanics of neocortical interactions (SMNI) which has been successful in calculating several important features of STM based on columnar structures in neocortex. This is taken as starting point to see how complementary processes at some larger and some smaller scales can be bridged to better understand STM

The next section describes the development of SMNI STM, followed by a section devoted to a summary of the mathematical development of SMNI. This helps to keep the rest of the paper relatively clear of some of these details, while still giving sufficient background to explain the development. The following section describes a larger context of STM, taking into account other work on smaller scales of neuronal as astrocyte interactions, as well as how the SMNI processes at columnar scales effects larger-scale regional activity. This discussion is conveniently described as bottom-up versus top-down processes. The following section deals with how SMNI processes at columnar scales, tuned to STM processing, can affect molecular scales of activity, via the electromagnetic vector potential, thereby describing a process that requires a casual threshold of columnar activity to influence ionic processes strongly implicated in STM at molecular levels. The last section is a conclusion emphasizing the importance of some top-down processes in STM phenomena.

2. SMNI STM

Neocortex has evolved to use minicolumns of neurons interacting via short-ranged interactions in macrocolumns, and interacting via long-ranged interactions across regions of macrocolumns (Buxhoeveden & Casanova, 2002; Mountcastle, 1978; Rakic, 2008). This common architecture processes patterns of information within and among different regions of sensory, motor, associative cortex, etc. The SMNI approach was the first physical application of a nonlinear multivariate calculus developed by other mathematical physicists in the late 1970's to define a statistical mechanics of multivariate nonlinear nonequilibrium systems (Graham, 1977; Langouche *et al.*, 1982).

SMNI builds minicolumnar, macrocolumnar, and regional interactions in neocortex. Since 1981, SMNI has been developed to model columns and regions of neocortex, spanning mm to cm of tissue, As depicted in Figure 1, SMNI develops three biophysical scales of neocortical interactions: (a)-(a*)-(a') microscopic neurons; (b)-(b') mesocolumnar domains; (c)-(c') macroscopic regions. SMNI has developed appropriate conditional probability distributions at each level, aggregating up from the smallest levels of interactions. In (a*) synaptic inter-neuronal interactions, averaged over by mesocolumns, are phenomenologically described by the mean and variance of a distribution Ψ. Similarly, in (a) intraneuronal transmissions are phenomenologically described by the mean and variance of Γ. Mesocolumnar averaged excitatory (E) and inhibitory (I) neuronal firings M are represented in (a'). In (b) the vertical organization of minicolumns is sketched together with their horizontal stratification, yielding a physiological entity, the mesocolumn. In (b') the overlap of interacting mesocolumns at locations r and r' from times t and $t+\tau$, τ on the order of 10 msec, is sketched. In (c) macroscopic regions of neocortex are depicted as arising from many mesocolumnar domains. (c') sketches how regions may be coupled by long-ranged interactions.

Most of these papers have dealt explicitly with calculating properties of STM and scalp EEG in order to test the basic formulation of this approach (Ingber, 1981, 1982, 1983, 1984, 1985a,b, 1986, 1991, 1992, 1994, 1995a,b, 1996a,b, 1997, 1998; Ingber & Nunez, 1990, 1995). The SMNI modeling of local mesocolumnar interactions (convergence and divergence between minicolumnar and macrocolumnar interactions) was tested on STM phenomena. The SMNI modeling of macrocolumnar interactions across regions was tested on EEG phenomena.

2.1. STM Capacity

SMNI studies have detailed that maximal numbers of attractors lie within the physical firing space of M^G, where $G = \{\text{Excitatory, Inhibitory}\}$ minicolumnar firings, consistent with experimentally observed capacities of auditory STM (Ericsson & Chase, 1982; Miller, 1956) and visual STM (Zhang & Simon, 1985), when a "centering" mechanism (CM), as detailed below, is enforced by shifting background noise in synaptic interactions, consistent with experimental observations under conditions of selective attention (Ingber, 1984, 1985b, 1994; Ingber & Nunez, 1995; Mountcastle *et al.*, 1981). This leads to all attractors of the short-time distribution lying along a diagonal line in M^G space, effectively defining a narrow parabolic trough containing these most likely firing states. This essentially collapses the two-dimensional M^G space down to a one-dimensional space of most importance. Thus, the predominant physics of STM and of (short-fiber contribution to) EEG phenomena takes place in a narrow "parabolic trough" in M^G space, roughly along a diagonal line (Ingber, 1984).

These calculations were further supported by high-resolution evolution of the two-variable short-time conditional-probability propagator using PATHINT (Ingber & Nunez, 1995). SMNI correctly calculated the stability and duration of STM, random access to memories within tenths of a second as observed, and the observed 7 ± 2 capacity rule of auditory memory (Miller, 1956) and the observed 4 ± 2 capacity rule of visual memory (Zhang & Simon, 1985).

Figure 2 shows the evolution of a Balanced Centered model (BC) after 500 foldings of $\Delta t = 0.01$, or 5 unit of relaxation time τ. Note the existence of ten well developed peaks or possible trappings of firing patterns (Ingber & Nunez, 1995). This seems to be able to describe the "7 ± 2" rule. The BC model is described in more detail below.

Figure 3 shows the evolution of a Balanced Centered Visual model (BCV) after 1000 foldings of $\Delta t = 0.01$, or 10 unit of relaxation time τ. Note the existence of four well developed peaks or possible trappings of firing patterns. Also note that other peaks at lower scales are clearly present, numbering on the same order as in the BC' model, as the strength

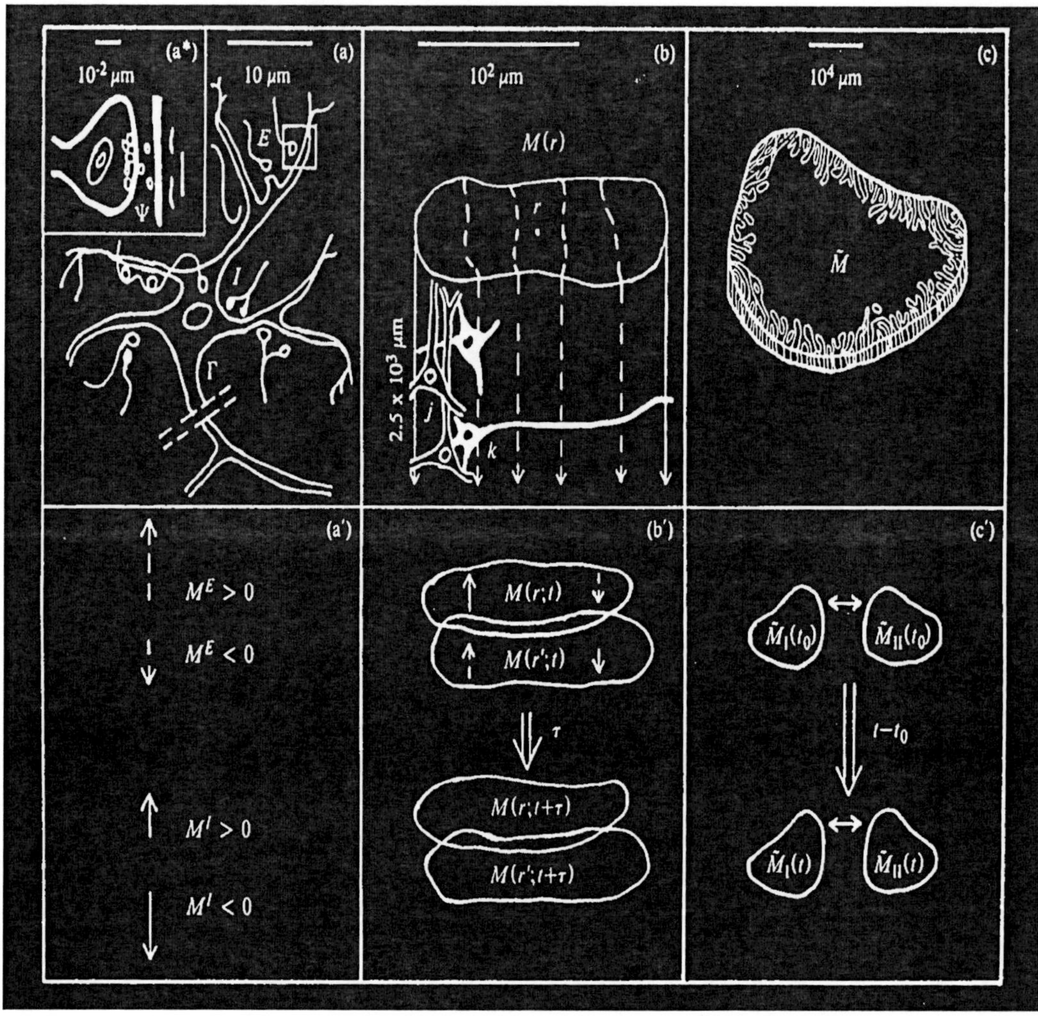

Figure 1. Illustrated are three biophysical scales of neocortical interactions: (a)-(a*)-(a') microscopic neurons; (b)-(b') mesocolumnar domains; (c)-(c') macroscopic regions. Reprinted with permission from (Ingber, 1983) by the American Physical Society.

in the original peaks dissipates throughout firing space, but these are much smaller and therefore much less probable to be accessed (Ingber & Nunez, 1995). This seems to be able to describe the "4 ± 2" rule for visual STM.

2.2. STM Duration

While early papers (Ingber, 1984, 1985b), suggested the possibility of sustenance of STM over epochs of tens of seconds just due to localized columnar interactions, it was clear that longer-ranged influences also are important to the development of the SMNI approach (Ingber, 1981, 1982, 1983). For example, calculations show that this duration of STM may not be possible if only localized columnar interactions are considered (Ingber, 1994;

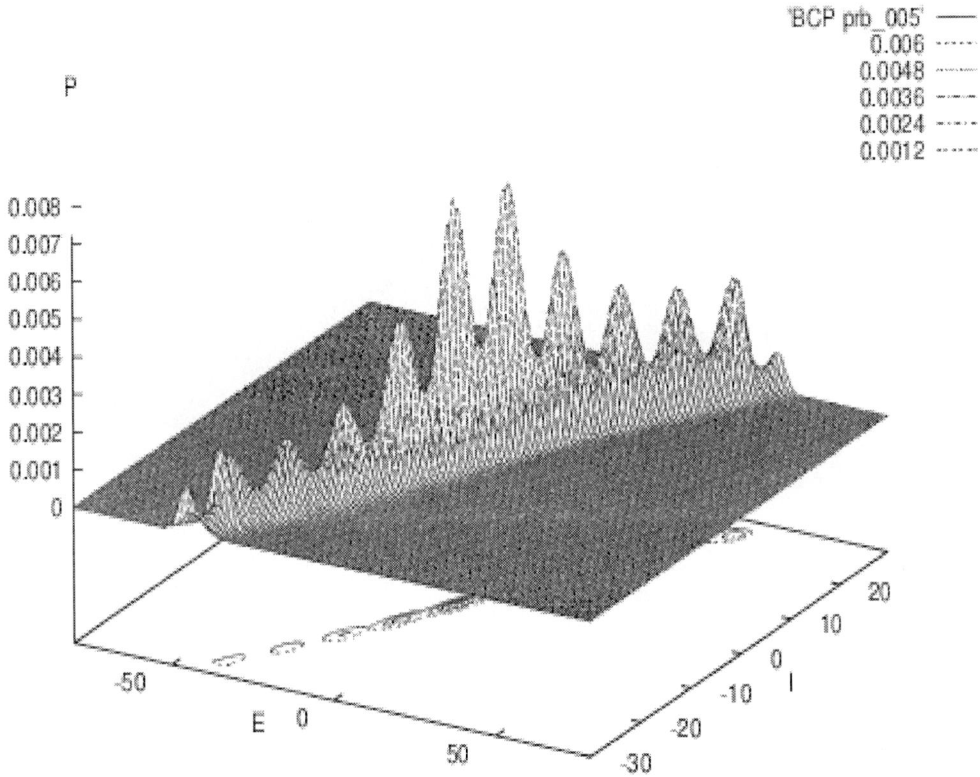

Figure 2. Illustrated is SMNI STM Model BC at the evolution at 5τ. Reprinted with permission from (Ingber & Nunez, 1995) by the American Physical Society.

Ingber & Nunez, 1995). After approximately 5τ, the clear separations between peaks of most-likely states in the evolving conditional probability distribution soon overlap. After approximately 10τ, the separations hardly exists. All four models considered, described below, representing dominant inhibition, dominant excitation, a "balanced" case in between these two (model BC' illustrated here), and the latter for the visual neocortex, exhibit similar decays of their peaks over these time scales. Future calculations, including all nonlinear SMNI effects might change this numerical result, but still the action of long-ranged neuron-neuron and diffuse neuromodulator interactions are known to be important to neocortical function, and they must be addressed.

2.3. Propagation of Information Across Minicolumns

In the sub-section below on Mathematical Development, it is noted that Euler-Lagrange (EL) equations are derived from the SMNI Lagrangian, the negative of the argument of the exponential describing the short-time conditional probability distribution of columnar firing states. Linearization of the EL equations permits the development of stability analyses and dispersion relations in frequency-wave-number space (Ingber, 1982, 1983, 1985a). It is noted in this regard that the corresponding wave propagation velocities pace interactions

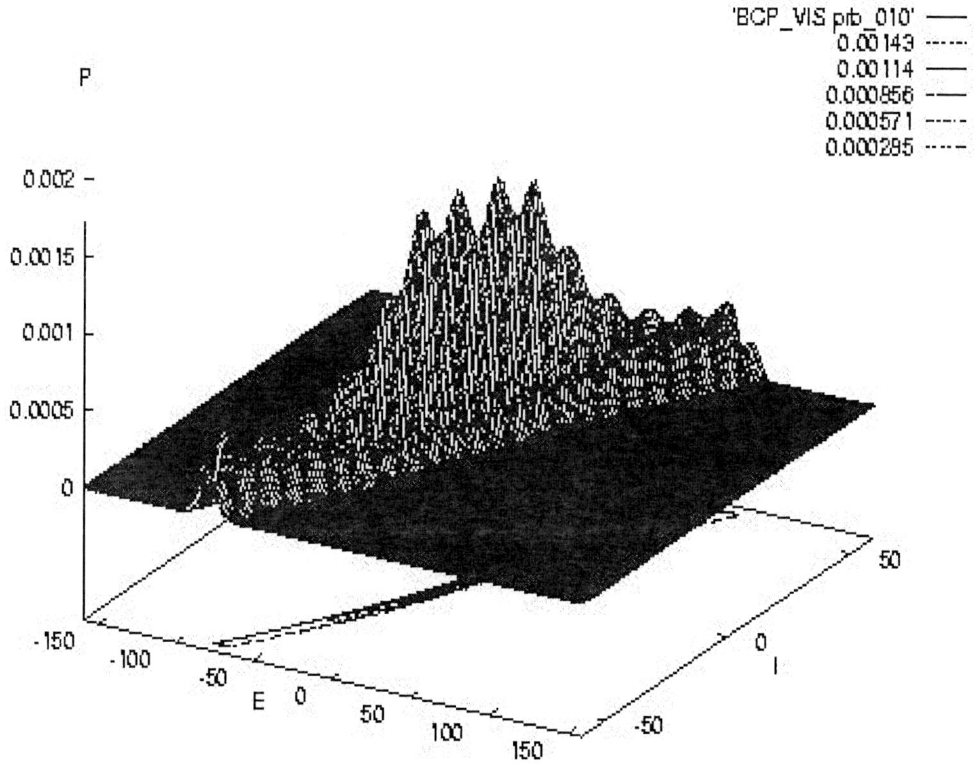

Figure 3. Illustrated is SMNI STM Model BCV at the evolution at 10τ. Reprinted with permission from (Ingber & Nunez, 1995) by the American Physical Society.

over several minicolumns, of magnitude sufficient to permit simultaneous information processing within about 10^{-1} sec with interactions mediated by long-ranged fibers possessing much greater propagation velocities about 600-900 cm/sec (Ingber, 1985a). E.g., detailed auditory and visual processing can feed information to the association cortex where it can be processed simultaneously, possibly giving feedback to the primary sensory regions. The propagation velocities calculated by SMNI, about 1 cm/sec, also are consistent with observed movements of attention (Tsal, 1983) and of hallucinations (Cowan, 1982) across the visual field. This strongly suggests that nearest-neighbor (NN) mesocolumnar interactions are an important mechanism in these movements.

2.4. Primacy Versus Recency Rule

Another phenomenon of STM capacity explained by the SMNI is the primacy versus recency effect in STM serial processing, wherein first-learned items are recalled most error-free, with last-learned items still more error-free than those in the middle (Murdock, 1983). The primacy versus recency rule is verified for acoustical STM, but visual or semantic STM typically requires longer times for rehearsal in a hypothesized articulatory loop of individual items (Zhang & Simon, 1985). In the SMNI approach, the basic assumption is made that a pattern of neuronal firing that persists for many τ cycles is a candidate to store the "memory" of activity that gave rise to this pattern. If several firing patterns can simultaneously exist, then there is the capability of storing several memories. The short-time conditional probability distribution derived for the neocortex is the primary tool to seek such firing patterns. The deepest minima of the Lagrangian, defined below, essentially the argument of this probability distribution, are more likely accessed than the others of this probability distribution, and these valleys are sharper than the others. I.e., they are more readily accessed and sustain their patterns against fluctuations more accurately than the relatively more shallow minima. The more recent memories or newer patterns may be presumed to be those having synaptic parameters more recently tuned and/or more actively rehearsed.

2.5. Hick's Law

SMNI supports random access to memories within tenths of a second as observed, and thereby helps to explain Hick's law of linearity of reaction time (RT) with STM information (Hick, 1952; Ingber, 1999; Jensen, 1987).

The RT necessary to "visit" the states under control during the span of STM can be calculated as the mean time of "first passage" between multiple states of this distribution, in terms of the probability P as an outer integral $\int dt$ (sum) over refraction times of synaptic interactions during STM time t, and an inner integral $\int dM$ (sum) taken over the mesocolumnar firing states M (Risken, 1989), which has been explicitly calculated to be within observed STM time scales (Ingber, 1984),

$$RT = -\int dt\, t \int dM \frac{dP}{dt}. \tag{1}$$

The probability distribution P is defined below.

As demonstrated by previous SMNI STM calculations, within tenths of a second, the conditional probability of visiting one state from another P, can be well approximated by a short-time probability distribution expressed in terms of the previously mentioned Lagrangian L as

$$P = \frac{1}{\sqrt{(2\pi dtg)}} \exp(-Ldt), \tag{2}$$

where g is the determinant of the covariance matrix of the distribution P in the space of columnar firings.

This expression for RT can be approximately rewritten as

$$RT \approx K \int dt \int dMP \ln P, \tag{3}$$

where K is a constant when the Lagrangian is approximately constant over the time scales observed. Since the peaks of the most likely M states of P are to a very good approximation well-separated Gaussian peaks (Ingber, 1984), these states may be treated as independent entities under the integral. This last expression is essentially the "information" content weighted by the time during which processing of information is observed.

The calculation of the heights of peaks corresponding to most likely states includes the combinatoric factors of their possible columnar manifestations as well as the dynamics of synaptic and columnar interactions. In the approximation that we only consider the combinatorics of items of STM as contributing to most likely states measured by P, i.e., that P measures the frequency of occurrences of all possible combinations of these items, we obtain Hick's Law, the observed linear relationship of RT versus STM information storage. For example, when the bits of information are measured by the probability P being the frequency of accessing a given number of items in STM, the bits of information in 2, 4 and 8 states are given as approximately multiples of $\ln 2$ of items, i.e., $\ln 2$, $2 \ln 2$ and $3 \ln 2$, resp. (The limit of taking the logarithm of all combinations of independent items yields a constant times the sum over $p_i \ln p_i$, where p_i is the frequency of occurrence of item i.)

2.6. STM Transference to LTM

SMNI also calculates how STM patterns (e.g., from a given region or even aggregated from multiple regions) may be encoded by dynamic modification of synaptic parameters (within experimentally observed ranges) into long-term memory patterns (LTM) (Ingber, 1983). This calculation simply shows how rates of firing can be encoded into synaptic parameters. It does not address any molecular mechanisms to cause such encodings, e.g., such as those referenced below.

2.7. SMNI Description of EEG

Using the power of the SMNI structure and the optimization algorithm Adaptive Simulated Annealing (ASA), sets of EEG and evoked potential data from an NIH study investigating genetic predispositions to alcoholism (Zhang *et al.*, 1995), were fitted to an SMNI model on a lattice of regional electrodes to extract brain "signatures" of STM (Ingber, 1997, 1998). Each electrode site was represented by an SMNI distribution of independent stochastic macrocolumnar-scaled M^G variables, interconnected by long-ranged circuitry with delays appropriate to long-fiber communication in neocortex. The global optimization algorithm ASA was used to perform maximum likelihood fits of Lagrangians defined by path integrals of multivariate conditional probabilities. Canonical momenta indicators (CMI) were thereby derived for individual's EEG data. The CMI give better signal recognition than the raw data, and were used to advantage as correlates of behavioral states. In-sample data was used for training (Ingber, 1997), and out-of-sample data was used for testing (Ingber, 1998) these fits.

These results gave strong quantitative support for an accurate intuitive picture, portraying neocortical interactions as having common algebraic physics mechanisms that scale across quite disparate spatial scales and functional or behavioral phenomena, i.e., describing interactions among neurons, columns of neurons, and regional masses of neurons.

Note that there are other models of EEG which also have sound experimental support. Some of the models can be shown to be indeed complementary to SMNI (Ingber & Nunez, 2010). Scalp potentials (EEG) are generated by synaptic current sources at small scales; each cubic millimeter of cortical tissue contains more than 100 million synapses. In contrast to this small scale activity, EEG data are recorded at macroscopic (centimeter) scales. All dependent variables are expressed as functions of time and cortical location. The basic approach ignores embedded network activity, although networks have been included in more advanced models (Jirsa & Haken, 1996; Nunez, 1989).

Below, some details of the SMNI approach lead to further confirmation of overlaps with some other approaches to EEG studies.

3. Mathematical Development

3.1. Neuronal Firings from Synaptic Aggregation

Figure 1 gives a visual representation of several stages of aggregation developed in SMNI (Ingber, 1982, 1983). Neocortical neurons typically have many dendrites that receive quanta of chemical postsynaptic stimulation from many other neurons. The distribution of quanta transmitted across synapses takes place on the scale of $10^{-2}\mu$m. Each quantum has thousands of molecules of chemical neurotransmitters that affect the chemically gated postsynaptic membrane. Chemical transmissions in the neocortex are believed to be either excitatory (E), such as glutamic acid, or inhibitory (I), such as γ aminobutyric acid. There exist many transmitters as well as other chemicals that modulate their effects, but it is assumed that after millions of synapses between hundreds of neurons are averaged over, then it is reasonable to ascribe a distribution function Ψ with a mean and variance for E and I interneuronal interactions.

Some neuroscientists do not accept the assumption that simple algebraic summation of excitatory depolarizations and inhibitory hyperpolarizations at the base of the inner axonal membrane determines the firing depolarization response of a neuron within its absolute and relative refractory periods (Shepherd, 1979), i.e., including the absolute refractory time after a firing during which no new spikes can be generated, and the relative refractory period during which spikes can be produced only at a decreased sensitivity (Sommerhoff, 1974). However, many other neuroscientists agree that this assumption is reasonable when describing the activity of large ensembles of neocortical neurons, each one typically having many thousands of synaptic interactions.

This same averaging procedure makes it reasonable to ascribe a distribution function Γ with a mean and variance for E and I intraneuronal interactions. A Gaussian Γ is taken to describe the distribution of electrical polarizations caused by chemical quanta impinging on the postsynaptic membrane. These polarizations give a resultant polarization at the base of the neuron, the axon. The base of the axon of a large fiber may be myelinated. However, smaller neurons typically lack these distinguishing features. Experimental techniques are not yet sufficiently advanced to attempt the explicit averaging procedure necessary to establish the means and variances of Ψ and Γ, and their parameters, *in vivo* (Vu & Krasne, 1992). Differential attenuations of polarizations from synapses to the base of an axon are here only phenomenologically accounted for by including these geometric and physiological effects into Γ.

With a sufficient depolarization of approximately 10 to 20 mV at the soma, within an absolute and relative refractory period of approximately 5 msec, an action potential is pulsed down the axon and its many collaterals, affecting voltage-gated presynaptic membranes to release quanta of neurotransmitters. Not detailed here is the biophysics of membranes, of thickness $\approx 5 \times 10^{-3}\mu$m, composed of biomolecular leaflets of phospholipid molecules (Caille' *et al.*, 1980; von der Heydt *et al.*, 1981; Scott, 1975). Ψ and Γ are taken to approximate this biophysics for use in macroscopic studies. Chemical independence of excitatory depolarizations and inhibitory hyperpolarizations are well established in the neocortex, and this independence is retained throughout SMNI.

It should be noted that experimental studies initially used to infer Ψ and Γ (e.g., at neuromuscular junctions) were made possible by deliberately reducing the number of quanta by lowering external calcium concentrations (Boyd & Martin, 1956; Katz, 1966). Ψ was found to be Poissonian, but in that system, where hundreds of quanta are transmitted *in vivo*, Ψ may well be otherwise; for example, Gaussian with independent mean and variance. Current research suggests a binomial distribution, having a Poisson limit (Ingber, 1982; Korn *et al.*, 1981; Perkel & Feldman, 1979). Note that some investigators have shown a Bernoulli distribution to be more accurate in some cases (Ingber, 1982; Korn & Mallet, 1984; Perkel & Feldman, 1979), and that the very concept of quantal transmission, albeit that good fits to experimental data are achieved with this concept, is under review. In the neocortex, probably small numbers of quanta are transmitted at synapses, but other effects, such as nonuniformity and nonstationarity of presynaptic release sites, and nonlinear summation of postsynaptic potentials, may detract from a simple phenomenological Poisson description (Shepherd, 1979).

This short description serves to point out possible differences in Ψ resulting from many sources. However, the derivation of synaptic interactions given here makes it plausible that for reasonable neuronal parameters, the statistical folding of Ψ and Γ is essentially independent of the functional form assumed for Ψ, just requiring specification of its numerical mean and variance.

The result of this analysis is to calculate the transition probability of the firing of neuron j, p_{σ_j}, given its interaction with its neighbors that also may fire or not fire. The result is given as the tabulated error function. Within the range where the total influences of excitatory and inhibitory firings match and exceed the average threshold potential of a given neuron, the probability of that neuron firing receives its major contribution to increase from 0 towards 1.

This is similar to mathematical results obtained by others (Little, 1974; Little & Shaw, 1978; Shaw & Vasudevan, 1974) who have modeled the neocortex after magnetic systems (Cragg & Temperley, 1954). However, in SMNI, this is derived more generally, and has the neural parameters more specifically denoted with different statistical significances given to Ψ and Γ, as described above.

Consider $10^2 < N < 10^3$ neurons, labeled by k, interacting with a given neuron j. Each neuron may contribute many synaptic interactions to many other neurons. A neuron may have as many as $10^4 - 10^5$ synaptic interactions. Within time $\tau_n \approx 5$ msec, Ψ is the distribution of q quanta of chemical transmitter released from neuron k to neuron j $(k \neq j)$ with mean a_{jk}, where

$$a_{jk} = A_{jk}(\sigma_k + 1)/2 + B_{jk}. \tag{4}$$

A_{jk} is the conductivity weighting transmission of polarization, dependent on k firing,

$$\sigma_k = \begin{cases} +1, & k \text{ fires} \\ -1, & k \text{ does not fire} \end{cases} \tag{5}$$

and B_{jk} is a background including some nonsynaptic and long-range activity. Of course, A and B are highly complicated functions of kj. This definition of σ_k permits a decomposition of a_{jk} into two different physical contributions.

Further SMNI development yields the conditional probability, p_{σ_j}, of neuron j firing given previous firings within τ of other neurons k:

$$p_{\sigma_j} = \pi^{-\frac{1}{2}} \int_{(\sigma_j F_j \sqrt{\pi}/2)}^{\infty} dz \exp(-z^2) \frac{1}{2} [1 - \text{erf}(\sigma_j F_j \sqrt{\pi}/2)],$$

$$F_j = \frac{V_j - \sum_k a_{jk} v_{jk}}{((\pi/2) \sum_{k'} a_{jk'} (v_{jk'}^2 + \phi_{jk'}^2))^{\frac{1}{2}}}. \quad (6)$$

"erf" is the tabulated error function, simply related to the normal probability function (Mathews & Walker, 1970). F_j is a "threshold factor," as p_{σ_j} increases from 0 to 1 between $\infty > \sigma_j F_j > -\infty$ sharply within the range of $F_j \approx 0$.

If

$$|\sigma_j F_j| < 1, \quad (7)$$

then an asymptotic expression for p_{σ_j} is

$$p_{\sigma_j} \approx \frac{\exp(-\sigma_j F_j)}{\exp(F_j) + \exp(-F_j)}. \quad (8)$$

3.2. Mesocolumns

The SMNI formulation of a multivariate nonlinear nonequilibrium system requires derivation in a proper Riemannian geometry to study proper limits of short-time conditional probability distributions. Prior to the late 1970's and early 1980's, many uses of path integrals for multivariate systems nonlinear in their drifts and diffusions were too cavalier in taking continuum limits. In general, results of derivations may be formally written as continuum limits, but these should be understood to be implemented as discrete in derivations as well as in numerical work (Langouche *et al.*, 1982; Schulman, 1981).

A sampling of these details can be seen in the context of SMNI. To properly deal with multivariate nonlinear multiplicative-noise systems, researchers have had to properly discretize the Feynman Lagrangian, L_F, in terms of the Feynman Action $\tilde{S}_F$, including Riemannian induced with the Stratonovich midpoint discretization (Langouche *et al.*, 1982). The Einstein convention of summing over factors with repeated indices is assumed. The Feynman probability distribution over the entire cortex, consisting of Λ mesocolumns spanning a total cortical area Ω, can be written formally, i.e., with discretization understood to be necessary in all derived uses and numerical calculations, as

$$\tilde{S}_F = \min \Lambda \Omega^{-1} \int dt' \int d^2 r \, L_F,$$

$$L_F = \frac{1}{2} N^{-1} (\dot{M}^G - h^G) g_{GG'} (M^{G'} - h^{G'}) - V,$$

$$h^G = g^G - \frac{1}{2} g^{-1/2} (g^{1/2} g^{GG'})_{,G'},$$

$$V = V' - (\frac{1}{2} h^G_{;G} + R/6)/N,$$
$$V' = V'^E + V'^I - M^G J_G/(2N\tau),$$
$$h^G_{;G} = g^{-1/2}(g^{1/2}h^G)_{,G},$$
$$g = ||g_{GG'}|| = \det(g_{GG'}) = g_{EE}g_{II},$$
$$g_{GG'} = (g^{GG'})^{-1},$$
$$R = g^{-1}(g_{EE,II} + g_{II,EE}) - \frac{1}{2}g^{-2} \times \{g_{II}[g_{EE,E}g_{II,E} + (g_{EE,I})^2] + g_{EE}[g_{II,I}g_{EE,I} + (g_{II,E})^2]\},$$
$$[\ldots]_{,G} \equiv (\partial/\partial M^G)[\ldots]. \tag{9}$$

The Riemannian curvature R arises from the nonlinear inverse variance $g_{GG'}$, which is a *bona fide* metric of this parameter space (Graham, 1978). The discretization of the determinant prefactor of the conditional probability distribution requires additional care (Langouche *et al.*, 1982).

Some of the algebra behind SMNI depicts variables and distributions that populate each representative macrocolumn in each region. While Riemannian terms were calculated when using the Stratonovich midpoint discretization of the probability distribution (Ingber, 1982, 1983), in order to explicitly deal with the multivariate nonlinearities, here it suffices to use the more readable Ito prepoint discretization, which is an equivalent numerical distribution when used consistently (Langouche *et al.*, 1982). Codes for all SMNI algebra were written in several languages and found to give the same numerical answers: algebraic languages Macsyma (and its later version Maxima) and Reduce, Fortran and C, and alphanumeric coding of magnetic strips for the hand calculator HP-41C.

A derived mesoscopic Lagrangian L_M defines the short-time probability distribution of firings in a minicolumn, composed of about 10^2 neurons, given its just previous interactions with all other neurons in its macrocolumnar surround. G is used to represent excitatory (E) and inhibitory (I) contributions. $\bar{G}$ designates contributions from both E and I.

$$P_M = \prod_G P^G_M[M^G(r;t+\tau)|M^{\bar{G}}(r';t)]$$
$$= \sum_{\sigma_j} \delta\left(\sum_{jE} \sigma_j - M^E(r;t+\tau)\right) \delta\left(\sum_{jI} \sigma_j - M^I(r;t+\tau)\right) \prod_j^N p_{\sigma_j}$$
$$\simeq \prod_G (2\pi\tau g^{GG})^{-1/2} \exp(-N\tau L^G_M),$$
$$P_M \simeq (2\pi\tau)^{-1/2} g^{1/2} \exp(-N\tau L_M),$$
$$L_M = L^E_M + L^I_M = (2N)^{-1}(\dot{M}^G - g^G)g_{GG'}(\dot{M}^{G'} - g^{G'}) + M^G J_G/(2N\tau) - V',$$
$$V' = \sum_G V''^G_{G'}(\rho\nabla M^{G'})^2,$$
$$g^G = -\tau^{-1}(M^G + N^G \tanh F^G), g^{GG'} = (g_{GG'})^{-1} = \delta^{G'}_G \tau^{-1} N^G \mathrm{sech}^2 F^G, \quad g = \det(g_{GG'}),$$
$$F^G = \frac{(V^G - a^{|G|}_{G'} v^{|G|}_{G'} N^{G'} - \frac{1}{2} A^{|G|}_{G'} v^{|G|}_{G'} M^{G'})}{((\pi/2)[(v^{|G|}_{G'})^2 + (\phi^{|G|}_{G'})^2](a^{|G|}_{G'} N^{G'} + \frac{1}{2} A^{|G|}_{G'} M^{G'}))^{1/2}}, \quad a^G_{G'} = \frac{1}{2} A^G_{G'} + B^G_{G'}, \tag{10}$$

where $A_{G'}^{G}$ and $B_{G'}^{G}$ are minicolumnar-averaged inter-neuronal synaptic efficacies, $v_{G'}^{G}$ and $\phi_{G'}^{G}$ are averaged means and variances of contributions to neuronal electric polarizations. $M^{G'}$ and $N^{G'}$ in F^G are afferent macrocolumnar firings, scaled to efferent minicolumnar firings by $N/N* \approx 10^{-3}$, where $N*$ is the number of neurons in a macrocolumn, about 10^5. Similarly, $A_{G}^{G'}$ and $B_{G}^{G'}$ have been scaled by $N*/N \approx 10^3$ to keep F^G invariant. V' is mesocolumnar NN interactions. Other values taken are consistent with experimental data, e.g., $V^G = 10$ mV, $v_{G'}^{G} = 0.1$ mV, $\phi_{G'}^{G} = 0.03^{1/2}$ mV. Note that these values and the factor $(\pi/2)^{1/2}$ in the denominator of F^G, give identical numerical values for F^G as in earlier papers with values of $\phi_{G'}^{G} = 0.1$ mV and a factor $\pi^{1/2}$.

It is notes that, as originally derived (Ingber, 1982, 1983), the numerator of F^G contains information derived from presynaptic firing interactions. The location of most stable states of this SMNI system is highly dependent on the interactions presented in this numerator. The denominator of F^G contains information derived from factors of presynaptic and postsynaptic neuromodular and electrical processing of these firings. The nonlinearities present in this denominator dramatically affect the number and nature of stable states at scales zoomed in at magnifications on the order of a thousand times, representing neocortical processing of detailed information within a sea of stochastic activity.

3.3. Inclusion of Macroscopic Circuitry

The most important features of this development are described by the Lagrangian L^G and the "threshold factor" F^G describing an important sensitivity of the distribution to changes in its variables and parameters.

To more properly include long-ranged fibers between macrocolumns, the J_G terms can be dropped, and more realistically replaced by a modified threshold factor F^G,

$$F^G = \frac{(V^G - a_{G'}^{|G|} v_{G'}^{|G|} N^{G'} - \frac{1}{2} A_{G'}^{|G|} v_{G'}^{|G|} M^{G'} - a_{E'}^{\ddagger E} v_{E'}^{E} N^{\ddagger E'} - \frac{1}{2} A_{E'}^{\ddagger E} v_{E'}^{E} M^{\ddagger E'})}{((\pi/2)[(v_{G'}^{|G|})^2 + (\phi_{G'}^{|G|})^2](a_{G'}^{|G|} N^{G'} + \frac{1}{2} A_{G'}^{|G|} M^{G'} + a_{E'}^{\ddagger E} N^{\ddagger E'} + \frac{1}{2} A_{E'}^{\ddagger E} M^{\ddagger E'}))^{1/2}},$$

$$a_{E'}^{\ddagger E} = \frac{1}{2} A_{E'}^{\ddagger E} + B_{E'}^{\ddagger E}. \qquad (11)$$

Here, afferent contributions from $N^{\ddagger E}$ long-ranged excitatory fibers, e.g., cortico-cortical neurons, have been added, where $N^{\ddagger E}$ might be on the order of 10% of N^*: Of the approximately 10^{10} to 10^{11} neocortical neurons, estimates of the number of pyramidal cells range from 2/3 up to 4/5 (Markram *et al.*, 2004). Nearly every pyramidal cell has an axon branch that makes a cortico-cortical connection; i.e., the number of cortico-cortical fibers is of the order 10^{10}. This development is used in the SMNI description of scalp EEG across regions.

3.4. Centering Mechanism (CM)

It was discovered that more minima of the static Lagrangian $\bar{L}$ are created, i.e., brought into the physical firing ranges, if the numerator of F^G contains terms only in $\bar{M}^G$, tending to center $\bar{L}$ about $\bar{M}^G = 0$ (Ingber, 1984). That is, B^G is modified such that the numerator of F^G is transformed to

$$F'^G = \frac{-\frac{1}{2} A_{G'}^{|G|} v_{G'}^{|G|} M^{G'}}{((\pi/2)[(v_{G'}^{|G|})^2 + (\phi_{G'}^{|G|})^2](a'^{|G|}_{G'} N^{G'} + \frac{1}{2} A_{G'}^{|G|} M^{G'}))^{1/2}},$$

$$a'^G_{G'} = \frac{1}{2} A^G_{G'} + B'^G_{G'}, \tag{12}$$

The most likely states of the centered systems lie along diagonals in M^G space, a line determined by the numerator of the threshold factor in F^E, essentially

$$A^E_E M^E - A^E_I M^I \approx 0, \tag{13}$$

noting that in F^I $I-I$ connectivity is experimentally observed to be very small relative to other pairings, so that $(A^I_E M^E - A^I_I M^I)$ is typically small only for small M^E.

Of course, any mechanism producing more as well as deeper minima is statistically favored. However, this particular CM has plausible support: $M^G(t+\tau) = 0$ is the state of afferent firing with highest statistical weight. I.e., there are more combinations of neuronal firings, $\sigma_j = \pm 1$, yielding this state than any other $M^G(t+\tau)$, e.g., $\approx 2^{N^G+1/2}(\pi N^G)^{-1/2}$ relative to the states $M^G = \pm N^G$. Similarly, $M^G(t)$ is the state of efferent firing with highest statistical weight. Therefore, it is natural to explore mechanisms which favor common highly weighted efferent and afferent firings in ranges consistent with favorable firing threshold factors $F^G \simeq 0$.

In general, B^G_E and B^G_I (and possibly A^G_E and A^G_I due to actions of neuromodulators, and J_G constraints from long-ranged fibers) are available to zero the constant in the numerator, giving an extra degree(s) of freedom to this mechanism. (If B'^G_E would be negative, this leads to unphysical results in the square-root denominator of F^G. In all examples where this occurs, it is possible to instead find positive B'^G_I to appropriately shift the numerator of F^G.) In this context, it is empirically observed that the synaptic sensitivity of neurons engaged in selective attention is altered, presumably by the influence of chemical neuromodulators on postsynaptic neurons at their presynaptic sites (Mountcastle *et al.*, 1981).

3.5. Prototypical Cases

Three Cases of neuronal firings were considered in the first introduction of STM applications of SMNI (Ingber, 1984). Below is a short summary of these details. Note that while it suffices to define these Cases using F^G, the full Lagrangian and probability distribution, upon which the derivation of the EL equations are based, are themselves quite nonlinear functions of F^G, e.g., via hyperbolic trigonometric functions, etc.

Since STM duration is long relative to τ, stationary solutions of the Lagrangian L, $\bar{L}$, can be investigated to determine how many stable minima $\ll \bar{M}^G \gg$ may simultaneously exist within this duration. Detailed calculations of time-dependent folding of the full time-dependent probability distribution supports persistence of these stable states within SMNI calculations of observed decay rates of STM (Ingber & Nunez, 1995).

A model of dominant inhibition describes how minicolumnar firings are suppressed by their neighboring minicolumns. For example, this could be effected by developing NN mesocolumnar interactions (Ingber, 1983), but here the averaged effect is established by inhibitory mesocolumns (Case I) by setting $A^I_E = A^E_I = 2A^E_E = 0.01N^*/N$. Since there appears to be relatively little $I-I$ connectivity, set $A^I_I = 0.0001N^*/N$. The background synaptic noise is taken to be $B^E_I = B^I_E = 2B^E_E = 10B^I_I = 0.002N^*/N$. As minicolumns are observed to have about 110 neurons (visual cortex appears to have approximately twice this density) (Mountcastle, 1978), and as there appear to be a predominance of E over I neurons

(Nunez, 1981), here take $N^E = 80$ and $N^I = 30$. Use $N^*/N = 10^3$, $\nu_{G'}^G$, and $\phi_{G'}^G$ as estimated previously. $\bar{M}^G$ represents time-averaged M^G. The threshold factors F_{I}^G for this I model are then

$$F_{\mathrm{I}}^E = \frac{(0.5\bar{M}^I - 0.25\bar{M}^E + 3.0)}{\pi^{1/2}(0.1\bar{M}^I + 0.05\bar{M}^E + 9.80)^{1/2}},$$

$$F_{\mathrm{I}}^I = \frac{(0.005\bar{M}^I - 0.5\bar{M}^E - 45.8)}{\pi^{1/2}(0.001\bar{M}^I + 0.1\bar{M}^E + 11.2)^{1/2}}. \tag{14}$$

In the prepoint-discretized deterministic limit, the threshold factors determine when and how smoothly the step-function forms $\tanh F_{\mathrm{I}}^G$ in $g^G(t)$ change $M^G(t)$ to $M^G(t+\tau)$. F_{I}^I will cause afferent $\bar{M}^I$ to fire for most of its values, as $\bar{M}^I \approx -N^I \tanh F_{\mathrm{I}}^I$ will be positive for most values of $\bar{M}^G$ in F_{I}^I, which is already weighted heavily with a term -45.8. Looking at F_{I}^E, it is seen that the relatively high positive values of efferent $\bar{M}^I$ require at least moderate values of positive efferent $\bar{M}^E$ to cause firings of afferent $\bar{M}^E$.

The centering effect of the I model, labeled here as the IC model, is quite easy for neocortex to accommodate. For example, this can be accomplished simply by readjusting the synaptic background noise from B_E^G to B'^G_E,

$$B'^G_E = \frac{[V^G - (\frac{1}{2}A_I^G + B_I^G)\nu_I^G N^I - \frac{1}{2}A_E^G \nu_E^G N^E]}{\nu_E^G N^G} \tag{15}$$

for both $G = E$ and $G = I$. In general, B_E^G and B_I^G (and possibly A_E^G and A_I^G due to actions of neuromodulators, and J_G constraints from long-ranged fibers) are available to zero the constant in the numerator, giving an extra degree(s) of freedom to this mechanism. (If B'^G_E would be negative, this leads to unphysical results in the square-root denominator of F^G. In all examples where this occurs, it is possible to instead find positive B'^G_I to appropriately shift the numerator of F^G.) In this context, it is empirically observed that the synaptic sensitivity of neurons engaged in selective attention is altered, presumably by the influence of chemical neuromodulators on postsynaptic neurons at their presynaptic sites (Mountcastle *et al.*, 1981).

By this CM, $B'^E_E = 1.38$ and $B'^I_I = 15.3$, and F_{I}^G is transformed to F_{IC}^G, Case IC,

$$F_{\mathrm{IC}}^E = \frac{(0.5\bar{M}^I - 0.25\bar{M}^E)}{\pi^{1/2}(0.1\bar{M}^I + 0.05\bar{M}^E + 10.4)^{1/2}},$$

$$F_{\mathrm{IC}}^I = \frac{(0.005\bar{M}^I - 0.5\bar{M}^E)}{\pi^{1/2}(0.001\bar{M}^I + 0.1\bar{M}^E + 20.4)^{1/2}}. \tag{16}$$

Note that, aside from the enforced vanishing of the constant terms in the numerators of F_{I}^G, the only other changes in F_{I}^G moderately affect the constant terms in the denominators.

The other extreme of normal neocortical firings is a model of dominant excitation, effected by establishing excitatory mesocolumns (Case E) by using the same parameters $\{B_{G'}^G, \nu_{G'}^G, \phi_{G'}^G, A_I^I\}$ as in the I model, but setting $A_E^E = 2A_E^I = 2A_I^E = 0.01N^*/N$. This yields

$$F_{\mathrm{E}}^E = \frac{(0.25\bar{M}^I - 0.5\bar{M}^E - 24.5)}{\pi^{1/2}(0.05\bar{M}^I + 0.10\bar{M}^E + 12.3)^{1/2}},$$

$$F_{\text{E}}^{I}=\frac{(0.005\bar{M}^{I}-0.25\bar{M}^{E}-25.8)}{\pi^{1/2}(0.001M^{I}+0.05M^{E}+7.24)^{1/2}}. \tag{17}$$

The negative constant in the numerator of F_{E}^{I} inhibits afferent $\bar{M}^{I}$ firings. Although there is also a negative constant in the numerator of F_{E}^{E}, the increased coefficient of $\bar{M}^{E}$ (relative to its corresponding value in F_{I}^{E}), and the fact that $\bar{M}^{E}$ can range up to $N^{E}=80$, readily permits excitatory firings throughout most of the range of $\bar{M}^{E}$.

Applying the CM to E, $B'^{E}_{I}=10.2$ and $B'^{I}_{I}=8.62$. The net effect in F_{EC}^{G}, Case EC, in addition to removing the constant terms in the numerators of F_{E}^{G}, is to change the constant terms in the denominators: 12.3 in F_{E}^{E} is changed to 17.2 in F_{EC}^{E}, and 7.24 in F_{E}^{I} is changed to 12.4 in F_{EC}^{I}.

Now it is natural to examine a balanced Case intermediate between I and E, labeled here as Case B. This is accomplished by changing $A_{E}^{E}=A_{E}^{I}=A_{I}^{E}=0.005N^{*}/N$. This yields

$$F_{\text{B}}^{E}=\frac{(0.25\bar{M}^{I}-0.25\bar{M}^{E}-4.50)}{\pi^{1/2}(0.050M^{E}+0.050M^{I}+8.30)^{1/2}},$$

$$F_{\text{B}}^{I}=\frac{(0.005\bar{M}^{I}-0.25\bar{M}^{E}-25.8)}{\pi^{1/2}(0.001M^{I}+0.050M^{E}+7.24)^{1/2}}. \tag{18}$$

Applying the CM to B, $B'^{E}_{E}=0.438$ and $B'^{I}_{I}=8.62$. The net effect in F_{BC}^{G}, Case BC, in addition to removing the constant terms in the numerators of F_{B}^{G}, is to change the constant terms in the denominators: 8.30 in F_{B}^{E} is changed to 7.40 in F_{BC}^{E}, and 7.24 in F_{B}^{I} is changed to 12.4 in F_{BC}^{I}.

Previously, calculations were performed for the three prototypical firing Cases, dominate excitatory (E), dominate inhibitory (I) and balanced about evenly (B). More minima were brought within physical firing ranges when a CM is invoked (Ingber, 1984), by tuning the presynaptic stochastic background, a phenomena observed during selective attention, giving rise to Cases EC, IC and BC. The states BC are observed to yield properties of auditory STM, e.g., the 7 ± 2 capacity rule and times of duration of these memory states (Ingber, 1984, 1985b).

It is observed that visual neocortex has twice the number of neurons per minicolumn as other regions of neocortex. In the SMNI model this gives rise to fewer and deeper STM states, consistent with the observed 4 ± 2 capacity rule of these memory states. These calculations are Cases ECV, ICV and BCV (Ingber, 1994).

3.6. Euler-Lagrange (EL)

To investigate dynamics of multivariate stochastic nonlinear systems, such as neocortex presents, it is not sensible to simply apply simple mean-field theories which assume sharply peaked distributions, since the dynamics of nonlinear diffusions in particular are typically washed out. Here, path integral representations of systems, otherwise equivalently represented by Langevin or Fokker-Planck equations, present elegant algorithms by use of variational principles leading to EL equations (Langouche *et al.*, 1982).

SMNI permits scaling to derive EL in several approximations which give insight into other phenomena that take advantage of the SMNI STM approach.

3.6.1. Columnar EL

The Lagrangian components and EL equations are essentially the counterpart to classical dynamics,

$$\text{Mass} = g_{GG'} = \frac{\partial^2 L}{\partial(\partial M^G/\partial t)\partial(\partial M^{G'}/\partial t)},$$

$$\text{Momentum} = \Pi^G = \frac{\partial L}{\partial(\partial M^G/\partial t)},$$

$$\text{Force} = \frac{\partial L}{\partial M^G},$$

$$\text{F} - \text{ma} = 0 : \ \delta L = 0 = \frac{\partial L}{\partial M^G} - \frac{\partial}{\partial t}\frac{\partial L}{\partial(\partial M^G/\partial t)}. \tag{19}$$

The EL equations are derived from the long-time conditional probability distribution of columnar firings over all cortex, represented by $\tilde{M}$, in terms of the Action S,

$$\tilde{P}[\tilde{M}(t)]d\tilde{M}(t) = \int \ldots \int D\tilde{M} \exp(-N\tilde{S}),$$

$$\tilde{M} = \{M^{G\nu}\}, \quad \tilde{S} = \int_{t_0}^{t} dt'\tilde{L}, \quad \tilde{L} = \Lambda\Omega^{-1}\int d^2r L, \quad L = L^E + L^I,$$

$$D\tilde{M} = \prod_{s=1}^{u+1}\prod_{\nu=1}^{\Lambda}\prod_{G}^{E,I}(2\pi dt)^{-1/2}(g_s^\nu)^{1/4} dM_s^{G\nu}\delta[M_t = M(t)][\delta[M_0 = M(t_0)], \tag{20}$$

where ν labels the two-dimensional laminar $\vec{r}$-space of $\Lambda \approx 5 \times 10^5$ mesocolumns spanning a typical region of neocortex, Ω, (total cortical area $\approx 4 \times 10^{11} \mu\text{m}^2$); and s labels the $u+1$ time intervals, each of duration $dt \leq \tau$, spanning $(t - t_0)$. At a given value of $(r;t)$, $M = \{M^G\}$.

The path integral has a variational principle, $\delta L = 0$ which gives the EL equations for SMNI (Ingber, 1982, 1983). The Einstein convention is used to designate summation over repeated indices, and the following notation for derivatives is used:

$$(\ldots)_{:z} = d(\ldots)/dz, z = \{x,y\},$$

$$(\ldots)_{,G} = \partial(\ldots)/\partial M^G, \ (\ldots)_{,\dot{G}} = \partial(\ldots)/\partial(dM^G/dt),$$

$$(\ldots)_{,G_{:z}} = \partial(\ldots)/\partial(dM^G/dz),$$

$$(\ldots)_{,\nabla G} = \hat{x}\partial(\ldots)/\partial(dM^G/dx) + \hat{y}\partial(\ldots)/\partial(dM^G/dy). \tag{21}$$

The EL equations are:

$$\delta L = 0,$$

$$\delta_G L = L_{,G} - \nabla \cdot L_{,\nabla G} - L_{,\dot{G}:t} = 0,$$

$$\nabla \cdot L_{,\nabla G} = L_{,G_{:z}:z} = (L_{,G_{:z}},_{G'})M^{G'}_{:z} + (L_{,G_{:z}},_{G'_{:z}})M^{G'}_{:zz}$$

$$L_{,\dot{G}:t} = (L_{,\dot{G}},_{G'})\dot{M}^{G'} + (L_{,\dot{G}},_{\dot{G}'})\ddot{M}^{G'}. \tag{22}$$

This exhibits the extremum condition as a set of differential equations in the variables $\{M^G, \dot{M}^G, \ddot{M}^G, M^G_{:z}, M^G_{:zz}\}$ in $r-t = (x,y,t)$ space, with coefficients nonlinear in M^G. Note that the V' term for NN interactions in the Lagrangian L will introduce spatial derivative terms that appear in these EL equations.

As noted above, linearization of the EL equations permit the development of stability analyses and dispersion relations in frequency-wave-number space (Ingber, 1982, 1983, 1985a), leading to wave propagation velocities of interactions over several minicolumns, consistent with experiments. This calculation first linearizes the EL, then takes Fourier transforms in space and time variables.

$$M^G = \Re M^G_{\text{osc}} \exp[-i(\xi \cdot r - \omega t)],$$

$$M^G_{\text{osc}}(r,t) = \int d^2\xi d\omega \hat{M}^G_{\text{osc}}(\xi,\omega) \exp[i(\xi \cdot r - \omega t)]. \tag{23}$$

For instance, a typical example (Ingber, 1985a). is specified by: extrinsic sources (used in earlier papers as a centering mechanism) $J_E = -2.63$ and $J_I = 4.94$, $N^E = 125$, $N^I = 25$, $V^G = 10$ mV, $A^E = 1.75$, $A^I = 1.25$, $B^G = 0.25$, $v^G 0.1$ mv, and $\phi^G = 0.03^{1/2}$ mV. The global minima is at $\bar{M}^E = 25$ and $\bar{M}^I = 5$. This set of conditions yields (dispersive) dispersion relations

$$\omega\tau = \pm\{-1.86 + 2.38(\xi\rho)^2; -1.25i + 1.51i(\xi\rho)^2\}, \tag{24}$$

where $\xi = |\xi|$. The propagation velocity defined by $d\omega/d\xi$ is about 1 cm/sec, taking typical wave-numbers ξ to correspond to macrocolumnar distances about 30ρ. Calculated frequencies ω are on the order of EEG frequencies of about 10^2 sec^{-1}. These mesoscopic propagation velocities permit processing over several minicolumns about 10^{-1} cm, simultaneous with processing of mesoscopic interactions over tens of cm via association fibers with propagation velocities about 600—900 cm/sec. I.e., both can occur within about 10^{-1} sec.

Note that this propagation velocity is not "slow": Visual selective attention moves at about 8 msec/degree (Tsal, 1983), which is about 1/2 mm/sec, if a macrocolumn of about mm^2 is assumed to span 180 degrees. This suggests that NN interactions play some part in disengaging and orienting selective attention.

3.6.2. Strings EL

The nonlinear string model was derived using the EL equation for the electric potential Φ measured by EEG, considering one firing variable along the parabolic trough of attractor states being proportional to Φ (Ingber & Nunez, 1990).

Since only one variable, the electric potential is being measured, is reasonable to assume that a single independent firing variable offers a crude description of this physics. Furthermore, the scalp potential Φ can be considered to be a function of this firing variable. (Here, "potential" refers to the electric potential, not any potential term in the SMNI Lagrangian.) In an abbreviated notation subscripting the time-dependence,

$$\Phi_t - \ll \Phi \gg = \Phi(M^E_t, M^I_t) \approx a(M^E_t - \ll M^E \gg) + b(M^I_t - \ll M^I \gg), \tag{25}$$

where a and b are constants, and $\ll \Phi \gg$ and $\ll M^G \gg$ represent typical minima in the trough. In the context of fitting data to the dynamic variables, there are three effective constants, $\{a, b, \phi\}$,

$$\Phi_t - \phi = aM_t^E + bM_t^I \tag{26}$$

The mesoscopic columnar probability distributions, P, is scaled over this columnar firing space to obtain the macroscopic conditional probability distribution over the scalp-potential space:

$$P_\Phi[\Phi] = \int dM^E dM^I P[M^E, M^I]\delta[\Phi - \Phi'(M^E, M^I)] \tag{27}$$

The parabolic trough described above justifies a form

$$P_\Phi = (2\pi\sigma^2)^{-1/2} \exp(-\Delta t \int dx L_\Phi),$$

$$L_\Phi = \frac{\alpha}{2}|\partial\Phi/\partial t|^2 + \frac{\beta}{2}|\partial\Phi/\partial x|^2 + \frac{\gamma}{2}|\Phi|^2 + F(\Phi),$$

$$\sigma^2 = 2\Delta t/\alpha, \tag{28}$$

where $F(\Phi)$ contains nonlinearities away from the trough, σ^2 is on the order of $1/N$ given the derivation of L above, and the integral over x is taken over the spatial region of interest. In general, there also will be terms linear in $\partial\Phi/\partial t$ and in $\partial\Phi/\partial x$.

Here, the EL equation includes variation across the spatial extent, x, of columns in regions,

$$\frac{\partial}{\partial t}\frac{\partial L}{\partial(\partial\Phi/\partial t)} + \frac{\partial}{\partial x}\frac{\partial L}{\partial(\partial\Phi/\partial x)} - \frac{\partial L}{\partial\Phi} = 0 \tag{29}$$

The result is

$$\alpha\frac{\partial^2\Phi}{\partial t^2} + \beta\frac{\partial^2\Phi}{\partial x^2} + \gamma\Phi - \frac{\partial F}{\partial\Phi} = 0 \tag{30}$$

The determinant prefactor g defined above also contains nonlinear details affecting the state of the system. Since g is often a small number, distortion of the scale of L is avoided by normalizing g/g_0, where g_0 is simply g evaluated at $M^E = M^{\ddagger E'} = M^I = 0$.

If there exist regions in neocortical parameter space such that $\beta/\alpha = -c^2$, $\gamma/\alpha = \omega_0^2$, i.e., as explicitly calculated using the Centering Mechanism (CM) and as derived in previous SMNI EEG papers,

$$\frac{1}{\alpha}\frac{\partial F}{\partial\Phi} = -\Phi f(\Phi), \tag{31}$$

then the nonlinear string model is recovered.

Note that if the spatial extent is extended across the scalp via long-ranged fibers connecting columns with $M^{\ddagger E'}$ firings, this leads to a string of columns.

3.6.3. Springs EL

For a given column in terms of the probability description given above, the above EL equations are represented as

$$\frac{\partial}{\partial t}\frac{\partial L}{\partial(\partial M^E/\partial t)} - \frac{\partial L}{\partial M^E} = 0,$$

$$\frac{\partial}{\partial t}\frac{\partial L}{\partial(\partial M^I/\partial t)} - \frac{\partial L}{\partial M^I} = 0 \tag{32}$$

Previous SMNI EEG studies had demonstrated that simple linearized dispersion relations derived from the EL equations support the local generation of frequencies observed experimentally as well as deriving diffusive propagation velocities of information across minicolumns consistent with other experimental studies. Then, the above equations can represent coupled springs. The earliest studies simply used a driving force $J_G M^G$ in the Lagrangian to model long-ranged interactions among fibers (Ingber, 1982, 1983). Subsequent studies considered regional interactions driving localized columnar activity within these regions (Ingber, 1996a, 1997, 1998).

A recent set of calculations examined these columnar EL equations to see if EEG oscillatory behavior could be supported at just this columnar scale, i.e., within a single column. At first, the EL equations were quasi-linearized, by extracting coefficients of M and dM/dt. The nonlinear coefficients were presented as graphs over all firing states (Ingber, 2009a). This exercise demonstrated that a spring-type model of oscillations was plausible. Then a more detailed study was performed, developing over two million lines of C code from the algebra generated by an algebraic tool, Maxima, to see what range of oscillatory behavior could be considered as optimal solutions satisfying the EL equations (Ingber, 2009b). The answer was affirmative, in that ranges of $\omega t \approx 1$ were supported, implying that oscillatory solutions might be sustainable just due to columnar dynamics at that scale. The full probability distribution was evolved with such oscillatory states, confirming this is true.

These results survive even with oscillatory input into minicolumns from long-ranged sources (Ingber & Nunez, 2010), since the CM is independent of firing states, and just depends on averaged synaptic values used in SMNI.

3.7. Computational Physics

3.7.1. Adaptive Simulated Annealing (ASA)

Adaptive Simulated Annealing (ASA) (Ingber, 1993) is used to optimize or importance-sample parameters of systems.

ASA is a C-language code developed to statistically find the best global fit of a nonlinear constrained non-convex cost-function over a D-dimensional space. This algorithm permits an annealing schedule for "temperature" T decreasing exponentially in annealing-time k, $T = T_0 \exp(-ck^{1/D})$. The introduction of re-annealing also permits adaptation to changing sensitivities in the multi-dimensional parameter-space. This annealing schedule is faster than fast Cauchy annealing, where $T = T_0/k$, and much faster than Boltzmann annealing, where $T = T_0/\ln k$. ASA has over 100 OPTIONS to provide robust tuning over many classes of nonlinear stochastic systems (Ingber, 2012a).

For example, ASA has ASA_PARALLEL OPTIONS, hooks to use ASA on parallel processors, which were first developed in 1994 when the author was Principal Investigator (PI) of a National Science Foundation grant, Parallelizing ASA and PATHINT Project (PAPP). Since then these OPTIONS have been used by people in various institutions.

3.7.2. PATHINT and PATHTREE

In some cases, it is desirable to develop a time evolution of a short-time conditional probability. Two useful algorithms have been developed and published by the author.

PATHINT (Ingber, 1994) motivated the development of PATHTREE (Ingber *et al.*, 2001), an algorithm that permits extremely fast accurate computation of probability distributions of a large class of general nonlinear diffusion processes.

The natural metric of the space is used to first lay down the mesh. The evolving local short-time distributions on this mesh are then dynamically calculated. The short-time probability density gives the correct result up to order $O(\Delta t)$ for any final point S', the order required to recover the corresponding partial differential equation. In fact, $O(\Delta t^{3/2})$ is available (Graham, 1978; Langouche *et al.*, 1979, 1982).

PATHINT and PATHTREE have demonstrated their utility in statistical mechanical studies in finance, neuroscience, combat analyses, neuroscience, and other selected nonlinear multivariate systems (Ingber, 2000; Ingber *et al.*, 1991; Ingber & Nunez, 1995). PATHTREE has been used extensively to price financial options (Ingber *et al.*, 2001).

3.8. Generic Mesoscopic Neural Networks (MNN)

SMNI was applied to a parallelized generic mesoscopic neural networks (MNN) (Ingber, 1992), adding computational power to a similar paradigm proposed for target recognition (Ingber, 1985c).

"Learning" takes place by presenting the MNN with data, and parameterizing the data in terms of the firings, or multivariate firings. The "weights," or coefficients of functions of firings appearing in the drifts and diffusions, are fit to incoming data, considering the joint "effective" Lagrangian (including the logarithm of the prefactor in the probability distribution) as a dynamic cost function. This program of fitting coefficients in Lagrangian uses methods of ASA.

"Prediction" takes advantage of a mathematically equivalent representation of the Lagrangian path-integral algorithm, i.e., a set of coupled Langevin rate-equations. A coarse deterministic estimate to "predict" the evolution can be applied using the most probable path, but PATHINT has been used. PATHINT, even when parallelized, typically can be too slow for "predicting" evolution of these systems. However, PATHTREE is much faster.

3.9. Ideas by Statistical Mechanics (ISM)

These kinds of applications of SMNI have obvious counterparts in an AI approach to Ideas by Statistical Mechanics (ISM). ISM is a generic program to model evolution and propagation of ideas/patterns throughout populations subjected to endogenous and exogenous interactions (Ingber, 2006, 2007, 2008). The program is based on SMNI, and uses the ASA code (Ingber, 1993) for optimizations of training sets, as well as for importance-sampling to apply the author's copula financial risk-management codes, TRD (Ingber, 2005, 2010), for assessments of risk and uncertainty. This product can be used for decision support for projects ranging from diplomatic, information, military, and economic (DIME) factors of propagation/evolution of ideas, to commercial sales, trading indicators across sectors of financial markets, advertising and political campaigns, etc.

It seems appropriate to base an approach for propagation of ideas on the only system so far demonstrated to develop and nurture ideas, i.e., the neocortical brain. Ultimately, ISM of course would not use functional relationships developed solely in neocortex, but rather those more appropriate to a given population. Following the SMNI structure, ISM develops subsets of macrocolumnar activity of multivariate stochastic descriptions of defined populations, with macrocolumns defined by their local parameters within specific regions and with parameterized endogenous inter-regional and exogenous external connectivities. Parameters of subsets of macrocolumns are to be fit using ASA to patterns representing ideas. Parameters of external and inter-regional interactions are to be determined that promote or inhibit the spread of these ideas.

4. Top-Down Versus Bottom-Up

In regard to neocortical information processing at the level of STM, there are two major paradigms that have not yet been reconciled, which is conveniently understood in terms of top-down versus bottom-up processes.

4.1. Bottom Up

There has been much work done, both experimentally and theoretically, detailing quite a few specific mechanisms at the level of individual neurons and glial processes and their interactions, that can explain information processing and codification of information that may be instrumental in STM (Amzica & Massimini, 2002). In particular, a class of glial cells, astrocytes, present in numbers greater than neurons in human neocortex, is of interest here (Oberheim *et al.*, 2009). For example, astrocytes in neocortical laminae 1 extend their mm processes across associative/computing laminae 1-3, afferent laminae 4, touching and communicating with other glia cells and neurons (Colombo *et al.*, 2005; Reisin & Colombo, 2002). Laminae 2-6 have larger astrocytes, and in laminae 5-6 with mostly efferent neuronal processes there are some astrocytes with varicose projections (Oberheim *et al.*, 2009). However, it appears that a primary means of communication among astrocytes (and other glial cells) is via Ca^{2+} waves, propagating at speeds up to 40 μm/s (Bellinger, 2005) over hundreds of mm of neuronal structures. They influence excitation and inhibition of neuromodulators, and recent research points to their direct effect on polarization thresholds via Ca^{2+} waves. For example, the influence of neuron firing on astroglial calcium ions may be caused by movement of sodium and potassium ions in and out the body and axon of neurons.

It should be noted that there are other mechanisms proposed, other than direct neuron-neuron interactions, to describe various aspects of neocortical information processing, e.g., soliton formation (Georgiev, 2003), and ephaptic excitation of neurons (Anastassiou *et al.*, 2011).

There are many approaches in this "bottom-up" context, including quantum computation in microtubles (Hagan *et al.*, 2002), nonlinear systems approaches to neural processes (Rabinovich *et al.*, 2006), magnetic processes within astrocytes (Banaclocha, 2005, 2007; Banaclocha & Banaclocha, 2010; Banaclocha *et al.*, 2010), pulsating Ca^{2+} waves in astrocytes (Goldberg *et al.*, 2010; Scemes *et al.*, 2000; Schipke *et al.*, 2002), neuron-astrocyte networks (Pereira & Furlan, 2009, 2010), including glutamate-specific Ca^{2+}-induced signaling processes between neurons and astrocytes (Postnov *et al.*, 2009), influences of blood flow on neuronal processes (Moore & Cao, 2008), and mathematical formulations of qualia based on neural information processing (Balduzzi & Tononi, 2009).

4.2. Top Down

There has been much theoretical work done at the level of columnar and regional neocortical activity, detailing correlations of experimental brain activity with behavioral observations (Buxhoeveden & Casanova, 2002; Rakic, 2008). For example, various imaging techniques, both intra-cranial and non-invasive, have demonstrated that specific brain activity often is correlated with STM as well as specific processing of information and attentional states (Nunez & Srinivasan, 2006).

There also has been much theoretical work trying to bridge brain activity across multiples scales, e.g., from neuronal to columnar to regional scales of activity, with detailed calculations defining STM (Ingber, 1981, 1983, 1984; Ingber & Nunez, 1995) and analyses of scalp EEG (Ingber, 1997, 2009b; Ingber & Nunez, 2010). Using SMNI, minicolumnar EEG has been demonstrated to scale up to EEG observed at regional scalp measurements. While minicolumnar EEG may not be the only source of scalp EEG, it is sufficient to scale for detailed fits to observed scalp EEG data.

It is reasonable to state that, while most neuroscientists believe that ultimately Bottom Up processing will explain all brain activity (Rabinovich *et al.*, 2006), some other neurophysiologists and psychologists believe that direct Top Down processes are important components of mammalian information processing, which cannot be solely explained by Bottom Up processes.

4.2.1. Smoking Gun

As yet, there does not seem to be any "smoking gun" for explicit Top to Down mechanisms that directly drive Bottom Up STM processes. Of course, there are many Top Down type studies demonstrating that neuromodulator (Silberstein, 1995) and neuronal firing states, e.g., as defined by EEG frequencies, can modify the milieu or context of individual synaptic and neuronal activity, which is still consistent with ultimate Bottom Up paradigms. However, there is a logical difference between Top Down milieu as conditioned by some prior external or internal conditions, and some direct Top Down processes that direct cause Bottom Up interactions specific to STM. Here, the operative word is "cause".

4.3. Support for Top-Down Electromagnetic Mechanism

There is a body of evidence that suggests a specific Top to Down mechanism for neocortical STM processing.

4.3.1. Magnetism Influences in Living Systems

An example of a direct physical mechanism that affects neuronal processing not part of "standard" sensory influences is the strong possibility of magnetic influences in birds at quantum levels of interaction (Kominis, 2009; Rodgers & Hore, 2009; Solov'yov & Schulten, 2009). It should be noted that this is just a proposed mechanism (Johnsen & Lohmann, 2008).

4.3.2. Neocortical Magnetic Fields

There are many studies on electric (Alexander *et al.*, 2006) and magnetic fields in neocortex (Georgiev, 2003; Irimia *et al.*, 2009; McFadden, 2007; Murakami & Okada, 2006).

At the level of a single neuron, electric field strengths can be as high as about 10V/m for a summation of excitatory or inhibitory postsynaptic potentials as a neuron fires. The electric field **D**

$$\mathbf{D} = \varepsilon \mathbf{E} \tag{33}$$

is rapidly attenuated as the dielectric constant ε seen by ions is close to two orders of magnitude times that in vacuum, ε_0 due to polarization of water (Nunez, 1981). Magnetic field strengths **H** in neocortex are generally quite small, even when estimated for the largest human axons at about 10^{-7}T, about 1/300 of the Earth's magnetic field, based on ferrofluid approximation to the microtuble environment with a magnetic permeability μ,

$$\mathbf{B} = \mu \mathbf{H} \tag{34}$$

about $10\mu_0$ (Georgiev, 2003). Thus, the electromagnetic fields in neocortex differ substantially from those in vacuum, i.e.,

$$\varepsilon_0 \mu_0 c^2 = 1 \tag{35}$$

where c is the speed of light. These estimates of magnetic field strengths appear to be reliable when comparisons between theoretical and experimental measurements are made in crayfish axons (Roth & Wikswo, 1985).

The above estimates of electric and magnetic field strengths do not consider collective interactions within and among neighboring minicolumns, which give rise to field strengths much larger as typically measured by noninvasive EEG and MEG recordings. While electrical activity may be attenuated in the neocortical environment, this is not true for magnetic fields which may increase collective strengths over relatively large neocortical distances. The strengths of magnetic fields in neocortex may be at a threshold to directly influence synaptic interactions with astrocytes, as proposed for long-term memory (LTM) (Gordon *et al.*, 2009) and short-term memory (STM) (Banaclocha, 2007; Pereira & Furlan, 2010) Magnetic strengths associated by collective EEG activity at a columnar level gives rise to even stronger magnetic fields. Columnar excitatory and inhibitory processes largely take place in different neocortical laminae, providing possibilities for more specific mechanisms.

4.3.3. Columnar EEG

Details of STM have been calculated in the SMNI papers. The Centering Mechanism (CM), associated in these calculations with changes in background inhibitory synaptic activity, drive the columnar system into multiple collective firing states. This CM leads to detailed calculations of STM capacity, duration and stability that agrees with experimental observations.

Future work must consider magnetic fields produced at different laminae due to collective minicolumnar firings as detailed by SMNI for STM processes. These magnetic fields may affect Ca^{2+} ion waves that are considered by some researchers as being vital processes for astrocyte-neural interactions that give rise to higher-order cognitive states (Bellinger, 2005; Nakano *et al.*, 2007).

The interactions between the momentum of these Ca^{2+} ions and minicolumnar magnetic fields can be approached classically, e.g., at a local minicolumnar scale, or quantum mechanically, e.g., considering possible entanglement across macrocolumnar scales.

4.4. Bottom-Up Complementary to SMNI STM

It is essential to recognize that, while SMNI STM has done well in calculating properties of STM, neuronal firing states are likely the just first fast stages of STM, and it must be appreciated that other molecular mechanisms are likely essential to understanding just how STM and LTM are processed and stored in some kind of coded neuronal-glial states.

A particularly plausible set of mechanisms has been proposed that reply on specific biomagnetic processes among neurons and astrocytes (Banaclocha, 2011; Banaclocha *et al.*, 2010). This proposal is that neurons synthesize and accumulate predominantly superparamagnetic magnetite, while astrocytes generate and accumulate preferentially single-domain magnetite nano-particles which have a permanent magnetic moment. This set of interacting mechanisms can plausibly code both STM and LTM. These mechanisms propose collective minicolumnar neuronal activity as possibly generating strong enough magnetic fields. Also, collective Ca^{2+} waves are invoked that may generate strong enough magnetic processes to develop astrocyte magnetic bubbles. These bubbles are a key concept in this proposal for processing information.

The section below on Vector Potential further details how SMNI STM can interface with electromagnetic processes affecting neuron-astrocyte interactions.

5. Vector Potential

To demonstrate that top-down influences can be appreciable, here a direct comparison is described between the momentum $\mathbf{p}$ of Ca^{2+}, ions which already have been established as being influential in STM and LTM, and an SMNI vector potential (SMNI-VP). The SMNI-VP is constructed from magnetic fields induced by neuronal electrical firings, at thresholds of collective minicolumnar activity with laminar specification, can give rise to causal top-down mechanisms that effect molecular excitatory and inhibitory processes in STM and LTM. A specific example might be causal influences on momentum $\mathbf{p}$ of Ca^{2+} ions by the SMNI-VP $\mathbf{A}$, as calculated by the canonical momentum $\mathbf{q}$

$$\mathbf{q} = \mathbf{p} - e\mathbf{A} \tag{36}$$

where e is the electron coulomb charge and $\mathbf{B} = \nabla \times \mathbf{A}$ is the magnetic field $\mathbf{B}$, which may be applied either classically or quantum-mechanically. Note that gauge of $\mathbf{A}$ is not specified here, and this can lead to important effects especially at quantum scales (Tollaksen *et al.*, 2010).

A can be calculated using the standard assumption that large-scale EEG is developed from oscillatory electrical dipole activity $\mathbf{p}\exp(-i\omega t)$, the first moment of the charge distribution density ρ giving rise to the dipole. The electromagnetic vector potential **A** (Jackson, 1962) is

$$\mathbf{A} = \frac{e^{i\omega r/c}}{cr} \int \mathbf{J} d^3x \tag{37}$$

for the electric current density **J**, which in the dipole approximation,

$$\mathbf{p} = \int \mathbf{x}\rho(\mathbf{x}) d^3x \tag{38}$$

gives rise to

$$\mathbf{A} = -\frac{i\omega \mathbf{p} e^{i\omega r/c}}{cr} \tag{39}$$

This is a dipole model for collective minicolumnar oscillatory currents, corresponding to top-down signaling, flowing in axons, not for individual neurons. The top-down signal is claimed to cause relevant effects on the surrounding milieu, but is not appropriate outside these surfaces due to strong attenuation of electrical activity. However, the vector potentials produced by these dipoles due to axonal discharges do survive far from the axons, and this can lead to important effects at the molecular scale, e.g., in the environment of ions (Feynman *et al.*, 1964; Giuliani, 2010).

Note that this is not necessarily the only or most popular description of electromagnetic influences in neocortex, which often describes dendritic presynaptic activity as inducing large scale EEG (Nunez, 1981), or axonal firings directly affecting astrocyte processes (McFadden, 2007). This work is only and specifically concerned with electromagnetic fields in collective axonal firings, directly associated with columnar STM phenomena in SMNI calculations, which create vector potentials influencing ion momenta just outside minicolumnar structures.

After fitting the electrical dipole moment **p** to minicolumnar electrical field near minicolumns, this value of **A** is then to be compared to the value of **p** for Ca^{2+}. Note that the magnetic field **B** derived from **A**,

$$\mathbf{B} = \nabla \times \mathbf{A} \tag{40}$$

is still attenuated in the glial areas where Ca^{2+} waves exist, but **A** derived near the minicolumns will be used there as well since it is not so attenuated.

The electrical dipole for collective minicolumnar EEG derived from **A** is

$$\mathbf{E} = \frac{ic}{\omega} \nabla \times \mathbf{B} = \frac{ic}{\omega} \nabla \times \nabla \times \mathbf{A} \tag{41}$$

which in a near-field approximation for minicolumns gives

$$\mathbf{E} = \frac{3\mathbf{n}(\mathbf{n} \cdot \mathbf{p}) - \mathbf{p}}{r^3}$$

$$\mathbf{B} = \frac{i\omega \mathbf{n} \times \mathbf{p}}{cr^2} \tag{42}$$

where $\mathbf{n}$ is the unit vector in the direction of $\mathbf{p}$. The far-field approximations are

$$\mathbf{E} = \mathbf{B} \times \mathbf{n}$$
$$\mathbf{B} = \frac{\omega^2 \mathbf{n} \times \mathbf{p} e^{i\omega r/c}}{(cr)^2} \tag{43}$$

The SMNI columnar probability distributions, derived from statistical aggregation of synaptic and neuronal interactions among minicolumns and macrocolumns, have established credibility at columnar scales by detailed calculations of properties of STM. Under CM conditions, they exhibit multiple columnar collective firing states. It must be stressed that these minicolumns are the entities which the above dipole moment is modeling. The Lagrangian of the SMNI distributions, although possessing multivariate nonlinear means and covariance, have functional forms similar to arguments of firing distributions of individual neurons, so that the description of the columnar dipole above is a model faithful to the standard derivation of a vector potential from an oscillating electric dipole.

The effective collective minicolumnar potential is estimated to be about 10 times as strong as a neuronal postsynaptic voltage of $10^{-3}V$, or 10^{-2} V, where V measures volts, equivalent to m^2-kg-/A-s^3 (A measures amperes). At a laminar thickness, r, within axons, of about 10^{-3} m, the $\mathbf{E}$ field density dimension is on the order of $10^{-2}/r$ V/m. This gives a dipole value on the order of $10^{-2}r^2$ C-m (C measures coulomb, measured by A-s) at the near field.

This yields an estimate for values of $|\mathbf{A}|$, for $\omega = 6.366$ cps, corresponding to EEG frequencies of 40 s^{-1} A-s/m^2, on the order of $10^{-10}r$ V-m at the near field of firing minicolumns. In SI units, as can be described by the Coulomb force, the equivalent units of $C = (\text{kg-m}^3/\text{s}^2)^{1/2}$, or eA will be in units of linear momentum. Taking r to be a laminae thickness gives an estimate of 10^{-13} V-m, which decreases as $1/r$ away from the near field, all measured within axons for the purposes of describing electrical activity.

The contribution of $\mathbf{A}$ to the canonical momentum is measured by $e\mathbf{A}$, where $e = 1.602 \times 10^{-19}$ C. This gives a momentum contribution from $\mathbf{A}$ on the order of 10^{-32} kg-m/s.

The mass of a Ca^{2+} ion is 1.33×10^{-25} kg. Assuming speeds of 40 μm/s, estimate the momentum of a single ion is estimated to be about 5×10^{-30} kg-m/s.

This comparison of $\mathbf{p}$ and $\mathbf{A}$ demonstrates it is possible for minicolumnar electromagnetic fields to influence important ions involved in cognitive and affective processes in neocortex. Our estimate of minicolumnar electric dipole is quite conservative, and a factor of 10 would make these effects even more dramatic. Since this effect acts on all Ca^{2+} ions, it may have an even greater effect on Ca^{2+} waves, contributing to their mean wave-front movement. Considering slower ion momenta $\mathbf{p}$ would make this comparison to $\mathbf{A}$ even closer.

Such a smoking gun for top-down effects awaits forensic in vivo experimental verification, requiring appreciating the necessity and due diligence of including true multiple-scale interactions across orders of magnitude in the complex neocortical environment.

Conclusion

For several decades the stated Holy Grail of chemical, biological and biophysical research into neocortical information processing has been to reduce such neocortical phenomena into specific bottom-up molecular and smaller-scale processes (Rabinovich *et al.*, 2006). Over the past three decades, with regard to short-term memory (STM) and long-term memory (LTM) phenomena, which themselves are likely components of other phenomena like attention and consciousness, the SMNI approach has yielded specific details of STM capacity, duration and stability not present in molecular approaches, but it is clear that most molecular approaches consider it inevitable that their reductionist approaches at molecular and possibly even quantum scales will yet prove to be causal explanations of such phenomena. The SMNI approach is a bottom-up aggregation from synaptic scales to columnar and regional scales of neocortex, and has been merged with larger non-invasive EEG scales with other colleagues – all at scales much coarser than molecular scales. As with many Crusades for some truths, other truths can be trampled. It is proposed that an SMNI vector potential (SMNI-VP) constructed from magnetic fields induced by neuronal electrical firings, at thresholds of collective minicolumnar activity with laminar specification, can give rise to causal top-down mechanisms that effect molecular excitatory and inhibitory processes in STM and LTM. Such a smoking gun for top-down effects awaits forensic in vivo experimental verification, requiring appreciating the necessity and due diligence of including true multiple-scale interactions across orders of magnitude in the complex neocortical environment.

This work simply shows that electromagnetic fields within neurons can have effects outside of them, e.g., on ions that mediate interactions between and among neurons and astrocytes (Pereira & Furlan, 2009, 2010). Other work has shown the important computational effects of such interactions, including consideration of magnetic influences per se (Banaclocha, 2007; Banaclocha *et al.*, 2010).

These minicolumnar processes of STM, as described by SMNI, as they affect and are affected by relatively regional macroscopic processes, and as they affect and are affected by relatively microscopic ionic processes, will be emphasized in other papers (Ingber, 2012b).

Acknowledgments

I thank Alfredo Pereira Jr and Marcos Banaclocha for several discussions and for references to relevant literature on astrocyte processes. I thank Paul Nunez for several discussions on electrical and magnetic fields in neocortex.

References

Alexander, J., Fuss, B., Colello, R. (2006). Electric field-induced astrocyte alignment directs neurite outgrowth. *Neuron Glia Biology* 2(2), 93–103.

Amzica, F., Massimini, M. (2002). Glial and neuronal interactions during slow wave and paroxysmal activities in the neocortex. *Cerbral Cortex* 12(10), 1101–1113.

Anastassiou, C., Perin, R., Markram, H., Koch, C. (2011). Ephaptic coupling of cortical neurons. *Nature Neuroscience* 14, 217–223.

Balduzzi, D., Tononi, G. (2009). Qualia: The geometry of integrated information. *PLoS Computational Biology* 5(8), 1–24.

Banaclocha, M. (2005). Magnetic storage of information in the human cerebral cortex: A hypothesis for memory. *International Journal of Neuroscience* 115(3), 329–337.

Banaclocha, M. (2007). Neuromagnetic dialogue between neuronal minicolumns and astroglial network: A new approach for memory and cerebral computation. *Brain Research Bulletin* 73, 21–27.

Banaclocha, M. (2011). Magnetic bubbles in brain neocortex: a new model for neurocognitive functions. Technical Report Report, Hospital Lluis Alcanyis, Jativa, Spain.

Banaclocha, M., Banaclocha, H. (2010). Spontaneous neocortical activity and cognitive functions: A neuron-astroglial bio-magnetic and self-organized process. *NeuroQuantology* 8(2), 191–199.

Banaclocha, M., Bóokkon, I., Banaclocha, H. (2010). Long-term memory in brain magnetite. *Medical Hypotheses* 74(2), 254–257.

Bellinger, S. (2005). Modeling calcium wave oscillations in astrocytes. *Neurocomputing* 65(66), 843–850.

Boyd, I., Martin, A. (1956). The end-plate potential in mammalian muscle. *Journal of Physiology (London)* 132, 74–91.

Buxhoeveden, D., Casanova, M. (2002). The minicolumn hypothesis in neuroscience. *Brain* 125(5), 935–951. URL http://tinyurl.com/bc2002brain.

Caille', A., Pink, D., de Verteuil, F., Zuckermann, M. (1980). Theoretical models for quasi-two-dimensional mesomorphic monolayers and membrane bilayers. *Canadian Journal of Physics* 58, 1723–1726.

Colombo, J., Reisin, H., Jones, M., Bentham, C. (2005). Development of interlaminar astroglial processes in the cerebral cortex of control and down's syndrome human cases. *Experimental Neurology* 193, 207–217.

Cowan, J. (1982). Spontaneous symmetry breaking in large scale nervous activity. *International Journal of Quantum Chemistry* 22, 1059–1082.

Cragg, B., Temperley, H. (1954). The organization of neurons: A cooperative analogy. *Electroencephalography Clinical Neurophysiology* 6, 85–92.

Ericsson, K., Chase, W. (1982). Exceptional memory. *American Scientist* 70, 607–615.

Feynman, R., Leighton, R., Sands, M. (1964). Chapter 15: The vector potential. In *The Feynman Lectures on Physics*, Addison-Wesley, Reading, MA, volume II. 1–16.

Georgiev, D. (2003). Electric and magnetic fields inside neurons and their impact upon the cytoskeletal microtubules. Technical Report Cogprints Report, Cogprints, U. Southampton, UK. http://cogprints.org/3190/.

Giuliani, G. (2010). Vector potential, electromagnetic induction and 'physical meaning'. *European Journal of Physics* 31(4), 871–880.

Goldberg, M., De Pittá, M., Volman, V., Berry, H., Ben-Jacob, E. (2010). Nonlinear gap junctions enable long-distance propagation of pulsating calcium waves in astrocyte networks. *PLoS Computational Biology* 6(8), 1–14.

Gordon, G., Iremonger, K., Kantevari, S., Ellis-Davies, G., MacVicar, B., Bains, J. (2009). Astrocyte-mediated distributed plasticity at hypothalamic glutamate synapses. *Neuron* 64, 391–403.

Graham, R. (1977). Covariant formulation of non-equilibrium statistical thermodynamics. *Zeitschrift für Physik* B26, 397–405.

Graham, R. (1978). Path-integral methods in nonequilibrium thermodynamics and statistics. In L. Garrido, P. Seglar, P. Shepherd (Eds.), *Stochastic Processes in Nonequilibrium Systems*, Springer, New York, NY. 82–138.

Hagan, S., Hameroff, R., Tuszyński, J. (2002). Quantum computation in brain microtubules: Decoherence and biological feasibility. *Physical Review E* 65(061901), 1–11.

Hick, W. (1952). On the rate of gains of information. *Quarterly Journal Experimental Psychology* 34(4), 1–33.

Ingber, L. (1981). Towards a unified brain theory. *Journal Social Biological Structures* 4, 211–224. URL http://www.ingber.com/smni81_unified.pdf.

Ingber, L. (1982). Statistical mechanics of neocortical interactions. i. basic formulation. *Physica D* 5, 83–107. URL http://www.ingber.com/smni82_basic.pdf.

Ingber, L. (1983). Statistical mechanics of neocortical interactions. dynamics of synaptic modification. *Physical Review A* 28, 395–416. URL http://www.ingber.com/smni83_dynamics.pdf.

Ingber, L. (1984). Statistical mechanics of neocortical interactions. derivation of short-term-memory capacity. *Physical Review A* 29, 3346–3358. URL http://www.ingber.com/smni84_stm.pdf.

Ingber, L. (1985a). Statistical mechanics of neocortical interactions. EEG dispersion relations. *IEEE Transactions Biomedical Engineering* 32, 91–94. URL http://www.ingber.com/smni85_eeg.pdf.

Ingber, L. (1985b). Statistical mechanics of neocortical interactions: Stability and duration of the 7+-2 rule of short-term-memory capacity. *Physical Review A* 31, 1183–1186. URL http://www.ingber.com/smni85_stm.pdf.

Ingber, L. (1985c). Statistical mechanics algorithm for response to targets (SMART). In *Workshop on Uncertainty and Probability in Artificial Intelligence: UC Los Angeles, 14-16 August 1985*, American Association for Artificial Intelligence, Menlo Park, CA. 258–264. URL http://www.ingber.com/combat85_smart.pdf.

Ingber, L. (1986). Statistical mechanics of neocortical interactions. *Bulletin American Physical Society* 31, 868.

Ingber, L. (1991). Statistical mechanics of neocortical interactions: A scaling paradigm applied to electroencephalography. *Physical Review A* 44(6), 4017–4060. URL http://www.ingber.com/smni91_eeg.pdf.

Ingber, L. (1992). Generic mesoscopic neural networks based on statistical mechanics of neocortical interactions. *Physical Review A* 45(4), R2183–R2186. URL http://www.ingber.com/smni92_mnn.pdf.

Ingber, L. (1993). Adaptive simulated annealing (ASA). Technical Report Global optimization C-code, Caltech Alumni Association, Pasadena, CA. URL http://www.ingber.com/#ASA-CODE.

Ingber, L. (1994). Statistical mechanics of neocortical interactions: Path-integral evolution of short-term memory. *Physical Review E* 49(5B), 4652–4664. URL http://www.ingber.com/smni94_stm.pdf.

Ingber, L. (1995a). Statistical mechanics of multiple scales of neocortical interactions. In P. Nunez (Ed.), *Neocortical Dynamics and Human EEG Rhythms*, Oxford University Press, New York, NY. 628–681. ISBN 0-19-505728-7. URL http://www.ingber.com/smni95_scales.pdf.

Ingber, L. (1995b). Statistical mechanics of neocortical interactions: Constraints on 40 hz models of short-term memory. *Physical Review E* 52(4), 4561–4563. URL http://www.ingber.com/smni95_stm40hz.pdf.

Ingber, L. (1996a). Statistical mechanics of neocortical interactions: Multiple scales of EEG. In R. Dasheiff, D. Vincent (Eds.), *Frontier Science in EEG: Continuous Waveform Analysis (Electroencephalography Clinical Neurophysiology Suppl. 45)*, Elsevier, Amsterdam. 79–112. Invited talk to Frontier Science in EEG Symposium, New Orleans, 9 Oct 1993. ISBN 0-444-82429-4. URL http://www.ingber.com/smni96_eeg.pdf.

Ingber, L. (1996b). Nonlinear nonequilibrium nonquantum nonchaotic statistical mechanics of neocortical interactions. *Behavioral and Brain Sciences* 19(2), 300–301. Invited commentary on Dynamics of the brain at global and microscopic scales: Neural networks and the EEG, by J.J. Wright and D.T.J. Liley. URL http://www.ingber.com/smni96_nonlinear.pdf.

Ingber, L. (1997). Statistical mechanics of neocortical interactions: Applications of canonical momenta indicators to electroencephalography. *Physical Review E* 55(4), 4578–4593. URL http://www.ingber.com/smni97_cmi.pdf.

Ingber, L. (1998). Statistical mechanics of neocortical interactions: Training and testing canonical momenta indicators of EEG. *Mathematical Computer Modelling* 27(3), 33–64. URL http://www.ingber.com/smni98_cmi_test.pdf.

Ingber, L. (1999). Statistical mechanics of neocortical interactions: Reaction time correlates of the g factor. *Psycholoquy* 10(068). Invited commentary on The g Factor: The Science of Mental Ability by Arthur Jensen. URL http://www.ingber.com/smni99_g_factor.pdf.

Ingber, L. (2000). High-resolution path-integral development of financial options. *Physica A* 283(3-4), 529–558. URL http://www.ingber.com/markets00_highres.pdf.

Ingber, L. (2005). Trading in risk dimensions (TRD). Technical Report Report 2005:TRD, Lester Ingber Research, Ashland, OR. URL http://www.ingber.com/markets05_trd.pdf.

Ingber, L. (2006). Ideas by statistical mechanics (ISM). Technical Report Report 2006:ISM, Lester Ingber Research, Ashland, OR. URL http://www.ingber.com/smni06_ism.pdf.

Ingber, L. (2007). Ideas by statistical mechanics (ISM). *Journal Integrated Systems Design and Process Science* 11(3), 31–54. Special Issue: Biologically Inspired Computing.

Ingber, L. (2008). AI and ideas by statistical mechanics (ISM). In J. Rabuñal, J. Dorado, A. Pazos (Eds.), *Encyclopedia of Artificial Intelligence*, Information Science Reference, New York. 58–64. ISBN 978-1-59904-849-9.

Ingber, L. (2009a). Statistical mechanics of neocortical interactions: Columnar EEG. Technical Report Report 2009:CEEG, Lester Ingber Research, Ashland, OR. URL http://www.ingber.com/smni09_columnar_eeg.pdf.

Ingber, L. (2009b). Statistical mechanics of neocortical interactions: Nonlinear columnar electroencephalography. *NeuroQuantology Journal* 7(4), 500–529. URL http://www.ingber.com/smni09_nonlin_column_eeg.pdf.

Ingber, L. (2010). Trading in risk dimensions. In G. Gregoriou (Ed.), *The Handbook of Trading: Strategies for Navigating and Profiting from Currency, Bond, and Stock Markets*, McGraw-Hill, New York. 287–300.

Ingber, L. (2012a). Asa options. In H. Oliveira, A. Petraglia, L. Ingber, M. Machado, M. Petraglia (Eds.), *Stochastic global optimization and its applications with fuzzy adaptive simulated annealing*, Springer, New York. (to be published). Invited Paper.

Ingber, L. (2012b). Computational algorithms derived from multiple scales of neocortical processing. In A. Pereira, Jr, E. Massad, N. Bobbitt (Eds.), *Pointing at Boundaries: Integrating Computation and Cognition on Biological Grounds* , Springer, New York. (to be published). Invited Paper.

Ingber, L., Chen, C., Mondescu, R., Muzzall, D., Renedo, M. (2001). Probability tree algorithm for general diffusion processes. *Physical Review E* 64(5), 056702–056707. URL http://www.ingber.com/path01_pathtree.pdf.

Ingber, L., Fujio, H., Wehner, M. (1991). Mathematical comparison of combat computer models to exercise data. *Mathematical Computer Modelling* 15(1), 65–90. URL http://www.ingber.com/combat91_data.pdf.

Ingber, L., Nunez, P. (1990). Multiple scales of statistical physics of neocortex: Application to electroencephalography. *Mathematical Computer Modelling* 13(7), 83–95.

Ingber, L., Nunez, P. (1995). Statistical mechanics of neocortical interactions: High resolution path-integral calculation of short-term memory. *Physical Review E* 51(5), 5074–5083. URL http://www.ingber.com/smni95_stm.pdf.

Ingber, L., Nunez, P. (2010). Neocortical dynamics at multiple scales: Eeg standing waves, statistical mechanics, and physical analogs. *Mathematical Biosciences* 229, 160–173. doi:10.1016/j.mbs.2010.12.003 URL http://www.ingber.com/smni10_multiple_scales.pdf.

Irimia, A., Swinney, K., Wikswo, J. (2009). Partial independence of bioelectric and biomagnetic field and its implications for encephalography and cardiography. *Physical Review E* 79(051908), 1–13.

Jackson, J. (1962). *Classical Electrodynamics*. Wiley & Sons, New York.

Jensen, A. (1987). Individual differences in the hick paradigm. In P. Vernon (Ed.), *Speed of Information-Processing and Intelligence*, Ablex, Norwood, NJ. 101–175.

Jirsa, V., Haken, H. (1996). Field theory of electromagnetic brain activity. *Physical Review Letters* 77(5), 960–963.

Johnsen, S., Lohmann, K. (2008). Magnetoreception in animals. *Physics Today* 61, 29–35.

Katz, B. (1966). *Nerve, Muscle, and Synapse*. McGraw-Hill, new York, NY.

Kominis, I. (2009). Zeno is pro darwin: quantum zeno effect suppresses the dependence of radical-ion-pair reaction yields on exchange and dipolar interactions. Technical Report arXiv:0908.0763v2 [quant-ph], University of Crete, Greece.

Korn, H., Mallet, A. (1984). Transformation of binomial input by the postsynaptic membrane at a central synapse. *Science* 225, 1157–1159.

Korn, H., Mallet, A., Faber, D. (1981). Fluctuating responses at a central synapse: n of binomial fit predicts number of stained presynaptic boutons. *Science* 213, 898–900.

Langouche, F., Roekaerts, D., Tirapegui, E. (1979). Discretization problems of functional integrals in phase space. *Physical Review D* 20, 419–432.

Langouche, F., Roekaerts, D., Tirapegui, E. (1982). *Functional Integration and Semiclassical Expansions*. Reidel, Dordrecht, The Netherlands.

Little, W. (1974). The existence of persistent states in the brain. *Mathematical Biosciences* 19, 101–120.

Little, W., Shaw, G. (1978). Analytic study of the memory storage capacity of a neural network. *Mathematical Biosciences* 39, 281–290.

Markram, H., Toledo-Rodriguez, M., Wang, Y., Gupta, A., Silberberg, G., Wu, C. (2004). Interneurons of the neocortical inhibitory system. *Nature Reviews* 5, 793–807.

Mathews, J., Walker, R. (1970). *Mathematical Methods of Physics, 2nd ed.* Benjamin, New York, NY.

McFadden, J. (2007). Conscious electromagnetic field theory. *NeuroQuantology* 5(3), 262–270.

Miller, G. (1956). The magical number seven, plus or minus two. *Psychology Review* 63, 81–97.

Moore, C., Cao, R. (2008). The hemo-neural hypothesis: On the role of blood flow in information processing. *Journal of Neurophysiology* 99, 2035–2047.

Mountcastle, V. (1978). An organizing principle for cerebral function: The unit module and the distributed system. In G. Edelman, V. Mountcastle (Eds.), *The Mindful Brain*, Massachusetts Institute of Technology, Cambridge. 7–50.

Mountcastle, V., Andersen, R., Motter, B. (1981). The influence of attentive fixation upon the excitability of the light-sensitive neurons of the posterior parietal cortex. *Journal of Neuroscience* 1, 1218–1235.

Murakami, S., Okada, Y. (2006). Contributions of principal neocortical neurons to magnetoencephalography and electroencephalography signals. *Journal of Physiology* 575(3), 925–936.

Murdock, Jr, B. (1983). A distributed memory model for serial-order information. *Psychology Review* 90, 316–338.

Nakano, T., Suda, T., Koujin, T., Haraguchi, T., Hiraoka, Y. (2007). Molecular communication through gap junction channels: System design, experiments and modeling. In *Proceedings 2nd International Conference on Bio-Insprired Models of Network, Information, and Computing Systems*, Institute for Computer Sciences, Social-Informatics and Telecommunications Engineering, Budapest, Hungary. 139–146.

Nunez, P. (1981). *Electric Fields of the Brain: The Neurophysics of EEG*. Oxford University Press, London.

Nunez, P. (1989). Generation of human EEG rhythms by a combination of long and short-range neocortical interactions. *Brain Topography* 1, 199–215.

Nunez, P., Srinivasan, R. (2006). *Electric Fields of the Brain: The Neurophysics of EEG, 2nd Ed.* Oxford University Press, London.

Oberheim, N., Takano, T., Han, X., He, W., Lin, J., Wang, F., Xu, Q., Wyatt, J., Pilcher, W., Ojemann, J., Ransom, B., Goldman, S., Nedergaard, M. (2009). Uniquely hominid features of adult human astrocytes. *Journal of Neuroscience* 29(10), 3276–3287.

Pereira, Jr, A., Furlan, F. (2009). On the role of synchrony for neuron-astrocyte interactions and perceptual conscious processing. *Journal of Biological Physics* 35(4), 465–480.

Pereira, Jr, A., Furlan, F. (2010). Astrocytes and human cognition: Modeling information integration and modulation of neuronal activity. *Progress in Neurobiology* 92, 405–420.

Perkel, D., Feldman, M. (1979). Neurotransmitter release statistics: Moment estimates for inhomogeneous bernoulli trials. *Journal of Mathematical Biology* 7, 31–40.

Postnov, D., Koreshkov, R., Brazhe, N., Brazhe, A., Sosnovtseva, O. (2009). Dynamical patterns of calcium signaling in a functional model of neuron-astrocyte networks. *Journal of Biological Physics* 35, 425–445.

Rabinovich, M., Varona, P., Selverston, A., Arbaranel, H. (2006). Dynamical principles in neuroscience. *Reviews Modern Physics* 78(4), 1213–1265.

Rakic, P. (2008). Confusing cortical columns. *Proceedings of the National Academy of Sciences* 105(34), 12099–12100. URL http://www.pnas.org/content/105/34/12099.full.

Reisin, H., Colombo, J. (2002). Considerations on the astroglial architecture and the columnar organization of the cerebral cortex. *Cellular and Molecular Neurobiology* 22(5/6), 633–644.

Risken, H. (1989). *The Fokker-Planck Equation: Methods of Solution and Applications*. Springer-Verlag, Berlin.

Rodgers, C., Hore, P. (2009). Chemical magnetoreception in birds: The radical pair mechanism. *Proceedings of the National Academy of Sciences* 106(2), 353–360.

Roth, B., Wikswo, Jr, J. (1985). The magnetic field of a single axon. *Biophysical Journal* 48, 93–109.

Scemes, E., Suadicani, S., Spray, D. (2000). Intercellular calcium wave communication via gap junction dependent and independent mechanisms. In *Current Topics in Membranes*, Academic Press, New York, NY, volume 49. 145–173.

Schipke, C., Boucsein, C., Ohlemeyer, C., Kirchhoff, F., Kettenmann, H. (2002). Astrocyte ca2+ waves trigger responses in microglial cells in brain slices. *Federation of American Societies for Experimental Biology Journal* 16, 255–257.

Schulman, L. (1981). *Techniques and Applications of Path Integration*. J. Wiley & Sons, New York.

Scott, A. (1975). The electrophysics of a nerve fiber. *Reviews Modern Physics* 47, 487–533.

Shaw, G., Vasudevan, R. (1974). Persistent states of neural networks and the random nature of synaptic transmission. *Mathematical Biosciences* 21, 207–218.

Shepherd, G. (1979). *The Synaptic Organization of the Brain*. 2nd ed. Oxford University Press, New York, NY.

Silberstein, R. (1995). Neuromodulation of neocortical dynamics. In P. Nunez (Ed.), *Neocortical Dynamics and Human EEG Rhythms*, Oxford University Press, New York, NY. 628–681.

Solov'yov, I., Schulten, K. (2009). Magnetoreception through cryptochrome may involve superoxide. *Biophysical Journal* 96(12), 4804–4813.

Sommerhoff, G. (1974). *Logic of the Living Brain*. Wiley, New York, NY.

Tollaksen, J., Aharonov, Y., Casher, A., Kaufherr, T., Nussinov, S. (2010). Quantum interference experiments, modular variables and weak measurements. *New Journal of Physics* 12(013023), 1–29.

Tsal, Y. (1983). Movements of attention across the visual field. *Journal of Experimental Psychology* 9, 523–530.

von der Heydt, I., von der Heydt, N., Obermair, G. (1981). Statistical model of current-coupled ion channels in nerve membranes. *Zeitschrift für Physik* 41, 153–164.

Vu, E., Krasne, F. (1992). Evidence for a computational distinction between proximal and distal neuronal inhibition. *Science* 255, 1710–1712.

Zhang, G., Simon, H. (1985). STM capacity for chinese words and idioms: Chunking and acoustical loop hypotheses. *Memory & Cognition* 13, 193–201.

Zhang, X., Begleiter, H., Porjesz, B., Wang, W., Litke, A. (1995). Event related potentials during object recognition tasks. *Brain Research Bulletin* 38(6), 531–538.

In: Short-Term Memory: New Research
Editors: Garifallia Kalivas and Sappho F. Petralia
ISBN: 978-1-62100-860-6

Chapter 3

SHARED OBJECT REPRESENTATIONS IN VISUAL SHORT-TERM MEMORY AND VISUAL ATTENTION

Philip C. Ko[1,*] ***and Adriane E. Seiffert***[2]
Departments of Neurology[1] and Psychology[2]
Vanderbilt University, Nashville TN, US

ABSTRACT

Visual short-term memory (VSTM) mediates the storage of visual information over a period of several seconds. Its relationship to visual attention has been the focus of much research. In this chapter we describe research investigating whether VSTM and visual attention share the same means of representing objects. First, we review the evidence and theories in the literature that relate visual attention and VSTM. From this review, we propose that VSTM and visual attention share the same object representations. Second, we describe new research investigating whether a process facilitating the perception of objects as being continuous over changes in space and time depend on both visual attention and VSTM. The tasks required participants to maintain the continuity of object representations as the display changed. The results suggested that periodically sampling visual information and matching it to representations in VSTM preserve object continuity. These experimental results support the claim that a critical link between VSTM and visual attention may be a shared means of representing objects.

INTRODUCTION

Objects surround us. The world that we see is not comprised of unrelated colors and edges. Instead, these elements are integrated into objects to which we attend, remember, and act upon. This experience is provided by our psychological representations of the world. When we attend to cars on the road, or when we search for a pen on our desks, we are attending to object representations. When we are recalling a stop sign that we just passed, or

* Corresponding Author: Philip C. Ko, PhD, Vanderbilt University, Department of Neurology, A-0118 Medical Center North, 1161 21st Avenue South, Nashville TN 37232-2551; p.ko@vanderbilt.edu.

remembering what we need from the grocery store, we are accessing memories about objects. To understand cognition is to understand how objects are represented and related.

In this chapter, we will review previous work on the role of object representations in visual attention and visual short-term memory (VSTM). In reviewing the objects of visual attention, we will show that the continuity of visual objects in attention may critically depend on interacting with VSTM. Similarly, in reviewing the objects of VSTM, we will show how maintaining objects may depend on interacting with visual attention. We will then propose that a critical link in the relationship between attention and memory is a shared means of object representation. Finally, we will present new data to support this proposal.

Objects in Visual Attention

Space and Objects

Attention is high-level processing of information in a capacity limited manner (Pashler, 1998). The consequences of this capacity limitation include the processing of some information at the cost of neglecting other information (James, 1890) and the inability to adequately perform two tasks simultaneously (Pashler, 1994). Visual attention refers to when an aspect of vision is the basis of this capacity limitation. For example, visual attention may select and process a small region of visual space at the cost of processing surrounding regions. Some early work in visual attention suggested that it shifted across a spatial representation in a manner like a "spotlight", processing all information within its scope (Posner, 1980). However, other work proposed that this spatial spotlight of attention served to bind the different visual features appearing in the same location, in order to make a single object representation (Treisman & Gelade, 1980). These ideas form the basis for contemporary theories of attention that describe both spatial and object-based properties (Bundesen, 1990; Desimone &Duncan, 1995; Itti & Koch, 2001; Treisman, 2006; Knudsen, 2007; Reynolds & Heeger, 2009; Chun, Golomb & Turk-Browne, 2011).

Early experimental evidence demonstrated the close relationship between visual attention and object representations with simple cognitive tasks such as visual search. Treisman and Gelade (1980) had participants search visual arrays containing a varying number of colored letters and report the presence of a target defined by a particular color and a letter identity (e.g. find the blue A). If the target differed from the other objects, usually called"distractors", by one unique feature, like color, then the search rate did not increase as a function of the number of objects present. It's easy to find the blue A in a group of all yellow letters. If the target could only be found from its conjunction of features, then the search rate increased with the number of items in the array. Finding the blue A amongst blue B's and yellow A's is more difficult. This data supported a two-stage model of cognitive function. At the first stage, prior to attentive processing, the elementary visual features of a scene are processed in a parallel manner. At the second stage, visual attention must be deployed to bind these features to perceive an object. Failure of attention results in an improperly bound object, i.e. an illusory conjunction (Treisman & Schmidt, 1982). Importantly, this implied attentional selection occurred at a stage earlier than that of object representation. Instead, object representation is the result of attentional selection. However, the way visual information is grouped into primitive forms, such as dots organized into horizontal rows or vertical columns, was found to profoundly affect attention (Prinzmetal, 1981; Kahneman & Henik, 1981). It is possible that some perceptual groups are formed with the same early vision process as feature analysis and could act as the basis of attentional selection (Treisman, 1982).

Duncan (1984) forwarded the idea of object-based attention even further by proposing that visual information was parsed into candidate objects in early vision to be selected by attention. In a divided attention task, participants briefly viewed two objects, a line and a box, that spatially overlapped and varied in appearance across trials. Participants reported two attributes of this stimulus on each trial. If visual attention operated on a purely spatial representation, there should be no difference in performance according to whether the two reported attributes appeared on one object or across two objects since they occupied the same space. In other words, attending to attributes across two objects should not divide attention. However, the results showed that participants reported two attributes from the same object performed better than those who reporting one attribute from each of two objects. These results showed clear evidence that visual information was grouped and represented as simple forms, or candidate objects, prior to attentional selection. Duncan's (1984) finding drove a wealth of research into understanding object-based attention. Some of the major investigations include whether objects of attention are represented within a spatial- or non-spatial frame of reference (Kramer & Jacobson, 1991; Vecera & Farah, 1994; Kramer, Weber & Watson, 1997; Logan, 1996), the automatic spread of attention within object boundaries (Egly, Driver & Rafal, 1994; Goldsmith & Yeari, 2003), and the visual properties of object representations (Watson & Kramer, 1994; Matsukura & Vecera, 2006). These investigations considered objects as spatial information that is organized into a visual formand treated by attention as a single unit.

Types and Tokens

The treatment of objects as specific visual forms has been investigated in terms of object types. An object type is the category and long-term memory representation of the object, containing semantic information and relational information about an object, such as how the object typically looks, how it is used, what the parts of the object are, and what other objects are usually associated with it. The definition of objects as types has been important in describing how the appearance of objects can drive attentional behavior. Desimone and Duncan (1995) proposed that perceived objects compete for representation at high-levels of cortical processing. Top-down signals, such as memory for the appearance of a target object, may bias the competition in favor of a specific object over other objects. Winning this competition results in the selection of one object over the others. In this way, object representations are a crucial determinant of attentional behavior – they are the units of attentional capacity limitations. Furthermore, Desimone and Duncan (1995) proposed one neural locus of competition to be the receptive fields in higher cortical areas of the ventral stream of cortical processing, which are known to represent the appearance of complex objects (Ungerleider & Mishkin, 1982). This means that the visual appearance of an object could be the primary input for attentional selection.

In contrast to defining a visual object's identity by its type, an object can be defined as a token, or its individuation from other objects. One way to consider object representations is as entities that must persist across time. A man walking towards you from the far end of the hall must be perceived as the same man from the time you first perceive him to when he reaches you. In other words, visual objects must be continuous or bound across time (Kanwisher, 1987; Kahneman, Treisman & Gibbs, 1992). In this way, the continuity of visual objects must somehow be related to the interactions between attention and memory. Pylyshyn (2001) noted there are instances of viewing an object in which visual appearance must be ignored or discarded in order to maintain the object's identity. For example, you might think that the person walking from the far end of the hall is Bill, but upon closer inspection you discover that the person is actually Betty. You perceived the person as the same object, even though yourrepresentation of their appearance changed.

One powerful demonstration of how objects can be individuated as different tokens independent of their appearance is the multiple object tracking (MOT) task (Pylyshyn & Storm, 1988; Cavanagh & Alvarez, 2005). In MOT, participants view several identical objects, some of which are indicated as targets. All of the objects move around the display during a motion period and participants must continually track the cued targets. Since the objects areidentical, discriminating the targets from non-targets as the objects move cannot rely on visual appearance. There is strong evidence for the role of attention in object tracking (Scholl, 2009). For example, Oksama and Hyona (2004) showed that individual differences in object tracking performance correlated with performance on other attentional tasks likeattentional switching. Also, Tombu and Seiffert (2008) showed that, in addition to visual attention, object tracking involves a general form of attention that is not specific to any modality.

Attention to Tracked Objects

During object tracking, object representations that continuously change spatial location across time must be attended. It is possible that spatial attention is focused over the entire area encompassed by the targets, but this is not supported by empirical evidence (Sears & Pylyshyn, 2000). Alternatively, Yantis (1992) proposed that participants attended to the group of multiple targets, by constructing them into a single object representation, such as how three points can be constructed into a triangle. A single focus of attention could be directed to this morphing object during tracking. This grouping strategy may also influence eye movement behavior during MOT (Fehd & Seiffert, 2008). However, evidence for the use of a grouped representation does not eliminate the representation of the individual targets. The use of the grouping strategy still demands the representation of each individual object in order to update the shape and position of the continuously morphing object (Pylyshyn, 2000). Knowing that the three targets make a triangle does not help differentiate between the targets and distractors, because distractors could also be grouped into equally-viable triangles. Grouping cannot be a full account of how attention is allocated during a tracking task.

As an alternative to the single-spotlight and grouping accounts of attention in MOT, Cavanagh and Alvarez (2005) proposed that MOT is accomplished by multiple foci of visual attention. Each focus of attention is centered over the location of each target and it outputs information about the target to higher-level processes. This information is used to spatially shift the focus of attention in order to remain centered on the moving target. Each focus of attention does not simply surround the space around a target but also adheres to the visual form of objects, as shown by the work of Scholl and colleagues. Scholl, Pylyshyn, and Feldman (2001) connected targets to distractors with lines so that the stimuli appeared like dumbbells and found that performance was impaired in these trials relative to trials without such groupings. This indicated that attention selected the entire object associated with the target, impairing the discrimination between the target and non-target. This ruled out an account of attention selecting the spatial region surrounding the target. In another study,

Scholl and Pylyshyn (1999) found that observers could continue to track objects in MOT even after the objects were briefly occluded, but this ability depended on specific visual cues during the occlusion. Tracking objects through occlusions was successful if the objects' visual appearance gradually deleted upon disappearance and gradually accreted upon reappearance, as if passing behind a solid object. Objects could not be tracked through occlusions if they suddenly disappeared and reappeared at the same points as the deletion/accretion condition. Van Marle and Scholl (2003) demonstrated that attention to tracked objects followed specific types of object boundaries. MOT performance was impaired when the tracked objects appeared to be liquid substances without a clear center of mass.

Another model of MOT critically involves discrete sampling of information and VSTM (Allen, McGeorge, Pearson &Milne, 2006; Oksama & Hyona, 2008). This model proposes that when the targets are cued prior to the motion period, information about the targets is sampled and stored in VSTM. While target information is stored in VSTM, another discrete sample of the visual display is taken at the next distinct time interval. Importantly, changes occurring between these sampling intervals do not affect the process. A central control mechanism compares the stored information to the newly sampled information, and if the two groups have similar attributes, the newly sampled information is stored and becomes the current representation of the targets. Successful target tracking depends on minimal discrepancy between memorized and perceived object information. This process is repeated throughout the motion period. This discrete sampling and memory account makes two important predictions. First, object continuity can be maintained even if an object disappears for a period of time. Second, object continuity depends on the consistency of information between samples.

Summary of Objects in Visual Attention

There is ample evidence that object representations can drive attention. Attention can be directed towards space but can also be directed toward and defined by the boundaries of objects. An object representation can be defined by its visual appearance or type, or by its individuation from other objects, or as a token. Object tracking exemplifies this latter brand of object-based attention because object representations must be sustained across time. Theories of how object tracking is accomplished describe an interaction between attention and visual memory. Object continuity critically depends on visual attention and memory.

Objects in Visual Memory

The Role of Visual Short-Term Memory (VSTM)

Visual memory has been described as a temporary storage of information that has some characteristics similar to visual perception. Sperling (1960) discovered that memory could be divided into two stages. The early, sensory stage is high in capacity and resolution, but short-lived and susceptible to masking. This was subsequently referred to as iconic memory (Neisser, 1967). A later stage is low in capacity, more enduring, and information is recoded to verbal information (see Coltheart, 1980). Phillips (1974) suspected the existence of another memory that resembled the latter stage, but represented information visually. Participants viewed a brief display of random visual patterns followed by a blank delay. Then, participants viewed another pattern and reported whether it was the same as the initial sample or different by some minor change. Using this change detection task, he concluded that visual memory could be delineated into two stages. The early stage resembled that of Sperling's iconic memory stage. The latter stage consisted of a visual representation that was relatively low in capacity, but it was more enduring and resistant to masking than iconic memory. This was called visual short-term memory (VSTM).

VSTM plays an important rolein maintaining the continuity of object representations as visual information changes. Evidence shows that detecting matchesbetween images across eye movements depends on VSTM (Irwin, 1991; Henderson & Hollingworth 2003). VSTM is also vital in correcting eye movements when they land inaccurately (Hollingworth, Richard & Luck, 2008; Hollingworth & Luck, 2009). The storage of visual information across eye movements is a crucial component of normal visual cognition since the retinal positions of objects shifts across saccades. This introduces a correspondence problem that demands the visual system to determine whether the image of an object projected onto one retinal region prior to a saccade is the same as another object projected on a different region after the saccade. The fulfillment of this role indicates that VSTM is important in maintaining the stability and continuity of visual objects across eye movements.

Features and Objects

What is stored in VSTM? There is strong evidence that VSTM storage capacity is limited by visual objects, which are defined as representations that are each composed of multiple visual features. For example, Irwin (1992) found that memory capacity in a spatial cueing task was limited to 3-4 letters. Using the same paradigm, Irwin and Andrews (1996) measured memory capacity for colored letters and found that it was similar for both color and letter information compared to letter information alone, which was interesting because colored letters carry twice as much information as letters alone. These results suggested that all the information within a location was integrated into and stored as an object. Luck and Vogel (1997) directly examined this hypothesis with a simple change detection task. Participants viewed displays of colored squares, black oriented bars, or bars that had both color and orientation. They were asked to report any change between two displays separated by a blank delay. The results showed that the number of items stored steadily increased with set-size, but did not continue to rise when there were more than four items in the display. This indicated a limitation in memory capacity at about four items. Importantly, there was no effect of stimulus type, indicating a similar memory capacity for simple features like colors and complex conjunctions like colored bars. This suggested that information was already integrated as objects by the time of storage in VSTM, and these objects were the units of capacity limitation in VSTM. Lee and Chun (2001) ruled out an alternative account that spatial representations were sufficient and confirmed that VSTM capacity was determined by the number of objects, not locations.

Research following Luck and Vogel's (1997; see also Vogel, Woodman & Luck, 2001) result seemed to qualify their findings by showing some memory cost related to the number of features stored in VSTM, but an overall benefit in storing information as objects. For example, Olson and Jiang (2002) showed that storing four colors and four orientations as four multi-feature conjunctions was easier than storing the same information as eight single-feature objects, but not as easy as storing two colors and two orientations as four single-feature objects. In other words, the benefit of storing information as objects was much less than expected if VSTM capacity was solely determined by the number of objects, but more than separate features alone. Olson and Jiang (2002) suggested that VSTM storage of objects was imperfect and that the number of features exerted some cost to VSTM storage. Similarly, Alvarez and Cavanagh (2004) proposed a role for complexity such that units of storage in memory would accept a minimal number of features that could be stored per object at an equal processing cost. When the number of features exceeded this minimum, objects would be stored with lower resolution, ultimately resulting in a lowered capacity.

Attention in VSTM

The imperfect integration of visual features into visual objects could indicate that a process separate from VSTM is involved in the integration. Wheeler and Treisman (2002) proposed that visual attention must be deployed throughout VSTM maintenance to bind together the separate features of each object in VSTM. In their experiments, they observed an impairment to change detection when the change trials involved colors between objects being swapped rather than replacing an old color with a new one. This indicated that bindings were not easily maintained, and sometimes failed, in VSTM. They also noticed worse change detection performance when memory was probed using a test array composed of all objects in the original display rather than a single item. They suggested that perception of the whole array at test demanded visual attention to properly bind all objects in the display. An impairment to memory in this condition may have been observed because attention was involved in VSTM storage, but had to be reassigned for perception of the test array. Together, these results suggested that bound objects were only represented in VSTM if attention was available to bind the features of each object.

The proposal that the storage of objects in VSTM depends on sustained visual attention has been investigated with experiments in which participants perform an attentionally demanding task during VSTM maintenance. The binding account predicts that, in such conditions, VSTM for features would be unaffected by the intervening task, but VSTM for conjunctions would be profoundly impaired since visual attention would be occupied with the intervening task. Some studies failed to show selective impairment for conjunctions under these conditions. For example, Johnson, Hollingworth and Luck (2006) showed that performing a visual search task during memory retention did not differentially affect memory for features or conjunctions. Also, Yeh, Yang and Chen (2005) showed no differential benefit of spatially cueing features or conjunctions during memory retention. Allen, Baddeley and Hitch (2006) showed that performance of a task demanding central attention did not differentially affect memory for features or conjunctions. However, it is possible that the tasks used in these studies were either not demanding enough to disrupt attentional binding of the object features (Johnson et al., 2008; Yeh et al., 2005) or did not require visual attention (Allen, Baddeley & Hitch, 2006). In response, Fougnie and Marois (2008) had participants perform MOT, which placed heavy demands on visual attention, during VSTM maintenance. The concurrent MOT performance resulted in severe impairment to memory for conjunctionscompared to single features, supporting the idea that visual attention is required for maintenance of feature binding in memory. In further support for a bound feature-based representation in VSTM, it has been shown that participants can selectively encode specific features of an object in memory (Woodman & Vogel, 2008). Furthermore, participants can selectively update a specific feature of an object in VSTM, while leaving the other features of that object unchanged (Ko & Seiffert, 2009).

Summary of Objects in VSTM

VSTM is a visual representation that is distinct from earlier sensory memories. It is low in capacity, but endures for several seconds and is robust to masking. The basic unit of storage in VSTM has been shown to be object representations but the means by which objects are represented has been a matter of debate. There is evidence that multi-feature objects are represented in VSTM when visual attention is available to bind the features of each object during the maintenance period. In other words, the storage of objects in VSTM may depend on an interaction with visual attention.

Object Continuity as a Product of Attention and Memory

In our review of the literature on how objects are represented in visual attention and visual memory, we have noted that some important aspects of object representation require both processes. Attention for the preservation of object continuity, as required by tasks like MOT, may require VSTM to store information. This process has been described as a cycle of sampling object information at discrete points in time and storing it for comparison to the next discrete sample of object information. Memory for the storage of complex objects, such as conjunctions of multiple features, may require sustained visual attention to keep object features bound together. These observations are consistent with the idea that visual attention and VSTM share the same means of representing objects. It is possible that the objects of attention and memory are the same.

The notion that visual attention and VSTM might share the same object representations resonates with object file theory (Kahneman, Treisman & Gibbs, 1992). Object file theory proposes that a single representation – called an object file – is used in the accrual and retention of visual information. An object file is created for each perceived object and it contains the features of the object while also retaining a history of information related to the object. The purpose of this representation is to maintain stability and continuity for the object. Detected changes in the visual input can also be related to objects that are already represented. If a change can be related to an object file, a single object could be perceived to be changing. If it cannot, a new file can be opened and the change could be perceived as a new object. Kahneman and colleagues (1992) proposed that object file continuity involved three operations: (1) a correspondence process determines whether a perceived object was previously seen or new, (2) if it was previous seen, a reviewing process retrieves previously viewed features of the object, and (3) an impletion process integrates current and reviewed information to produce the perception of a single object changing, rather than separate events involving distinct objects. The original research on object files focused on the reviewing process. Kahneman and colleagues (1992) presented participants with two boxes containing two different letters. After the letters disappeared, the boxes shifted location. Participants were asked to name the letter that subsequently appeared inside one of the boxes. Letter naming was facilitated if the letter appeared inside the same box as at the beginning of the trial, compared to the same letter appearing in a different box, or compared to a new letter. In other words, repetition priming was greater if the object continuity was maintained. This object-specific preview benefit suggested that information related to an object at one point in time remains linked to it, even if the object changes across time and space. Further work with this paradigm showed that some of the variance in performance could be attributed to priming independent of the perceived objects under some conditions (Henderson & Anes, 1994). Other studies have shown the content of object files can also contain abstract semantic information (Gordon & Irwin, 2000) and purely episodic information (Mitroff, Scholl & Noles, 2007).

In the following sections of this chapter, we will describe experiments examining how visual attention and visual memory support object representations. The experiments examined predictions derived from memory-based theories of MOT that propose a discrete sampling and memory cycle. Specifically, we examined whether the consistency of object color could interfere with this process, as well as whether object continuity could survive long pauses between samples. The results supported the memory-based theories of MOT, indicating that both visual attention and VSTM may be necessary to preserve object continuity.

Empirical Investigation of How Attention Preserves Object Continuity

This section examines the process by which objects are perceived to be continuous. Object continuity is important in object tracking tasks where participants are required to follow targets moving amongst distractors. Despite the continual change in objects' positions, participants must perceive the targets as the same enduring entities throughout tracking. Memory-based theories (Allen, McGeorge et al., 2006; Oksama & Hyona, 2008) propose that object tracking is accomplished by discretely sampling visual information across time. When targets are cued, information related to them is sampled and stored in VSTM. When the objects begin to move, the visual system begins to sample spatial and featural information in a discrete and periodic manner and compare it to target information stored in VSTM. Sampled information that matches the contents of VSTM within a certain degree isconsidered to belong to targets. The sampled information is then used to update the target properties in VSTM. This updated information is used for comparison to the next sample. If sampled information from distractors matches just as well or better than the information from targetsor if it differs too much from information stored in VSTM, the targets are confused with distractors or lost.

Results from previous work are consistent with the idea that a sampling mechanism could facilitate object tracking. Experiments have employed a target recovery (TR) task, which is just like the MOT task in that participants track the positions of multiple moving targets, but it differs from MOT because the display briefly disappears while participants are tracking (Alvarez, Horowitz, Arsenio, DiMase &Wolfe, 2005; Horowitz, Birnkrant, Fencik, Tran & Wolfe, 2006). Keane and Pylyshyn (2006) manipulated the duration of this blank and the post-blank object positions in a TR task. In some trials, the objects paused during the blank, so that the pre-blank object positions matched the post-blank positions. In other trials, the objects moved during the blank, so that the pre-blank and post-blank positions became increasingly discrepant as the blank duration increased. Performance was high when objects paused during the blank and remained high across all blank durations. However, performance declined when objects moved during the blank and became more impaired as the blank duration increased. These results showed that accuracy declined as the spatial discrepancy increased between the object locations prior to and after the blank. These results support the memory-based accounts of MOT (Horowitz et al., 2006) including sampling models of object tracking (Oksama & Hyona, 2008). As the duration of the blank increases, so does the discrepancy between pre- and post-blank positions, and so it would degrade the match between the stored location and the newly indexed location. The sampling account of TR is also appealing because performance is not impaired by the blank in the display, but by the consistency of information across the blank.

A memory-based sampling mechanism may account for TR performance, but does it apply to multiple-object tracking without a blank? One way to examine this is by testing whether performance at the MOT and TR tasks is similarly affected by consistency of the same kind of target information. In this section, we examined whether the consistency of color affected performance in MOT and TR. The role of surface features in MOT has been controversial (Bahrami, 2003; Horowitz, Klieger, Fencsik, Yang, Alvarez & Wolfe, 2007), but there is a facilitative effect of surface features on MOT (Makovski & Jiang, 2009a, 2009b). This observation prompted us to determine whether consistent colors also facilitated TR. In a pilot experiment, we asked sixteen participants to track objects appearing in different task-irrelevant colors in a TR task. Color consistency was manipulated so that, in half of the trials, color was the same across the blank, while in the other half of trials the color was different. Importantly, the objects continued moving during the blank so that they were in different positions when they reappeared. TR performance was superior when the object colors were consistent before and after the blank, $t(15) = 6.89$, $p < 0.001$ ($d = 1.7$). Color information, therefore, was used to facilitate target recovery, just as it had been shown to facilitate object tracking. In the experiments that follow in this section, we examined the relationship between MOT and TR more closely to detail the similar benefits of color consistency. The goal was to determine whether a similar process is used to solve the TR and MOT tasks, which would be consistent with the notion that visual attention to objects, for object tracking, and visual memory of objects, for target recovery, share the same object representations.

Experiment 1: Color Consistency in MOT and TR

In this experiment, we examined whether color consistency effects were similar in MOT and TR. In order to compare the tasks directly, MOT and TR trials were mixed within blocks; the absence or presence of a blank varied randomly across trials. Importantly, the consistency of colors was manipulated to examine the effects of consistency on behavior related to MOT and TR. In MOT trials (blank absent), the effect of color consistency was assessed by manipulating the consistency of colors across motion periods. In TR trials (blank present), the effect of color consistency was assessed by manipulating the consistency of colors across the blank. If a common process mediates both MOT and TR, then the effect of color consistency should be the same in both tasks. If distinct processes mediate both MOT and TR, then the effect of color consistency should be different across tasks.

Method

Participants, Apparatus and Stimuli

Twelve Vanderbilt undergraduate students participated for course credit (mean age = 18.58, s = 0.9). They were tested in accordance with Vanderbilt University's Policy for the Protection of Human Subjects and the APA 2002 Code of Ethics. The stimuli were presented on an eMac G4 using MATLAB and the Psychophysics Toolbox extension (Brainerd, 1997; Pelli, 1997). Observers sat 60 cm from the monitor. The visual display consisted of ten items within a white frame subtending 19 x 19 degrees visual angle (hereafter °) on a black background. Each dot was 0.8°in diameter. The initial directions of motion for each dot were randomly selected from 0 to 360 degrees in 5 degree steps. At each step, the direction of motion changed randomly from –20 to +20 degrees from the previous direction. The direction of a dot was shifted if it came close to the edges of the tracking area. The dots also repulsed each other by a factor scaled according to the proximity of the surrounding dots, such that closer dots were weighted more heavily. These factors produced some variability in speed and changes in direction. The average velocity of a dot was 9.15 degrees of visual angle per second (°/s).

Procedure

As shown in Figure 1, participants viewed 2 vertically aligned digits for 500 ms and were instructed to repeatedly recite these digits aloud into a microphone until the end of the dot motion. A 200 ms interstimulus interval (ISI) followed. The square white frame then appeared for 500 ms, followed by nine dots, including the 3 circled targets, for 2000 ms. The circle cues disappeared, and after 200 ms, the dots randomly moved for 6000 ms. The blank was absent in half of the trials and present in the other half of the trials, indicating MOT and TR trials, respectively. In the TR trials, all of the dots disappeared at 1, 2, 3 or 4 seconds after the start of the dot motion for 200 ms. The dots continued to move during the blank in all trials. In order to find conditions under which MOT and TR could be equated for task difficulty, the average speed of the dots' motion was varied to be 9.38, 12.42, 15.49, or 18.56°/s. At the end of the trial, all the dots remained still on the screen during the participants' response. Participants selected targets by moving a box on the display with the computer mouse over an object and clicking the mouse button. An uninformative tone accompanied each selection. After participants selected three objects, the targets appeared red for 200 ms before the blank intertrial interval.

Color Manipulation

Nine unique colors assigned to each dot at the beginning of each trial. The colors were randomly chosen without replacement from a set of 12 equidistant color coordinates on an imaginary circle (radius = 0.09 *u'v'* units) centered on the white spot in 1976 CIE $L^*u^*v^*$ color space (CIE, 1986). The mean luminance of the colors was 29.88 cd/m^2 (s = 0.88). In half of all the trials, the dot colors were consistent across motion periods, while in the other half they were made inconsistent across periods by swapping between dots at a random point in each period. Motion periods were 500 ms, so there were 12 swaps in the 6 second duration of motion. The dot colors were inconsistent across the blank in half of the TR trials, and consistent across the blank in the other half of TR trials.

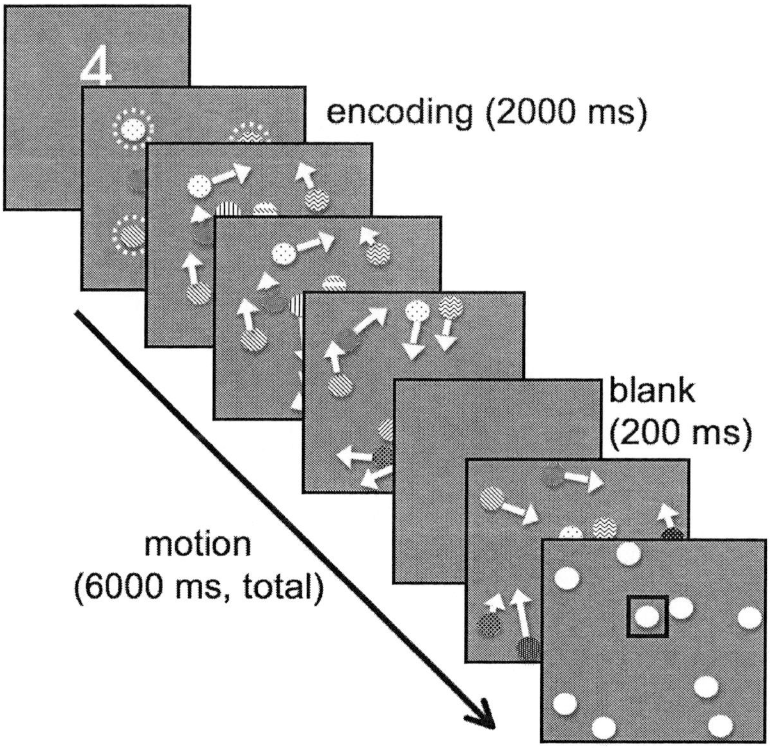

Figure 1. A schematic of the procedure for target recovery (TR) trials when colors were inconsistent across periods in Experiment 1. First, participants were shown two digits for the articulatory suppression task. Next, different colored dots appeared for 2000 ms with the targets cued by circles. Next, the dots started to move and change colors. The blank appeared at 1, 2, 3 or 4 seconds from the beginning of the 6000 ms motion duration. Multiple-object tracking (MOT) trials were similar except that the blank was absent.The actual display used colored dots (not textured) on a black background (not gray).

Results

Accuracy was measured as the proportion of correct target selections averaged across trials. We directly compared the consistent color benefits on MOT and TR performance by examining the difference in accuracy between trials when color was consistent and inconsistent across motion periods and across the blank, respectively. For TR, only trials with consistent colors across motion periods were considered for analysis. The data were submitted to a 3-way ANOVA to examine the effects of Speed (9.38, 12.42, 15.49, 18.56°/s) x Task (MOT, TR) x Consistency (inconsistent, consistent). There were main effects of Speed, $F(3,33) = 98.4$, $p< 0.001$ ($\eta_p^2 = 0.899$), Task, $F(1,11) = 168.5$, $p< 0.001$ ($\eta_p^2 = 0.94$), and Consistency, $F(1,11) = 39.08$, $p< 0.001$ ($\eta_p^2 = 0.78$). These results replicated previous work in that performance declined with faster motion, when a blank was present (TR) and when the colors were inconsistent. There was no Speed x Consistency interaction, $F(3,33) = 1.27$, $p = 0.3$. However, there was a Speed x Task interaction, $F(3,33) = 5.5$, $p< 0.01$ ($\eta_p^2 = 0.33$), likely due to the stronger effect of speed in the TR task than the MOT task because MOT accuracy was close to or at ceiling performance. There was also a Task x Consistency interaction, $F(1,11) = 26.96, p < 0.001$ ($\eta_p^2 = 0.71$), which was likely due to the smaller effect of color consistency in the MOT task, again because MOT accuracy was at ceiling. The three-way interaction was significant, $F(3,33) = 3.19, p < 0.05$, $\eta_p^2 = 0.22$ (see Figure 2A).

The goal of the speed manipulation was to observe the effects of color consistency in both MOT and TR under conditions in which MOT performance was in a similar range as TR performance. To do this, we selected the speeds that produced similar accuracy in MOT and TR when the colors were consistent. On average, MOT accuracy ($\overline{X} = 0.77$, $SEM = 0.03$) when the object speed was 18.56°/s was similar to TR accuracy ($\overline{X} = 0.72$, $SEM = 0.04$) when the object speed was 15.49°/s, $t(11) = 1.06$, $p = 0.31$. Importantly, this MOT performance was not at ceiling, as it was significantly lower than MOT performance in color-consistent trials when the object speed was 9.38°/s, $t(11) = 3.78, p < 0.001$ ($d = 1.44$). We then examined the effects of color consistency for both tasks at these speeds. These data showed main effects of Task, $F(1,11) = 14.93$, $p = 0.01$ ($\eta_p^2 = 0.58$), and Consistency, $F(1,11) = 27.62, p < 0.001$ ($\eta_p^2 = 0.72$), but no interaction, $F(1,11) = 3.47, p = 0.09$ ($\eta_p^2 = 0.24$). Paired comparisons showed superior performance in consistent trials compared to inconsistent trials for both MOT, $t(11) = 3.27, p < 0.01$ ($d = 1.14$), and TR, $t(11) = 4.9, p < 0.001$ ($d = 2.08$). The lack of interaction observed in this analysis suggests a similar use of surface features in both tasks (Figure 2B).

Discussion

The results of Experiment 1 showed that consistent object colors facilitated performance in both MOT and TR, supporting the hypothesis that a common process mediates both MOT and TR. These results accord with a sampling model of object continuity, which predicts that performance is determined the consistency of information related to the target objects (Allen, McGeorge, et al., 2006; Oksama & Hyona, 2008). The decrease in accuracy due to inconsistent colors can be accounted for if the mismatch between the memory of the target colors and new input impaired object correspondence. Observing the same effect of color consistency in both MOT and TR suggests that the same mechanism is common to both tasks.

Experiment 2: Color representation in MOT and TR

The consistent-color benefit was observed in Experiment 1 despite the use of a concurrent articulatory suppression task in both MOT and TR. This suggested that the information about colors was not stored as a verbal code, but instead stored in VSTM. The consistent-color benefit observed in the MOT task with concurrent articulatory suppression suggests that color information in MOT may also be maintained in VSTM, which agrees with previous research (Makovski & Jiang, 2009b). However, unlike TR, the objects in MOT are always visible so it is possible that the color representation is sustained in the visual system without relying on VSTM. Experiment 2 was designed to test another property of color consistency effects in MOT and TR to further examine the notion that the same object representations are used in MOT and TR. VSTM is known to be a low resolution representation (Olsson & Poom, 2005; Awh, Barton & Vogel, 2007) and is robust to effects of visual masking (Vogel, Woodman & Luck, 2006). We predicted that a low-resolution representation in VSTM would enable participants to detect large changes in color, but less able to detect small changes in color. Because the TR task requires object continuity, this predicts better performance when changes are small because they are less detectable. This experiment also employed a full-screen mask just prior to the blank in TR trials to exclude visual representations that were not sustained in VSTM.

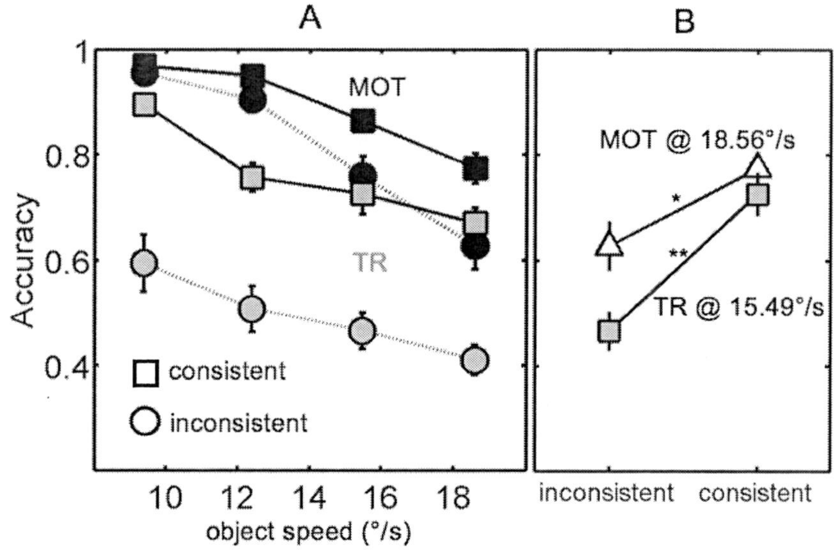

Figure 2. The results of Experiment 1 are depicted above. (A) Accuracy is plotted as a function of object speed in terms of degrees per second (°/s). The results of MOT trials are depicted as black symbols, while the results of TR are depicted as gray symbols. The results of trials with consistent colors are depicted as squares, while those with inconsistent colors are depicted as circles. (B) A direct comparison between MOT trials brought below ceiling performance and TR is depicted, using data from (A). MOT performance at the fastest object speed (18.56°/s) was shown to be comparable to that of TR at a slower speed (15.49°/s) when object color was consistent ($p = 0.31$). Consistent-color benefits were observed for both MOT (* $p < 0.01$) and TR (** $p < 0.001$). Error bars show standard error of the mean for each condition.

Method

Sixteen Vanderbilt undergraduate students participated for course credit (mean age = 19.4, $s = 1.18$). The apparatus and stimuli were identical to that of Experiment 1, except that the blank was preceded by a full screen mask composed of 36 discs appearing in randomly selected colors drawn from the same color set described above. The procedure was identical to that of Experiment 1, except the color changes were either small or large. Small color changes involved changing the color of a dot to one of two 2nd neighbors in our set of 12 colors, such as between two shades of blue. Large color changes involved changing the current color to one of two 5th neighbors in our color set, such as between blue and red. In addition, we only used the 500 ms motion period duration. We added a factor of speed to equate task difficulty between MOT and TR, so that the dots moved at 9.5°/s or 18.36°/s.

Results and Discussion

The trials were sorted as inconsistent or consistent, just as in Experiment 1. The data were then submitted to a 4-way ANOVA to examine the effects of Speed (9.5, 18.36°/s) x Magnitude (Small, Large) x Task (MOT, TR) x Consistency (consistent, inconsistent). The results revealed main effects of Speed, $F(1,15) = 114.01$, $p < 0.001$ ($\eta_p^2 = 0.88$), Task, $F(1,15) = 154.71$, $p < 0.0001$ ($\eta_p^2 = 0.91$), and Consistency, $F(1,15) = 114.9$, $p < 0.0001$ ($\eta_p^2 = 0.906$), replicating Experiment 1. The significant main effect of Magnitude, $F(1,15) = 14.23$, $p < 0.01$ ($\eta_p^2 = 0.49$), indicated that accuracy was better when color changes were small than when they were large. The data showed several significant interactions that justified further analysis. There were two-way interactions between Speed x Task, $F(1,15) = 5.92$, $p < 0.05$ ($\eta_p^2 = 0.28$), Magnitude x Task, $F(1,15) = 9.42$, $p < 0.01$ ($\eta_p^2 = 0.386$), Task x Consistency, $F(1,15) = 27.23$, $p < 0.001$ ($\eta_p^2 = 0.64$), and Magnitude x Consistency, $F(1,15) = 8.29$, $p < 0.05$ ($\eta_p^2 = 0.36$). The other interactions were not significant (F's < 1). The only significant three-way interaction was Speed x Task x Consistency, $F(1,15) = 11.97$, $p < 0.01$ ($\eta_p^2 = 0.44$). While the Speed x Magnitude x Task interaction was approaching significance, $F(1,15) = 3.9$, $p = 0.067$ ($\eta_p^2 = 0.206$), the others were not close to significance (F's < 2.3). The 4-way interaction was also significant, $F(1,15) = 8.92$, $p < 0.01$ ($\eta_p^2 = 0.37$). We investigated the source of these interactions with simple effects ANOVAs and planned comparisons.

The results of performance at 9.5°/s showed that the magnitude of color change modulated performance in TR, but not MOT performance (Figure 3A). For MOT at 9.5°/s, a simple effects analysis revealed no main effect of Magnitude, $F(1,15) = 0.27$, $p = 0.6$ ($\eta_p^2 = 0.018$), however there was an effect of Consistency, $F(1,15) = 4.73$, $p < 0.05$ ($\eta_p^2 = 0.24$), which revealed higher performance when colors were consistent ($\overline{X} = 0.94$, $SEM = 0.015$) compared to when they were inconsistent ($\overline{X} = 0.87$, $SEM = 0.04$). There was no Magnitude x Consistency interaction, $F(1,15) = 0.72$, $p = 0.41$ ($\eta_p^2 = 0.045$). Performance was very high for MOT at this speed, so the results are likely affected by the performance ceiling. For TR at 9.5°/s, there were main effects of Magnitude, $F(1,15) = 18.58$, $p < 0.001$ ($\eta_p^2 = 0.55$), and Consistency, $F(1,15) = 110.99$, $p < 0.001$ ($\eta_p^2 = 0.88$), and a significant interaction, $F(1,15) = 13.76$, $p < 0.01$ ($\eta_p^2 = 0.48$). This interaction was confirmed with difference scores, constructed by subtracting performance in the inconsistent trials from the consistent trials, showed a larger difference for large color changes compared to small color changes in TR, $t(15) = 3.71$, $p < 0.01$ ($d = 1.08$).

The purpose of the speed manipulation was to examine whether the magnitude of color change affected MOT performance once it was brought down from ceiling. Contrasting MOT performance at 9.5°/s to 18.36°/s revealed significantly lower performance at 18.36°/s, $t(15) = 8.99$, $p < 0.001$ ($d = 1.66$), confirming that MOT performance was lower than ceiling at the faster speed. For MOT at 18.36°/s, a simple effects analysis revealed a main effect of Consistency, $F(1,15) = 36.1$, $p < 0.001$ ($\eta_p^2 = 0.71$), which showed higher performance when colors were consistent ($\overline{X} = 0.76$, $SEM = 0.03$) compared to when they were inconsistent ($\overline{X} = 0.62$, $SEM = 0.05$). However, there was no effect of Magnitude, $F(1,15) = 3.87$, $p = 0.068$ ($\eta_p^2 = 0.20$), and no interaction, $F(1,15) = 0.7$, $p = 0.42$ ($\eta_p^2 = 0.04$). For TR at 18.36°/s, a simple effects analysis revealed a main effect of Consistency, $F(1,15) = 77.82$, $p < 0.001$ ($\eta_p^2 = 0.84$), which showed higher performance when colors were consistent ($\overline{X} = 0.54$, $SEM = 0.02$) compared to when they were inconsistent ($\overline{X} = 0.33$, $SEM = 0.016$). There was no effect of Magnitude, $F(1,15) = 4.0$, $p = 0.06$ ($\eta_p^2 = 0.21$), and no interaction, $F(1,15) = 0.3$, $p = 0.59$ ($\eta_p^2 = 0.02$). When speed was 18.36°/s, we still did not observe an effect of color change magnitude in MOT, even though MOT performance was brought down from ceiling (Figure 3B). We also did not observe effects of color change magnitude in TR at this speed, but this may have been because performance in the inconsistent trials was at floor (Figure 3B). Together, it seems that color representation in TR was sensitive to the magnitude of change, while color representation in MOT was not.

These results showed that while the color consistency effect in MOT was not sensitive to the magnitude of color change, the color consistency effect in TR was. This may indicate that color representations in TR are mediated by VSTM, but are represented differently in MOT. It is possible that VSTM mediates color representation in MOT (Makovski & Jiang, 2009b), but it can be buttressed by other systems, such as iconic memory or sensory persistence, which were not eliminated in the MOT task. Extra precision in the representation of color afforded by iconic memory may provide greater sensitivity to the small color changes during MOT. In summary, the results support the notion that color is represented differently in TR and MOT.

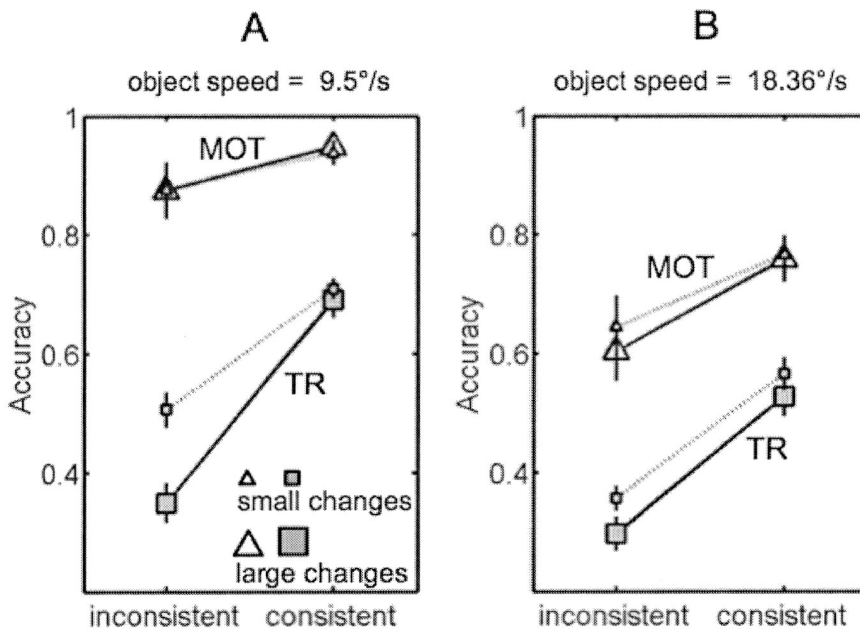

Figure 3. The results of Experiment 2 are depicted to the right. (A) At 9.5°/s, TR performance was modulated by the magnitude of color change, while ceiling performance in MOT may have obscured effects of magnitude. (B) At 18.36°/s, MOT performance was brought down from ceiling (see text for analysis), but no effect of color change magnitude was observed. Error bars show standard error of the mean for each condition.

Experiment 3: Color-based Correspondence in TR Is Not Object-Specific

In this experiment, we examined whether the process of matching colors between each sample was specific to each object. An alternative account is that participants stored a list of the target colors without remembering which color belonged to which object. We contrasted these accounts by manipulating whether the targets swapped colors with other targets or with non-targets. The object-specific account predicts that task performance would drop in both conditions, because each specific object's color would be inconsistent. The alternative account predicts that task performance would only drop in the latter condition. If participants remembered target colors without making a correspondence to each object, then the matching process would not consider swaps between targets to be inconsistent, but it would consider swaps with non-targets to be inconsistent.

Method

Participants were 11 Vanderbilt undergraduates, including 5 females (mean age = 18.63, s = 1.02). The apparatus and stimuli were identical to that of Experiment 2. The procedure was identical to that of Experiment 2, except that we did not manipulate the magnitude of the color change or object speed. Instead, we manipulated how the colors were swapped in the inconsistent trials. In half of the trials, targets swapped colors with other targets, while non-targets swapped colors with other non-targets. In other words, the colors were swapped within groups. In the other half, the targets swapped colors with non-targets, so that colors were swapped across groups. Finally, participants tracked four out of eight objects. There were 8 trials per condition, resulting in 128 trials in total.

Results and Discussion

The data were categorized as consistent or inconsistent, as in Experiment 1, and submitted to a 3-way ANOVA to examine the effects of Group (within, across) x Task (MOT, TR) x Consistency (inconsistent, consistent). This revealed main effects of Group, $F(1,10) = 7.18$, $p< 0.05$ ($\eta_p^2 = 0.42$), Task, $F(1,10) = 269.05$, $p< 0.001$ ($\eta_p^2 = 0.96$), and Consistency, $F(1,10) = 19.67$, $p< 0.01$ ($\eta_p^2 = 0.66$). There was no Group x Task interaction, $F(1,10) = 2.28$, $p = 0.16$. However, there was a significant Group x Consistency interaction, $F(1,10) = 13.93$, $p< 0.01$ ($\eta_p^2 = 0.58$), and a Task x Consistency interaction, $F(1,10) = 9.06$, $p< 0.05$ ($\eta_p^2 = 0.47$). The three-way interaction was significant, $F(1,10) = 10.14$, $p< 0.01$ ($\eta_p^2 = 0.5$). The results of the three-way interaction suggested that consistency effects were observed when the changes were made across groups rather than within groups. This was confirmed by paired comparisons made between inconsistent and consistent trials for each task and each level of the grouping manipulation. Of these four *t*-tests, a significant effect was found only in TR when changes were made across groups, $t(10) = 5.77$, $p< 0.001$ (all other *t*'s < 1.3).

Color-based Errors

We conducted further analyses to pursue the possibility that participants are using a color-based strategy involving memorizing a list of target colors and using it for recovery when a target is lost. We examined the number of response errors made in TR trials when colors were consistent across motion periods, across levels of Group (Within, Across) and consistency across the blank (inconsistent, consistent). A 2-way ANOVA revealed main effects of Group, $F(1,10) = 5.36$, $p< 0.05$ ($\eta_p^2 = 0.35$), and Consistency, $F(1,10) = 17.78$, $p< 0.01$ ($\eta_p^2 = 0.64$), and a significant interaction, $F(1,10) = 16.42$, $p< 0.01$ ($\eta_p^2 = 0.62$). Paired comparisons revealed that more errors were made in inconsistent trials compared to consistent trials Across Groups, $t(10) = 5.77$, $p< 0.001$, but not Within Groups, $t(10) = 0.55$, $p = 0.59$. Of the errors made in the inconsistent trials of the Across Groups condition, we calculated how often participants selected a non-target whose post-blank color matched that of a pre-blank color of a missing target. These errors accounted for 57% of the errors in that condition.

These results show that the consistent-color benefits that we observed in previous experiments are not object-specific. That is, a one-to-one object correspondence is not necessary to maintain consistency. At a glance, these results seem to support the idea that participants strategically remember a list of target colors. If the targets are lost, as in target recovery, they simply recover objects appearing colors belonging to that list, regardless of the objects' positions. In trials where targets swap colors with other targets, selection errors would be less likely since participants using this strategy would recover other targets. In trials where targets swap colors with other targets, participants using this strategy would mistakenly recovery non-targets, leading to more selection errors. This predicts no performance impairment in within-group trials, but does predict impairment in across-group trials. However, this idea is not supported by the error analysis in TR, which showed that mistakenly recovering non-targets that appeared in the same colors as targets prior to the blank only accounted for a little over half of the total errors. There could be other kinds of information, such as motion or position (Fencsik, Klieger & Horowitz, 2007), which contribute to object correspondence along with color. An alternative account is that due to attention being divided between several targets, some target colors were mistakenly bound to targets other than the ones the colors were originally assigned. In other words, participants could have formed illusory conjunctions (Treisman & Schmidt, 1982), and misbind target relevant information.

Objects in Attention and Memory

Discussion of Empirical Results

This chapter explored the idea that attending to objects and remembering features of objects uses the same representations. The experiments presented here employed object tracking and target recovery tasks to investigate how people attend to and remember visual features of changing objects. The theory that was tested was that a sampling process mediates the ability to track objects. Visual information about target objects is selected by attention so that it is sampled at discrete moments in time, then stored in visual short-term memory for later use. Successful object tracking occurs when new samples of objects match target information stored in memory appropriately, even though changes in object properties, such as position, occur between samples. The idea of a sampling mechanism makes two general predictions. First, objects can be tracked across a visual discontinuity. This is because no information is processed between samples, and this is supported by findings in TR (Alvarez et al., 2005; Horowitz et al., 2006). Second, preservation of object continuity is dependent upon the consistency of information between samples. The experiments reported here test this second prediction.

We examined whether performance related to two tasks, multiple object tracking (MOT) and target recovery (TR), was similarly affected by the consistency of objects' colors. The sampling mechanism predicts that performance would be facilitated by consistent object information and impaired by inconsistent object information. The results demonstrated a consistent color benefit in both the MOT and TR tasks. Experiment 1 directly compared the effects of color consistency in MOT and TR. It was hypothesized that if a common process mediated MOT and TR, then there would be similar effects of color consistency across both tasks. If distinct processes mediated MOT and TR, there would be different effects of color consistency across both tasks. The results of Experiment 1 showed a consistent-color benefit in both MOT as well as TR, which agreed with the prediction of the common process hypothesis. The results of Experiments 2 showed the consistent-color benefits were modulated by the magnitude of the color change in TR, but not MOT. Finally, the results of Experiment 3 showed that the consistent color benefit was not object-specific. Accurate tracking did not depend on there being a one-to-one correspondence between the target objects and their colors. Instead, target recovery was successful and object continuity was maintained if any target appeared in any target color.

Together, these results suggest that object continuity is preserved by a process that is sensitive to the consistency of object color for both objects that remain continuously visible, as in MOT, and objects that are briefly invisible, as in TR. This could be a process that periodically samples information and compares it to other samples across discrete time intervals. We offer the observation that both MOT and TR are similarly affected by the consistency of color information as evidence that the object correspondence process is uses a sampling mechanism. Furthermore, our results suggest that a higher-resolution representation of color may be available when objects are visible. This may be because in addition to the use of VSTM, color representation for visible objects may be buttressed by iconic memory or another kind of sensory memory. Regardless, these observations are consistent with the notion that attention and memory work together to sustain object continuity for the sake of target tracking and recovery. As such, these observations provide support for the theory that visual attention and visual memory share object representations.

Does a Common Process Mediate Both MOT and TR?

The results of this chapter suggest that a common process could support the preservation of object continuity for both MOT and TR, and that this process may involve a periodic sampling mechanism. Previous work using MOT had suggested that location information about the targets was sampled and compared in an iterative process (Allen et al., 2006; Oksama & Hyona, 2008). Not only does this account for the effects of speed on MOT performance (Oksama & Hyona, 2008), but it also accounts for the results of TR (Keane & Pylyshyn, 2006). The current results extend this theory by suggesting that the sampling process is sensitive to color. Manipulating the consistency of object colors in our tasks affected behavior, such that inconsistent colors impaired performance of both MOT and TR. These results support the idea that color information is sampled from objects during tracking and stored for comparison during the next interval of sampling. The goal of this comparison is to find a match based on position and color – matches preserve object continuity, while mismatches impair object continuity.

The idea of periodically sampling information is not restricted to tracking tasks such as MOT and TR. Other types of research on visual attention have demonstrated that information is not apprehended in a continuous manner. The type of attention that can be drawn transiently to a spatial location is not the same as the type of attention used to sustain it in one location (Nakayama & Mackeben, 1989). Van Rullen, Carlson and Cavanagh (2007) provided some psychophysical evidence that attention processes information in a periodic manner, even when only one object is attended. Observers viewed four discs of random noise, and were cued to one or more locations in order to detect a brief change in contrast. Performance was compared to computational models that assumed either a continuous accrual of information or a periodic sampling of information. When stimuli had a lower overall contrast, the results were more consistent with the sampling model, suggesting that visual attention operated in a periodic sampling manner under some viewing conditions. Also, Van Rullen, Reddy and Koch (2005) made similar conclusions by testing the wagon-wheel illusion. The wagon-wheel illusion refers to the misperception of a wheel's spokes rotating in the opposite direction to that of the wheel. This has been attributed to a mechanism that discretely samples position information of a moving object and computes motion based on the smallest spatial displacements in the display. The illusion arises because the mechanism samples at a sub-optimal rate, so that the smallest displacements between samples are not in the wheel's direction of motion, but in the opposite direction of motion. They showed that observers misperceived the direction of motion when the elements of a wagon-wheel stimulus cycled around 10 Hertz. However, this misperception was eliminated when observers divided their attention between the wagon-wheel task and another concurrent task, providinga rare demonstration that fullattention could impair psychophysical performance. Together, these results suggested that visual attention was the source of discrete sampling of information in this illusion.

Though visual attention samples visual information, another system is required for storage.The storage of sampled information may be mediated by VSTM, as suggested by Allen and colleagues (2006) and Oksama and Hyona (2008). During object tracking, the storage of position information can account for previous results of TR studies (Keane & Pylyshyn, 2006), as well as findings of how speed affects MOT (Oksama & Hyona, 2008). Our results extend this account by suggesting that color information may also be stored in VSTM during TR. Makovski and Jiang (2009b) showed that color information, when used to facilitate MOT performance, was stored in VSTM. Tracking performance benefited when the objects were uniquely colored compared to when they were homogenously colored, but this benefit was not observed when participants concurrently performed a one-back color memory task during tracking. The results of the current study suggested that the color representation used during MOT was of higher resolution than what is expected of VSTM. However, they do not refute the results of Makovski and Jiang (2009b), since it is possible that color representation for visible objects may benefit from additional types of memory, like iconic memory.

Could the attentional sampling mechanism account for the observation that color correspondence is not object-specific? It is possible that attention to the multiple objects stems from a single, common resource. Divided attention could have resulted in binding errors that produced illusory conjunctions (Treisman & Schmidt, 1982). All of the target colors and locations could have been sampled and accurately retained, but improperly matched to information in memory. The comparison mechanism would recognize a match for any previously retained color, regardless of what object previously appeared in that color. The conditions of the task could have increased the probability for illusory conjunctions, because the colors were not task relevant.

The Role of Spatiotemporal and Surface Features in Object Continuity

Object continuity depends on making a correspondence between different states of perception with some form of information in memory. What kind of information mediates object continuity? In its original form, object file theory proposed that correspondence is based on spatiotemporal continuity, while appearance is allowed to vary greatly (Kahneman, Treisman & Gibbs, 1992). In other words, the way an object is considered to be the same object even when the visual information changes is determined by its place in space and time, not by its appearance. In accordance with the original version of object file theory, some research has shown that object continuity is based primarily on spatial and temporal information, rather than appearance (Scholl, 2001; Mitroff & Alvarez, 2007; Flombaum, Scholl & Santos, 2009). For example, motion of a single object can be perceived between two spatially- and temporally-distinct events, even when the object changes appearance (Cavanagh, Arguin & von Grunau, 1989; Kolers & Pomerantz, 1971; Kolers & von Grunau, 1976). Visual masking occurring on the level of object representations may reflect the integration of two differently appearing objects into a single representation (Enns & Di Lollo, 1997; Lleras & Moore, 2003). Also, an object passing through a tunnel in a smooth motion path is perceived as a single object, even if it appears dramatically different between entering and exiting the tunnel (Flombaum, Kundey, Santos & Scholl, 2004).

However, other studies have shown that appearance can have an important role in preserving object continuity. Memory for appearance can be important for preserving object continuity across saccades (Hollingworth, Richard & Luck, 2008). Apparent motion perception can be facilitated with consistent spatial frequency (Green, 1986; Ramachandran, Ginsburg & Anstis, 1983) or color (Green, 1989; Dobkins & Albright, 1993). Appearance information is also crucial in determining the perception of an object's motion path when spatiotemporal information is made ambiguous (Feldman & Tremoulet, 2006). A moving object changing in appearance can be perceived as multiple objects rather than different states of the same object (Moore & Enns, 2004; Moore, Mordkoff & Enns, 2007).

The results of the current study do not speak to whether spatiotemporal information or surface features are dominant in preserving object continuity, but they do support the idea that both play a role. Tracking tasks like MOT and TR are inherently spatial, but the results of the current study as well as others (Horowitz et al., 2007; Oksama & Hyona 2004, 2008; Makovski & Jiang, 2009a, 2009b) have provided evidence that surface features facilitate tracking, and can play a role in successful object correspondence processes.

CONCLUSIONS

The goal of this chapter was to discuss the link between visual attention and visual short-term memory in relation to object representations. By reviewing previous work, we showed an important relationship between object representations in visual attention and visual short-term memory (VSTM). The continuity of visual objects in attention seems to critically depend on temporary storage in VSTM. Maintaining objects in memory seems to depend on binding features with visual attention. The critical link in the relationship between attention and memory may be a shared means of object representation. The results of experiments described in this chapter suggest that attentively tracking objects seems to be mediated by periodically sampling information for storage in visual short-term memory. This work moves the field forward in understanding how people use attention and memory to support solve dynamic tasks and maintain an integrated experience of objects in the world around them.

References

Allen, R., McGeorge, P., Pearson, D., & Milne, A. (2006). Multiple-target tracking: A role for working memory? *Quarterly Journal of Experimental Psychology, 59*(6), 1101 - 1116.

Allen, R. J., Baddeley, A. D., & Hitch, G. J. (2006). Is the binding of visual features in working memory resource-demanding? *Journal of Experimental Psychology: General, 135*(2), 298-313.

Alvarez, G. A., & Cavanagh, P. (2004). The capacity of visual short-term memory is set both by visual information load and by number of objects. *Psychological Science, 15*(2), 106-111.

Alvarez, G. A., Horowitz, T. S., Arsenio, H. C., DiMase, J. S. & Wolfe, J. M. (2005). Do multielement visual tracking and visual search draw continuously on the same visual attention resources? *Journal of Experimental Psychology: Human Perception and Performance. 31*(4), 643 - 667.

Awh, E., Barton, B., & Vogel, E. K. (2007). Visual working memory represents a fixed number of items regardless of complexity. *Psychological Science, 18*(7), 622 - 628.

Bahrami, B. (2003). Object property encoding and change blindness in multiple object tracking. *Visual Cognition, 10*(8), 949-963.

Brainerd, D. H. (1997). The psychophysics toolbox. *Spatial Vision, 10*(433-436).

Bundesen, C. (1990) A theory of visual attention. *Psychological Review, 97*, 523 – 547.

Cavanagh, P., & Alvarez, G. A. (2005). Tracking multiple targets with multifocal attention. *Trends in Cognitive Science, 9*(7), 349-354.

Cavanagh, P., Arguin, M., & von Grunau, M. (1989). Interattribute apparent motion. *Vision Research, 29*(9), 1197 - 1204.

Chun, M. M., Golomb, J. D., Turk-Browne, N. B. (2011) A taxonomy of external and internal attention. *Annual Reviews in Psychology, 62*, 73-101.

CIE (1986) Publication 15.2 (E-1.3.1) Colorimetry, 2nd Edition, Central Bureau of the CIE, PO Box 169, A-1033 Vienna, Austria.

Coltheart, M. (1980). Iconic memory and visible persistence. *Perception and Psychophysics, 27*(3), 183-228.

Desimone, R., & Duncan, J. (1995). Neural mechanisms of selective visual attention. *Annual Review of Neuroscience, 18*, 193-222.

Dobkins, K. R., & Albright, T. D. (1993). What happens if it changes color when it moves? Psychophysical experiments on the nature of chromatic input to motion detectors. *Vision Research, 33*(8), 1019 - 1036.

Duncan, J. (1984). Selective attention and the organization of visual information. *Journal of Experimental Psychology: General, 113*, 501-517.

Egly, R., Driver, J., & Rafal, R. D. (1994). Shifting visual attention between objects and locations: Evidence from normal and parietal lesion subjects. *Journal of Experimental Psychology General, 123*, 161-177.

Enns, J. T., & Di Lollo, V. (1997). Object substitution: A new form of masking in unattended visual locations. *Psychological Science, 8*(2), 135 - 139.

Fehd, H. M., & Seiffert, A. E. (2008). Eye movements during multiple object tracking: Where do participants look? *Cognition, 108*(1), 201 - 209.

Feldman, J., & Tremoulet, P. D. (2006). Individuation of visual objects over time. *Cognition, 99*(2), 131-165.

Fencsik, D. E., Klieger, S. B., & Horowitz, T. S. (2007). The role of location and motion information in the tracking and recovery of moving objects. *Perception and Psychophysics, 69*(4), 567 - 577.

Flombaum, J. I., Kundey, S. M., Santos, L. R., & Scholl, B. J. (2004). Dynamic object individuation in rhesus macaques. *Psychological Science, 15*(12), 795 - 800.

Flombaum, J. I., Scholl, B. J., & Santos, L. R. (2009). Spatiotemporal priority as a fundamental principle of object persistence. In B. H. L. Santos (Ed.), *The Origins of Object Knowledge.* (pp. 135 - 164): Oxford University Press.

Fougnie, D., & Marois, R. (2008). Attentive tracking disrupts feature binding in visual working memory. *Visual Cognition, 17*(1/2), 48 - 66.

Goldsmith, M., & Yeari, M. (2003). Modulation of object-based attention by spatial focus under endogenous and exogenous orienting. *Journal of Experimental Psychology: Human Perception and Performance, 29*(5), 897 - 918.

Gordon, R. D., & Irwin, D. E. (2000). The role of physical and conceptual properties in preserving object continuity. *Journal of Experimental Psychology: Learning Memory and Cognition, 26*(1), 136-150.

Green, M. (1986). What determines correspondence strength in apparent motion? *Vision Research, 26*(4), 599 - 607.

Green, M. (1989). Color correspondence in apparent motion. *Perception and Psychophysics, 45*(1), 15 - 20.

Henderson, J. M., & Anes, M. D. (1994). Roles of object-file review and type priming in visual identification within and across eye fixations. *Journal of Experimental Psychology: Human Perception and Performance, 20*(4), 826 - 839.

Henderson, J. M., Hollingworth, A. (2003). Eye movements and visual memory: detecting changes to saccade targets in scenes. *Perception and Psychophysics 65*(1), 58-71.

Hollingworth, A., Richard, A. M., & Luck, S. J. (2008). Understanding the function of visual short-term memory: Transsaccadic memory, object correspondence, and gaze correction. *Journal of Experimental Psychology: General, 137*(1), 163 - 181.

Hollingworth, A., Luck, S. J. (2009). The role of visual working memory (VWM) in the control of gaze during visual search.*Attention, Perception & Psychophysics, 71*(4), 936-49.

Horowitz, T. S., Birnkrant, R. S., Fencsik, D. E., Tran, L., & Wolfe, J. M. (2006). How do we track invisible objects? *Psychonomic Bulletin and Review, 13*(3), 516 - 523.

Horowitz, T. S., Klieger, S. B., Fencsik, D. E., Yang, K. K., Alvarez, G. A., & Wolfe, J. M. (2007). Tracking unique objects. *Perception and Psychophysics, 69*(2), 172 - 184.

Irwin, D. E. (1991). Information integration across saccadic eye movements. *Cognitive Psychology, 23*, 420 - 456.

Irwin, D. E. (1992). Memory for position and identity across eye movements. *Journal of Experimental Psychology: Learning, Memory and Cognition, 18*(2), 307 - 317.

Irwin, D. E., & Andrews, R. V. (1996). Integration and accumulation of information across saccadic eye movements. In T. Inui & J. L. McClelland (Eds.), *Attention and Performance XVI: Information Integration in Perception and Communication.* Cambridge, MA: MIT Press, Bradford Books.

Itti, L., Koch, C. (2001) Computational modelling of visual attention. *Nature Reviews Neuroscience, 2*(3), 194-203.

James, W. (1890) *The Principles of Psychology, Volume 1.* New York: Dover Publications, Inc.

Johnson, J. S., Hollingworth, A., & Luck, S. J. (2008). The role of attention in the maintenance of feature bindings in visual short-term memory. *Journal of Experimental Psychology: Human Perception and Performance, 34*(1), 41 - 55.

Kahneman, D., & Henik, A. (1981). Perceptual organization and attention. In M. Kubovy & J. R. Pomeranz (Eds.), *Perceptual Organization* (pp. 181 - 211). Hillsdale, NJ: Erlbaum.

Kahneman, D., Treisman, A., & Gibbs, B. J. (1992). The reviewing of object files: Object-specific integration of information. *Cognitive Psychology, 24*(174-219).

Kanwisher NG (1987) Repetition blindness: type recognition without token individuation. *Cognition 27*, 117 – 143.

Keane, B. P., & Pylyshyn, Z. W. (2006). Is motion extrapolation employed in multiple object tracking? Tracking as a low-level non-predictive function. *Cognitive Psychology, 52*(4), 346 - 368.

Knudsen EI. (2007). Fundamental components of attention. *Annual Reviews in Neuroscience, 30*, 57-78.

Ko, P. C. & Seiffert, A. E. (2009) Updating objects in visual short-term memory is feature selective. *Memory and Cognition, 37*(6), 909 - 923.

Kolers, P. A., & Pomeranz, J. R. (1971). Figural change in apparent motion. *Journal of Experimental Psychology, 87*(1), 99 - 108.

Kolers, P. A., & von Grunau, M. (1976). Shape and color in apparent motion. *Vision Research, 16*, 329 - 335.

Kramer, A. F., & Jacobson, A. (1991). Perceptual organization and focused attention: The role of objects and proximity in visual processing. *Perception and Psychophysics, 50*(3), 267 - 284.

Kramer, A. F., Weber, T. A., & Watson, S. E. (1997). Object-based attentional selection - grouped arrays or spatially invariant representations? Comment on Vecera and Farah (1994). *Journal of Experimental Psychology: General, 126*(1), 3 - 13.

Lee, D., & Chun, M. M. (2001). What are the units of visual short-term memory, objects or spatial locations? *Perception and Psychophysics, 63*(2), 253-257.

Lleras, A., & Moore, C. M. (2003). When the target becomes the mask: Using apparent motion to isolate the object-level component of object substitution masking. *Journal of Experimental Psychology: Human Perception and Performance, 29*(1), 106-120.

Logan, G. D. (1996). The code theory of visual attention: An integration and space-based and object-based attention. *Psychological Review, 103*(4), 603 - 649.

Luck, S. J., & Vogel, E. K. (1997). The capacity of visual working memory for features and conjunctions. *Nature, 390*(6657), 279-281.

Makovski, T., & Jiang, Y. V. (2009a). Feature binding in attentive tracking of distinct objects. *Visual Cognition, 17*(1/2), 180 - 194.

Makovski, T., & Jiang, Y. V. (2009b). The role of visual working memory in attentive tracking of unique objects. *Journal of Experimental Psychology: Human Perception and Performance, 35*(6), 1687 - 1697.

Matsukura, M., & Vecera, S. P. (2006). The return of object-based attention: Selection of multiple-region objects. *Perception and Psychophysics, 68*(7), 1163 - 1175.

Mitroff, S. R., & Alvarez, G. A. (2007). Space and time, not surface features, guide object persistence. *Psychonomic Bulletin and Review, 14*(6), 1199 - 1204.

Mitroff, S. R., Scholl, B. J., & Noles, N. S. (2007). Object files can be purely episodic. *Perception, 36*, 1730 - 1735.

Moore, C. M., & Enns, J. T. (2004). Object updating and the flash-lag effect. *Psychological Science, 15*(12), 866-871.

Moore, C. M., Mordkoff, J. T., & Enns, J. T. (2007). The path of least persistence: Object status mediates visual updating. *Vision Research, 47*, 1624 - 1630.

Nakayama, K., & MacKeben, M. (1989). Sustained and transient components of focal visual attention. *Vision Research, 29*(11), 1631 - 1647.

Oksama, L., & Hyona, J. (2004). Is multiple object tracking carried out automatically by an early vision mechanism independent of higher-order cognition? An individual difference approach. *Visual Cognition, 11*(5), 631-671.

Oksama, L., & Hyona, J. (2008). Dynamic binding of identity and location information: A serial model of multiple identity tracking. *Cognitive Psychology, 56*, 237 - 283.

Olson, I. R., & Jiang, Y. (2002). Is visual short-term memory object based? Rejection of the "strong-object" hypothesis. *Perception and Psychophysics, 64*(7), 1055-1067.

Olsson, H., & Poom, L. (2005). Visual memory needs categories. *Proceedings of the National Academy of Sciences USA, 102*(24), 8776-8780.

Pashler, H. (1998). *The Psychology of Attention.* Cambridge, MA: MIT Press.

Pelli, D. G. (1997). The videotoolbox software for visual psychophysics: Transforming numbers into movies. *Spatial Vision, 10*(437-442).

Phillips, W. A. (1974). On the distinction between sensory storage and short-term visual memory. *Perception and Psychophysics, 16*(2), 283-290.

Posner, M. I. (1980). Orienting of attention. *Quarterly Journal of Experimental Psychology, 32*, 3 - 25.

Prinzmetal, W. (1981). Principles of feature integration in visual perception. *Perception and Psychophysics, 30*, 330 - 340.

Pylyshyn, Z. W. (2000). Situating vision in the world. *Trends in Cognitive Science, 4*(5), 197-207.

Pylyshyn, Z. W. (2001). Visual indexes, preconceptual objects, and situated vision. *Cognition, 80*, 127-158.

Pylyshyn, Z. W., & Storm, R. W. (1988). Tracking multiple independent targets: Evidence for a parallel tracking mechanism. *Spatial Vision, 3*, 179-197.

Ramachandran, V., Ginsburg, A., & Anstis, S. M. (1983). Low spatial frequencies dominate apparent motion. *Perception, 12*, 457 - 473.

Reynolds, J. H.& Heeger, D. J. (2009). The normalization model of attention. *Neuron. 61*(2):168-85.

Scholl, B. J.& Pylyshyn, Z. W. (1999). Tracking multiple items through occlusion: clues to visual objecthood. *Cognitive Psychology, 38*(2), 259 – 90.

Scholl, B. J. (2001). Objects and attention: The state of the art. *Cognition, 80*, 1-46.

Scholl, B. J., Pylyshyn, Z. W., & Feldman, J. (2001). What is a visual object? Evidence from target merging in multiple object tracking. *Cognition, 80*, 159-177.

Sears, C. R., & Pylyshyn, Z. W. (2000). Multiple object tracking and attentional processing. *Canadian Journal of Experimental Psychology, 54*(1), 1-14.

Sperling, G. (1960). The information available in brief visual presentations. *Psychological Monographs, 74*(1-29).

Tombu, M., & Seiffert, A. E. (2008). Attentional costs in multiple-object tracking. *Cognition, 108*(1), 1-25.

Treisman, A. (1982). Perceptual grouping and attention in visual search for features and for objects. *Journal of Experimental Psychology: Human Perception and Performance, 8*(2), 194 - 214.

Treisman, A. (2006). How the deployment of attention determines what we see. *Visual Cognition, 14*(4/5/6/7/8), 411 - 443.

Treisman, A., & Schmidt, H. (1982). Illusory conjunctions in the perception of objects. *Cognitive Psychology, 14*, 107 - 141.

Treisman, A. M., & Gelade, G. (1980). A feature-integration theory of attention. *Cognitive Psychology, 12*(1), 97-136.

Ungerleider, L. G., & Mishkin, M. (1982). Two cortical visual systems. In J. Ingle, M. A. Goodale & R. J. W. Mansfield (Eds.), *Analysis of Visual Behavior*. Cambridge, MA: MIT Press.

vanMarle, K., & Scholl, B. J. (2003). Attentive tracking of objects versus substances. *Psychological Science, 14*(5), 498-504.

VanRullen, R., Carlson, T., & Cavanagh, P. (2007). The blinking spotlight of attention. *Proceedings of the National Academy of Sciences, USA, 104*(49), 19204 - 19209.

VanRullen, R., Reddy, L., & Koch, C. (2005). Attention-driven discrete sampling of motion perception. *Proceedings of the National Academy of Sciences, USA, 102*(14), 5291 - 5296.

Vecera, S. P., & Farah, M. J. (1994). Does visual attention select objects or locations? *Journal of Experimental Psychology: General, 123*(2), 146-160.

Vogel, E. K., Woodman, G. F., & Luck, S. J. (2001). Storage of features, conjunctions, and objects in visual working memory. *Journal of Experimental Psychology: Human Perception and Performance, 27*(1), 92-114.

Vogel, E. K., Woodman, G. F., & Luck, S. J. (2006). The time course of consolidation in visual working memory. *Journal of Experimental Psychology: Human Perception and Performance, 32*(6), 1436 - 1451.

Watson, S. E., & Kramer, A. F. (1999). Object-based visual selective attention and perceptual organization. *Perception and Psychophysics, 61*(1), 31 - 49.

Wheeler, M. E., & Treisman, A. M. (2002). Binding in short-term visual memory. *Journal of Experimental Psychology: General, 131*(1), 48-64.

Woodman, G. F., & Vogel, E. K. (2008). Selective storage and maintenance of an object's features in visual working memory. *Psychonomic Bulletin and Review, 51*(1), 223 - 229.

Yantis, S. (1992). Multielement visual tracking: Attention and perceptual organization. *Cognitive Psychology, 24*(3), 295-340.

Yeh, Y.-Y., Yang, C.-T., & Chiu, Y.-C. (2005). Binding or prioritization: The role of selective attention in visual short-term memory. *Visual Cognition, 12*(5), 759-799.

In: Short-Term Memory: New Research
Editors: Garifallia Kalivas and Sappho F. Petralia
ISBN: 978-1-62100-860-6

Chapter 4

Neuron-Astroglial Communication in Short-Term Memory: Bio-Electric, Bio-Magnetic and Bio-Photonic Signals?

Marcos Arturo Martínez Banaclocha[1]* and Helios Martínez Banaclocha[2]
[1]Servicio de Patología, Hospital Lluis Alcanyis, Játiva, Spain
[2]Servicio de Inmunología, Hospital Virgen de la Arrixaca, Murcia, Spain

To María Banaclocha Marqués, in memoriam

Abstract

It is thought that there is a very close structure-function relationship in cerebral neocortex and present neurobiological concepts regarding short-term and long-term memory are based on synaptic neurotransmission and plasticity. However, the diversity and complexity of neurocortical connections, circuits, maps and their relationships with superior cognitive functions are not fully understood requiring a re-evaluation of the classical approach. It is proposed that cerebral neocortex is organized fundamentally in two functionally complementary and closely interrelated three-dimensional structures formed by the neuronal and the astroglial networks, which in addition to chemical and electrical signals may communicate with each other through magnetic fields and electromagnetic waves. If ultra-weak electromagnetic waves (bio-photons) generated as cellular by-products of reactive oxygen species and reactive nitrogen species could play a biological function in information processing and short-term memory it must be under the driving of neuron-astroglial interactions. There is evidence that changes of bio-photonic activity is related to consciousness and other neuro-cognitive functions, suggesting that bio-photons may play some role in the function of the nervous system. Moreover, the

* Correspondence to: Marcos A. Martínez Banaclocha, MD, PhD. Urbanización Tiro de Pichón 77, 46740 Carcagente, Valencia. Spain. E-mail address: martinez_marben@gva.es.

discovery that human brain has magnetite nano-particles has opened new possibilities about the role of these nano-crystals in information processing and memory at quantum level. Neuro-electrophysiological data have shown a close correlation between external magnetic pulses and neural activity, which have been explained based on mechanical, chemical and specific spin-electronic mechanisms. This chapter reviews recent discoveries concerning the ability of neuronal cells to perceive and process electro-magnetic information, and put forward the possible role of bio-photons generated as consequence of neuronal and astroglial metabolisms in short-term memory. A final discussion concerns relationship between the bio-photonic activity and bio-electro-magnetic activity in the neocortex. Our present concept suggests that in the human cerebral cortex there is an electro-magnetic interplay between neurons and astrocytes that allows the generation of innumerable bio-phonic-mediated nano-holograms, which are based on magnetite-compounds associated to neuronal and astroglial membranes. In the present chapter we put forward that bio-photons generated by neuronal and astroglial metabolism may produce holographic pictures explaining retrieval of short-term and long-term memories as well as other neuro-cognitive representations such as dreams produced during sleep. Our hypothesis proposes that interactions between bio-electric, bio-magnetic and bio-photonic activities in neurons and astrocytes in the human neocortex may play important roles in cognitive functions, providing new perspectives for better understand complex functions of the central nervous system such as short-term memory.

Keywords: Memory; magnetite; memory bubble; bio-photon; astroglial matrix; self-organization; holography; attractor

1. INTRODUCTION

The knowledge how memories are physically fixed in the brain is fundamental to understand almost all cognitive processes from thinking to creativity and dreams. It is widely accepted that neocortical functions are accomplished solely through utilisation of complex networks of neuronal connections, which integrate a huge number of input from multiple peripheral organs and internal brain activity itself. However, despite theoretical and experimental efforts to model neuronal networks, the origin of memory, neuro-computation and neuro-cognitive representations remain a mystery.

New theoretical and experimental works have opened new perspectives for understand complex cognitive functions such as sort-term (STM) and long-term memory (LTM) focused in the possibility that bio-electric, bio-magnetic and even bio-photonic signals may play a role in these crucial cognitive functions. Human brain grows exponentially directed by patterns of information codified in DNA, but neuro-blasts need the contribution of a matrix of glial cells that provide the scaffolding for neurocortical organization (Rakic, 1995). After birth, the immature neocortex is exposed to the external information through the sense organs, which allow processing of environmental information, learning and memory. Today, it is accepted that billions of synaptic connections among neurons, constructed in response to specific sensorial information, enables the mature neocortex to learn and store the necessary information to perform all superior cognitive functions. However, the intimate mechanisms by which these superior functions are accomplished are not fully understood yet.

Recently we have proposed that cerebral neocortex is organized fundamentally in two functionally complementary and closely inter-related three-dimensional (3-D) physical structures formed by the neurocortex and the gliocortex, which in addition to chemical and electrical signals may communicate with each other through magnetic fields (Banaclocha, 2002; 2004; 2005; 2007). In this chapter we review the scientist literature regarding the possible role of ultra-weak electromagnetic waves in superior cognitive functions and put forward the hypothesis that if ultra-weak electromagnetic waves (bio-photons) generated into the cells could play a biological function in information processing and short-term memory it must be under the direction of neuron-astroglial interactions.

The use of highly sensitive and low-noise cooled camera and other very sensitive and recently developed technologies have shown weak emission of light from cells, living organisms and even into the brain. A bio-photon theory for information processing based on the evidence of its coherence (high degree of order with an extremely stable intensity) suggests that bio-photons may operate as a biological laser, able to manage a network of information in the organism as well as to form electromagnetic field patterns (Bischof, 2005).

Information processing, memory fixation and retrieval in the human neocortex are unresolved problems that need a reinterpretation of our knowledge about neuro-cognitive functions based on physical principles. For instance we have recently proposed that memory-associated and derived neuro-cognitive representations are physical processes supported by the close electric and magnetic interaction between the neurocortex and the gliocortex that may work like a complex magnetic-bubble memory device (Banaclocha and Banaclocha, 2011). In this chapter, we suggest that bio-photonic signals generated by neurons and astroglial cells may contribute to neocortical representations through holographic pictures generated under the cyto-architectonic arrangement of neurons and astrocytes.

2. Bio-Electric, Bio-Magnetic and Bio-Electromagnetic Fields in Neocortex

2.1. Bio-Electric Fields

EEG activity is a reflection of the electrophysiological functions of the brain. However the exact origin of EEG and its functional significance is not completely understood. Multiple theories have been developed but EEG recording seems to be the summation of the synchronous activity of thousands of neurons that have perpendicular orientation to the scalp. The amplitude of spontaneous activity measured by the EEG is about 100 μV when measured on the scalp and about 1-2 mV when measured on the surface of the brain. The bandwidth of this signal is from < 1 Hz to about 50 Hz. Evoked potentials are those components of the EEG that arise in response to a stimulus (electric, auditory, visual signals). Single-neuron behavior can be examined through the use of microelectrodes which impale the cells of interest. Through studies of single neurons properties and neuronal microcircuits, we may build models of cell network that will reflect actual tissue properties but these models are always a simplification of the real biological ground.

The number of neurons in the brain has been estimated to be on the order of 10^{11}. Cortical neurons are widely interconnected through 10^3-10^6 synapses (Nunez, 1981). The resting voltage of a neuron is around -70 mV, and the peak of the action potential is positive with amplitude of about 100 mV and 1 ms of duration. Bio-electric current density associated with neuronal activation produces an electric field, which can be measured on the surface of the head or directly on the brain tissue. The basis for the impressed current density is the propagating action potential while EEG signals appear to arise from the action of neurotransmitters on postsynaptic cortical neurons. Today it is assumed that the addition of the actions caused by localized depolarization (excitatory postsynaptic potential, EPSP) and hyper-polarization (inhibitory postsynaptic potential, IPSP) are integrated for generate local field potentials (LFPs), which reflect the state of synchronized neurons containing more information than do single action potentials. This would explain information processing and neuro-computation. Indeed, statistical mechanics of neocortical interactions (SMNI) studies based on EEG data, have developed probabilistic distributions at microscopic (neurons), mesoscopic (minicolumns) and macroscopic (neocortical areas) scales in agreement with the architectural organization developed by Nature in mammalian neocortex (Ingber, 1984; 2009; 2011a,b) giving strong support for describing interactions among neurons, mini-columns and different areas of the neocortex.

Previous theoretical approaches suggested that short-term memory may be supported for sufficient long periods of time by 'bubbles' of neuronal activity created by external input in suitably connected sheets of neurons (Taylor, 2003). Such possible localized bubbles of neuronal activities were originally explored in one dimensional (Amari, 1977) and two-dimensional (Taylor, 2000) extremely simple mathematical models of neural connectivity. Moreover, bubbles of neuronal activity have been modeled for various paradigms (Taylor, 1997) including for achieving motor guidance (Stringer et al., 2003). However, if multiple bubbles of neuronal activities represent the real information present in the environment; multiple active bubbles are required at the same time resulting in the blurring of the different representations. To resolve this problem, Stringer and co-workers suggested that a further cellular network would be able to decode these representations in the overlapping sheet of neurons, reducing the noise in the whole representation (Stringer et al., 2004). However, this further cellular network has not been suggested yet.

More recently, ephaptic coupling of cortical neurons has been demonstrated suggesting that endogenous electrical activity can affect neural function through field effects under physiological conditions (Anastassiou et al., 2011). This means that extracellular electric fields as low as 0,5mV can modulate de activity of neighboring neurons.

2.2. Bio-Magnetic Fields

Maxwell's equations connect time-varying electric and magnetic fields, so that when there are bio-electric fields there are also bio-magnetic fields, and vice versa (Maxwell, 1865). The physiological phenomenon that generates bio-magnetic signals is the electric activity of the brain. Then, the source for the magneto-encephalogram (MEG) is the electric activity of the neurons, as it is the source of electro-encephalogram (EEG). The theoretical difference between the bio-magnetic and bio-electric signals is the difference in the sensitivity distribution of these measurements, represented by the form of their mathematical equations. The magnetic field arises from the curl and the electric field from the divergence of the source

(Malmivuo and Plonsey, 1995). Besides, bio-magnetic signal may also arise from magnetic material because such material exists in brain tissues (Kirschvink et al., 1992).

David Cohen was the first scientist to detect the magnetic alpha rhythm, using an induction coil magnetometer in a magnetically shielded room (Cohen, 1968). A few years later he was also the first scientist to detect the MEG (Cohen, 1972) with amplitudes under 0.5pT and frequency range similar to that of the EEG. These magnetic fields had very low amplitude compared to the ambient noise fields and even the most sensitive induction coil magnetometer built for bio-magnetic measurement purposes was not sensitive enough to detect the MEG for clinical use (Estola and Malmivuo, 1982). Therefore, the Superconducting Quantum Interference Device (SQUID) is the only non-invasive instrument that is sensitive enough for high-quality bio-magnetic field measurements.

Although it has been known for a long time that neurons and astrocytes have associated magnetic fields, they have not been seriously considered as plausible signals in information processing, memory and other neuro-cognitive functions. Based on the finding that neuronal and astroglial activities have associated magnetic fields and on the conjecture that in addition to anatomical, bio-chemical and bio-electrical relationships, neurons and astrocytes are interconnected by magnetic forces generated by themselves, we have developed a neuron-astroglial complex 3-D magnetic-bubble memory model (Banaclocha and Banaclocha, 2011). As it has been described previously, neuronal activities produce extremely low time-varying magnetic fields. The amplitude of magnetic fields associated with an axonal impulse is about 0,4 nT (Bradley and Wikswo, 1985) but a more real estimation of the strength of the magnetic fields associated to axons in the neocortex of humans is at least two orders of magnitude higher than that previously reported. Georgiev (2003) has calculated magnetic field strength (B) in the largest human myelinated axons, which have a diameter (d) of 25×10^{-6} m. Having in account a current intensity (I) of 10 μA (Katz, 1966), an effective magnetic permeability $\mu_{eff} = 10$ and a magnetic permeability of the vacuum (μ_0) of $4\pi \times 10^{-7}$ H/m, he obtained an axonal magnetic field:

$$B = \mu_{eff}\, \mu_0\, I / \pi d = 10 \times 4 \times 10^{-7}\ \mathrm{H.m^{-1}} \times 10^{-6}\ \mathrm{A} / 25 \times 10^{-6}\ \mathrm{m} = 1.6 \times 10^{-7}\ \mathrm{T}$$

However, non-myelinated axons in neocortex range in diameter from 0.3 to 1.2 μm, which give us an axonal magnetic field strength from 1.3×10^{-5} T to 0.3×10^{-5} T when a biologically-realistic current (I) of 1μA for neocortical neurons is used. These axonal magnetic fields result in about five orders of magnitude greater than the experimentally measured magnetic field ($B = 10^{-10}$ T) in frog sciatic nerve (diameter = 600μm) at 1.3 mm from the nerve surface, using SQUID magnetometer (Wikswo et al., 1980).

Moreover, the above estimations do not consider the collective magnetic interactions among neighboring neurons within a mini-column (around 100 neurons) or the fact that in neocortex non-myelinated axons are closely adjacent to the astrocytic processes, which are likely to communicate directly with neurons via cell–cell adhesion junctions (Spacek and Harris, 1998) and intercellular calcium signaling (Parpura et al., 1994), suggesting that neuronal activity-associated magnetic fields may directly influence astrocytic Ca^{2+} waves and their role in tripartite synaptic interactions (Ingberg, 2011b). In addition, unlike electric potentials, cellular magnetic fields, although attenuated somewhat (Georgiev, 2003), are not obliterated by the conductivity of the extracellular medium or membranes and do not require direct contact with molecules or cells to produce physical effects.

On the other hand, although astrocytes cannot generate action potentials, these cells show two main forms of excitation. One that is generated by chemicals signals in neighbouring neuronal circuits, and the other that occurs independently of neuronal inputs (spontaneous activity) (Haydon, 2001; Bezzi and Volterra, 2001). Astroglial activity has been observed in acute brain slices as well as in *in vivo* studies, and it is related to Ca^{2+} release from intracellular stores and additional influx of extra-cellular Ca^{2+} (Aguado et al., 2002). Astroglial oscillations are a common feature of developing and adult resting astrocytes in all brain regions and can recruit dozens of neighbouring astrocytes showing synchronisation with spontaneous neuronal activity (Aguado et al., 2002). This bio-electrical activity of astrocytes with Ca^{2+} waves propagating at speeds around 30-40μm/s may generate magnetic fields that may behave like magnetic bubbles forming 3-D magnetic domains with a direction of magnetization in the opposite direction to its surrounding background.

Mathematical approaches have estimated that magnetic strengths associated with EEG activities may affect Ca^{2+} ion momenta outside neurons leading to important effects at the molecular level into astrocytes, which in virtue of the close proximity between neurons and astrocytes in the neocortex may influence astroglial electro-magnetic fields (Ingber, 2011b). Since a single astrocyte can make contact with hundreds of synapses from both neighboring and distant neurons, it is proposed that multiple axonal and dendritic magnetic fields can induce changes in the resting astrocytic magnetic fields. The arrangement of intralaminar and interlaminar neocortical astroglia allows the interaction and self-organization among innumerable astrocytic magnetic fields, resulting in 3-D magnetic bubbles that presumably may contribute to neocortical computation and memory. Besides, magnetic domains and bubbles tend to form stable closed loops and other complex constructs by self-organization when they are bound to physical structures (Boncheva et al., 2005). These characteristics were fundamental for the construction and development of the present model (Banaclocha, 2007; Banaclocha and Banaclocha, 2010), suggesting that the human neocortex has the necessary cyto-architectonic organization and sufficient bio-physical mechanisms to behave like a very complex 3-D magnetic-bubble memory device.

2.3. Bio-Electromagnetic Waves (Bio-Photons)

The embryologist Alexander Gurwitsch introduced the concept of “morphogenetic field” suggesting the existence of a coherent activity of embryonic cells regulated by optical interference. Gurwitsch observed that cells division in the tip of one onion root influenced the division of cell in another root when the medium used to isolate each root was a quartz glass but no when the medium was an ordinary glass (Gurwitsch, 1926). Thus, he concluded this phenomenon was a “mitogenetic radiation” in the ultraviolet range suggesting that the life process was somehow entangled in a “morphogenetic field” (Gurwitsch, 1988).

The use of new developed photomultipliers showed that very weak photon emissions in the spectral range from 400-700nm was possible from living tissues (Popp et al., 1984). In quantum physics a photon is the term used to designate a quantum of electromagnetic radiation. Then, bio-photons refer to photons emitted by biological systems not restricted to the infrared range but generally between 200-800nm to ultraviolet spectra. It is known that the intensity of bio-photon from living organism is about 10^{-16} W/cm^2 (Popp, 1979; Kobayashi et al., 1999 a, b).

The major characteristics of bio-photons have been summarized as follow (Bischof, 2005): (a) non-linear property; (b) low radiation strength; (c) flat spectral distribution of strength without major peaks; (d) delayed luminescence decay following a hyperbolic decay; (e) probability of recording n photons in a time following Poison distribution; (f) extreme sensitivity of bio-photon emission to environmental factors. Bio-photonic coherence can be tapped via a hyperbolic decay pattern that is independent of the emitted wavelength, which is in contrast to incoherent systems such as radioactive decay that follow an exponential pattern.

Bio-photons are associated to energy-matter interactions since absorbed electromagnetic radiation results in an excited atomic state (quantum jumps) and vice versa (VanWijk, 2001). In solid state, electrons may fall to a lower still excited state without the emission of visible light, or they may start to move generating an electric current, or they may be involved in chemical reactions. However, in biological systems an excited electron-hole pair can propagate over long distances within the system before releasing their energy by emitting a photon, being the basis of their implications in energy transduction mechanisms as well as in their propagation as bio-communicators (Bischof, 2005; Popp et al., 2002; Van Wijk 2001).

The physicist Masaki Kobayashi has defined bio-photon as a spontaneous photon emission, without any external photo-excitation, that originates in the chemical excitation of molecules undergoing oxidative metabolism. It is distinct from thermal radiation arising from the body temperature (Kobayashi et al., 1999 a, b). Bio-photon emission must be associated with biological and physiological functions, showing sensitivity to environmental changes (Popp et al., 1984; Devaraj et al., 1997) and high coherence (Bischof, 2005). Coherence means that the photon particles or waves released by the cells form a whole interlinked system working as a synchronic electromagnetic field. The high degree of order in such light reflects its laser-like properties and because of its coherence it has been proposed that bio-photons are able to generate, keep order and transmit information among cells (Bischof, 2005).

It has been suggested two sources of bio-photon emission. One mechanism is based on the coherent field theory (Popp, 1979; Popp et al., 2002; Popp and Yan, 2002) in which, bio-photons are stable and spontaneously emitted by DNA in the cells without external photon or chemical stimulus. The other mechanism suggests that bio-photon emission depend on the biochemical reactions in living organisms (Kobayashi et al., 1999a, b), principally reactive oxygen species (ROS) and reactive nitrogen species (RNS) produced by the metabolic activity of cells (Inaba et al., 1979).

Cell to cell communication by bio-photons has been demonstrated in plants, bacteria and animal cells as well as under physiological and pathological conditions such as mechanical, thermal and chemical stresses, mitochondrial respiration and cancer growth (Amano et al., 1995; Kataoka et al., 2001; Nakano, 1989; Niggli, 1993; Slawinsk et al., 1992; Tilbury, 1992; Van Wijk et al., 2005; Yoon et al., 2005). Moreover, in humans there is evidence suggesting that bio-photon emission is related to various conscious states (Van Wijk et al., 2005) and also that it varies following a circadian rhythm (Kobayashi et al., 2009).

2.3.1. Bio-Photons and Neurons

Recently it has been described a new method called *in situ* bio-photon autography similar to a histochemical staining technique using $AgNO_3$ (Sun et al., 2010). The method is based on the finding that bio-photonic activity induces an Ag^+ to Ag transformation due to electron transfer and consequently Ag deposits in the cells. Deposited dark Ag granules are insoluble in water and organic solvents such as alcohol and xylene, and they can be viewed and localized morphologically under common light microscopes. To investigate whether bio-photons could serve as neural communication signals in the nervous system light emitting diode resources, including infrared, red, yellow, green, blue and white sources, in a dark room were used for 30 min at one end and observed the effect from the other end of spinal nerve roots. The optical density of the deposited Ag granules, representing the bio-photonic signals, at the segment of the spinal motor or sensory nerve roots immersed in 10% $AgNO_3$ during light stimulation was measured by an imaging analysis system after the assay was complete. It was found that various light stimulations had a significant increase in the nerve bio-photonic activity. Besides procaine, an anesthetic that block neural conduction, and the use of 2-deoxy-D-glucose plus sodium azide for inhibit oxidative metabolism largely inhibited bio-photonic activity, suggesting that the observed bio-photonic signals after light stimulation have an action and a background bio-photon components (Sun et al., 2010). A possible explanation for this observation is that external light stimulation might generate action bio-photons that are conducted along the neural fibers resulting in an increase in bio-photonic activity at the other end of the spinal nerve root. Another explanation of action bio-photonic activity is that action potentials and associated magnetic fields generated as the result of light stimulation at one end of the nerve roots would result in bio-photonic generation at the other nerve ends by transduction of action potentials into electro-magnetic waves. On the other hand, background bio-photons are generated *in situ*, principally by mitochondrial oxidative metabolism due to the lipid peroxidation of mitochondrial membranes initiated by the action of the respiratory electron transport chain. Although these experiments have shown that bio-photons can be generated by external light stimulation and conducted along neural fibers, implying that bio-photons might serve as neural signals in information processing, there are some important unresolved questions yet. In regard to the mechanisms of bio-photons conduction along neuronal processes, a mechanism called protein–protein bio-photonic interaction has been proposed based on previous studies showing that certain proteins, such as fluorescent proteins, have unique characteristics of light absorption and emission (Shaner et al., 2005; Shu et al., 2009). Two different proteins may achieve bio-photonic conduction if one protein absorbs bio-photons at certain wave-length and emits bio-photons at another wave-length (Benninger et al., 2008). Since the wave-length emitted is longer (low energetic photons) than the wave-length absorbed it has been proposed that active bio-photons emitted from proteins and background bio-photons generated from mitochondrial oxidative metabolism are simultaneously absorbed allowing protein-protein conduction. Likewise, mitochondrial networks in neuronal processes can be electrically coupled, and can coordinate and synchronize each other (Skulachev, 2001; Dedov and Roufogalis, 1999) allowing that bio-photons can be guided along microtubules and mitochondrial networks inside neurons (Thar and Kühl, 2004). Thus, protein–protein bio-photonic interactions, as well as microtubule-mitochondrial interaction networks, may contribute to bio-photonic conduction inside neuronal processes.

As previously mentioned, it is accepted that information processing by neurons is mediated by their electrical activity, which is generated by the movement of ions carrying electrical charges, raising the question about the possible relationship between bio-electric, bio-magnetic and bio-photonic activities in neuronal cells. Some studies have shown that increased bio-photonic activity is related to the depolarization induced by high potassium concentrations in the medium, and the removal of extracellular Ca^{2+}. Besides, suppressed neural activity by tetrodotoxin, a voltage-dependent sodium channel inhibitor, decreased the bio-photon activity in hippocampus slices (Kataoka et al., 2001). In vivo imaging of the spontaneous bio-photonic activity in the brain of animals correlated with EEG activity, cerebral metabolism and oxidative stress (Isojima et al., 1995; Kobayashi et al. 1999a, b). Likewise, pulsed electric excitation of frog sciatic nerve has been reported to cause photon emission (Artem'ev et al., 1967), and it has been demonstrated a significant correlation between the bio-photon emission and the strength of alpha wave production in the brain (Van Wijk, 2001; Van Wijk et al., 2008).

On the other hand, it was found that focused infrared light alters membrane potential and activates individual neural processes (Wininger et al., 2009) and the application of a 60 Hz AC magnetic field on Madin-Darby canine kidney (MDCK) cells showed a sharp peak at the initial stage of the decay suggesting that a decay of bio-photon intensity has taken a different path following exposure to the magnetic field. The origin of the sharp peak was not explained by the authors but the experiment demonstrates an unequivocal effect of AC magnetic fields on bio-photon emission by living cells (Cheun et al., 2007).

Previous mentioned data indicate that bio-electric, bio-magnetic and bio-photonic activities in the nervous system are not independent bio-physical phenomena suggesting that the interactions among these signals may contribute to information exchange in the neocortex. Then, bio-electric activity is only one of the interchangeable signals necessaries for transfer and processing information in the brain that support learning, memory and other cognitive functions. In agreement with this concept Wang and co-workers recently presented experimental proofs for the existence of spontaneous bio-photon emission and visible light induced delayed ultra-weak photon emission in *in vitro* freshly isolated rat's whole eye, lens, vitreous humor and retina (Wang et al., 2010). As a consequence of their findings the authors proposed that the photochemical source of retinal discrete noise, as well as retinal phosphenes, may originate from bio-photons within the eyes (Bókkon, 2009; Bókkon et al., 2010).

Recently it has been suggested that there may be an interaction between bio-photons and bio-molecules inside the neurons for explain EEG coherence and its relationship with cognitive functions (Rahnama et al., 2010). When the eyes start to be opened, the incident numbers of photons into the eyes increases and the amplitudes of EEG waves are reduced. Although the authors have not been able to find an exact relationship between the EEG diagrams and their theoretical fluctuation function, they argued that the synchronous and coherent vibrations of billions electric dipoles of bio-molecules cannot be ignored in the EEG diagrams suggesting in agreement with Hameroff and Penrose (1996) that microtubules inside the neurons are the best candidate for long coherence and large synchrony into the brain. They suggested a correlation between the alpha-EEG activity and microtubules activities through the fluctuation function in response to the intensity of photons that reach the brain through the retina, but a mathematical relation between the fluctuation function in microtubules and the electric potential in neurons has not be accomplished yet. Alternatively, we have suggested that neuronal synchronization in neocortex, reflected in the coherence of EEG registers, depend on the close magnetic interplay between neurons and neighboring astroglial matrix (Banaclocha, 2004, 2005; 2007) and then, bio-photon emission by neurons and astrocytes must regulate and play a physiological function under the driving of electrical and magnetic interactions.

2.3.2. Mitochondria and Bio-Photons

Bio-photons are generated by radical and non-radical reactions of ROS and RNS, which derive principally from the oxidative metabolism of mitochondria (Inaba et al., 1979; Kobayashi et al., 1999a, b; Tuszynski and Dixon, 2001). Although the generation of ROS and RNS seem to be byproducts of biochemical reactions they can be linked to precise signaling pathways. ROS and RNS have been implicated in multiple cellular processes including gene expression, apoptosis and cell growth, synaptic plasticity, neurotransmission and memory formation (Volterra et al. 1994, Kishida and Klann, 2007). Consequently, it has been proposed that the generation of ROS and RNS during natural oxidative metabolism may be used to produce bio-photons within neurons, contributing to information processing in the brain (Wang et al., 2010; Sun et al., 2010).

2.3.3. DNA and Bio-Photons

Experiments made with Drosophila embryos exposed to weak electrical and magnetic fields have shown that they interact with the MGF and induce malformations, which result in missing extremities, twisted body axis, or even phenotypic expression of ancestral traits that are already extinct (Ho, 2003). This has been suggested to be related with the finding that at least 75% of bio-photonic activity originates from the DNA into the cell, but when DNA is purified and isolated it becomes bio-photonically inactive. That is, photons may be trapped and condense in time into living systems, known in physics as Bose-Einstein-Condensate (BEC) phenomenon. In fact, the DNA molecule itself is considered to be an excited duplex, in which photons are effectively stored between the two DNA strands. Hence, living systems emit light from processes taking place all over the cell (Ho, 2003; Bischof, 2005). The BEC may play an essential role in the formation of the MGF that is basically a chemic-mechanic-electro-magnetic field that exerts its action at nanometer scale but resulting in effects on molecules, cells, tissues, organs and organisms. On the other hand, the cytoplasm seems to provide a fraction of the bio-photonic activity (VanWijk, 2001). However, the microtubules of the cytoplasm seem to play an important role in the propagation of bio-photons that originate in the nucleus, which along neuronal processes and through gap-junctions can be conducted to neighboring cells and to the extra-cellular matrix.

3. Tree-Dimensional (3-D) Structure of the Neocortex

Whatever the model, hypothesis or theory constructed for explain superior cognitive functions, including memory, learning and computation it must consider the exquisite cyto-architecture of the human neocortex. Despite it has been observed a considerable diversity of cell types, laminar organization, functional architecture and connectivity, cerebral neocortex is composed by innumerable neuronal and glial cells organized fundamentally in two closely interrelated 3-D structures (Figure 1). One formed by the neurocortex, organized in neuronal layers and columns (Buxhoeveden and Casanova, 2002; De Felipe et al., 2002; Helmstaedter et al., 2007; Hubel and Wiesel, 1969; Livingstone et al., 1995; Livingstone and Hubel, 1984; Lorente De Nó, 1949; Marin-Padilla, 1992; Mountcastle, 1957; Ramon y Cajal, 1897); the other by the astroglial syncytium or gliocortex (Mugniani, 1986). This fundamental binary organization of the neocortex has been proposed as the central concept for understand information processing, short-term and long-term memory (Banacclocha, 2004, 2005, 2007) and it is now considered essential for the present hypothesis.

3.1. Neurocortex

In addition to layers and columns, mammal neurocortex shows a more complex organization. For instance, the striate neurocortex is organized in three overlapping subsystems (the ocular-dominance columns, orientation-preference bands, and the cytochrome oxidase blobs) (Livingstone and Hubel, 1984; Polimeni et al., 2005). However, although the intrinsic connectivity within the visual cortex is very similar among mammals, the exact layout and relationships between blobs, iso-orientation domains, and ocular-dominance columns have not been clearly determined yet (Adams and Horton, 2006; Horton and Adams, 2005; Van Hooser, 2007). Furthermore, stereotypic pyramidal neurons into neurocortical columns do not preferentially contact with dendrites of specific neighboring neurons. Instead, axons and dendrites are profusely branched forming an all-to-all geometrical matrix from which a multitude of functional microcircuits can potentially be formed (Kalisman et al., 2005). The formation of neurocortical circuits is driven by the transformation of pre-existing geometrical touches into synaptic connections, which seem to be dependent on the electrical activity of the pre- and post-synaptic neurons. This process result in the fact that only a small fraction of touch sites are used to form functional connections, explaining neurocortical plasticity.

Neurocortical layers seem to play specifics roles inside the monotonous and repetitive organization of minicolumns (Buxhoeveden and Casanova, 2002). Layers 2 and 3 have associational functions sending projections into these layers to neighboring minicolumns, ipsilateral cortex and corpus callosum. Layer 4 may be considered the sensory cortex since afferent inputs from the thalamus arrive preferentially to this layer. Layer 4 send inputs to layers 3 and 2, which in turn send connections to layers 5 and 6, the efferent or motor layers. These layers send back the response to other neocortical areas, the thalamus and other sub-cortical nucleus. However, today we do not have a full understanding of how and why neurocortical organization is necessary from a functional point of view.

3.2. Gliocortex

Astrocytes are the largest, most numerous and most elaborated of all glial elements in the neocortex. It seems that astrocytes concentrate around synapses at different proportion depending on the specific cortical area and different cortical layers. Indeed, the ratio of astrocytes to neurons increases exponentially through phylogeny (Haydon, 2001) being approximately 3:2 in humans (Nedergaard et al., 2003). In addition to responding and releasing neurotransmitters, astrocytes are viewed as active partners of the pre-synaptic and post-synaptic terminals in the elaboration of tripartite synaptic structures (Haydon, 2001).

Moreover, astrocytes parcel the cortical neuropil into small domains isolating neuronal dendrites, axons and synapses within specific geometric compartments, which prevent axon terminals from influencing neighboring and unrelated receptive neuronal surfaces (Nedergaard et al., 2003). Each astrocytic domain can integrate and modulate many thousands of synapses under specific neocortical regions (Santello and Volterra, 2010). Only the most peripheral astrocytic processes overlap with each other and interconnect through gap junctions, providing channels for the movement of ionic currents among astrocytes, forming a functional and anatomical syncytium (Mugniani, 1986).

Increasing number and organization of astrocytes in neocortex implicates a role for these cells in the evolution of increasingly complex brain functions. Indeed, recent studies in primates have shown that interlaminar astrocytes from the neocortical layer 1, extend vertical processes that traverse several cortical layers running parallel to apical dendrites within the supra-granular neocortex (above layer 4). This organization of the astroglial network provides an extra-parcellation of the supra-granular neuropil by alternating high and low-density spaces of astroglial processes, enclosing neuronal minicolumns (Reisin and Colombo, 2002; Oberheim et al., 2009). Therefore, it seems that, at least in primates, the organization of the gliocortex has a well defined 3-D configuration that interpenetrate and parcellate the 3-D (columns and layers) neurocortex (Figure 1).

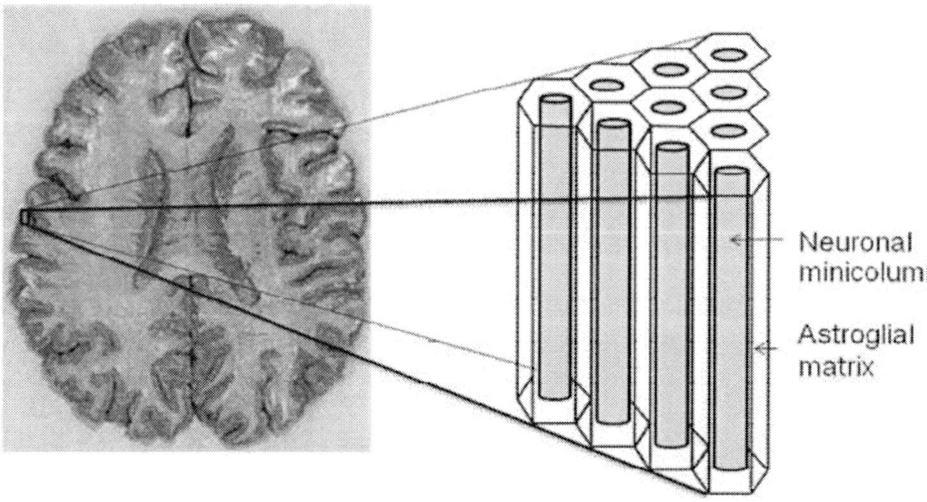

Figure 1. Three-dimensional organization of the human neocortex. Schematic representation of the astroglial matrix (hexagonal network) that interpenetrate and parcellate neuronal columns (cylinders) and layers.

4. Role of Magnetite in STM

Magnetite was discovered in the human brain by Kirschvink's group (1992) and later confirmed in human hippocampus (Dobson and Grassi, 1996). Brain magnetite is produced by *in situ* bio-mineralization and it is diffusely and homogeneously distributed over all cerebral lobes, cerebellum, basal ganglia and midbrain. The particles found in human brain are frequently below 100 nm. Morphologically, the nano-particles are similar to those found in magnetotactic bacteria and are present in clusters. Bio-magnetite crystallize in the prismatic or isometric system (crystallographic axes of equal length at 90° to each other), and is made from alternating lattices of Fe^{2+} and Fe^{3+}. This alternation of lattices and their corresponding differences in the number of unpaired electron spins supplies magnetite its strong magnetization (Kirschvink, 1989). Single-domain magnetite chains are formed by individual crystals with the faces of adjacent crystals lying perpendicular to the chain axes having a permanent magnetic moment that can twist into alignment with an external magnetic field (Kirschvink, 1989). A magnetic pulse anti-parallel to the magnetization direction of single-domain magnetite causes the magnetic moment to reverse direction. Then, the controlled application of weak magnetic fields may cause the rotation of single-domain magnetite, which may be transduced into other physiological functions resulting in the modulation of the transmembrane potential (Kirschvink, 1989; Sonnier and Marino, 2010).

In addition, bio-magnetite also exists in a form called superparamagnetic magnetite (around 10 nm) that has different magnetic properties than single-domain nano-crystals. Superparamagnetic crystals do not have a permanent magnetic moment in the absence of an external magnetic field (Shcherbakov and Winklhofer, 1999), but in the presence of an external magnetic field these nano-particles develop a magnetic moment that track the direction of the local magnetic fields without rotation of the crystal itself. Thus, superparamagnetic magnetite tends to track the direction of an external magnetic field, whereas the magnetic axis of single-domain magnetite is fixed and stable under the same conditions. However, under external magnetic fields, superparamagnetic magnetite may generate fields strong enough to attract or repel adjacent crystals providing the basis for possible transduction mechanisms (Davila et al., 2003; Fleissner et al., 2003; Kirschvink and Gould, 1981; Shcherbakov and Winklhofer, 1999; Sonnier and Marino, 2010).

Magnetite bio-mineralization has been proposed to playa central role in short-term and long-term memory since this process can integrate long time and iterative magnetic signals produced into specific neocortical areas. In virtue of the physico-chemical properties of magnetite nano-particles and its interaction to membrane proteins and phospholipids, it has been proposed that neuro-magnetic and glio-magnetic fields can drive magnetite bio-mineralization in neuronal and astroglial membranes, not only in cytoplasmic membranes but also in intracellular membranes. For instance, magnetite nano-particles synthesis and distribution in the neocortex would be viewed as a specific and very controlled process (Banaclocha et al., 2010). Moreover, we have conjectured that the neocortical magnetic dialogue between neuronal and astroglial networks may have quantum scale effects on brain bio-magnetite biogenesis and distribution (Banaclocha and Banaclocha, 2010). We have proposed that bio-magnetite nanoparticles play a key role in the transduction of magnetic signals produced inside the neocortex itself by neurons and astrocytes. In virtue of their physico-chemicals properties, magnetite nano-crystals could be distributed in neuronal and astroglial membranes in a bio-controlled manner, supporting the bidirectional magnetic interplay necessary for short-term, long-term and memory retrieval at quantum level. These effects would depend on the specific distribution and quantum biomechanical actions of single-domain and/or super-paramagnetic bio-magnetite in the cellular components of the neocortex and the controlled manipulation of their magnetic moments (Banaclocha et al., 2010). Then, the growing structural complexity of the bio-cellular organization (with physical sizes in the µm-to-mm range) allows the greatest control of the strength, range and selectivity of physical interactions including quantum bio-mechanics entanglement. In this way, physical information at microscopic and mesoscopic scales is sufficient massive that it is unaffected by thermal noise.

Having in account that cells generate the strongest magnetic fields into the brain (Brem et al., 2006), we have suggested that neuronal activity-associated magnetic fields (NAAMFs) may drive the synthesis and distribution of magnetite nano-crystals in neurons, which would result in a non-random bio-mineralization of these crystals in neuronal membranes and their organelles. If magnetic fields associated with neuronal activities drive magnetite nano-particles distribution on their own cytoplasmic and mitochondrial membranes, each neuron would have a specific bio-magnetite hallmark depending on their activity and connectivity (Banaclocha and Banaclocha, 2010). These magnetite signatures would be modulated depending on the long time activity of each specific neurocortical circuit, constituting a dynamic process. Moreover, neurons have many mitochondria to support the high energetic demand necessary to the cellular work. If mitochondria are ancestors of magnetotactic bacteria in eukaryotic cells, they might conserve some proteins and phospholipids associated with the machinery necessary to support magnetite bio-mineralization in the inner mitochondrial membrane (Arakaki et al., 2008; Wang and Liang, 2009). This would contribute to the neuronal magnetic hallmark and then, to the mechanism of magnetite bio-mineralization previously suggested (Banaclocha and Banaclocha, 2011).

We have proposed that non-random but specific synthesis and distribution of magnetite on neuronal and astroglial cells have a central role in the processing, fixation, retrieval and representation of information (Banaclocha 2007, 2010).

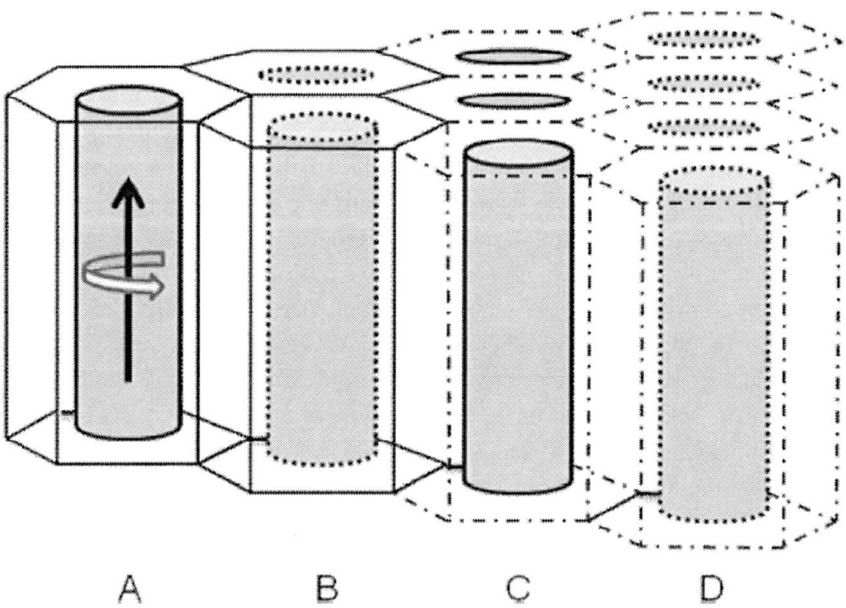

Figure 2. Schematic representation of magnetite bio-mineralization and distribution in neuro-cortex and glio-cortex. A) Cylinders represent minicolumns and hexagons the astroglial matrix. B) Superparamagnetic magnetite is accumulated principally in neuronal membranes as the result of neuronal-activity associated magnetic fields. C) Single-domain magnetite bio-mineralization occurs preferentially in astroglial membranes depending on and modulating magnetic-bubbles. D) Neuron-astroglial bio-magnetic cross-talk.

In agreement with magnetite magnetic properties (Kirschvink et al., 1992; Dobson and Grassi, 1996) we have predicted that magnetite nano-particles distributed in cytoplasmic and mitochondrial neuronal membranes must be composed principally from superparamagnetic crystals, which track the magnetic direction of NAAMFs without the rotation of the crystals themselves (Banaclocha et al., 2010). In this way, neuronal superparamagnetic magnetite may amplify neuronal potentials and generate magnetic fields strong enough to induce, after an iterative process, astroglial magnetic-bubbles (Banaclocha and Banaclocha, 2011). These magnetic bubbles may drive single-domain magnetite nano-particle synthesis and distribution in astroglial membranes being the basis for long-term memory in the neocortex. Then, it was proposed that neurons synthesize and accumulate predominantly superparamagnetic magnetite while astrocytes generate and accumulate preferentially single-domain magnetite nano-particles, which have a permanent magnetic moment and can work in the proposed model storing magnetic representations (Banaclocha and Banaclocha, 2011). This single-domain magnetite would form stable complex structures by self-organization when they are bound to the physical structures formed by the astroglial matrix, constituting a fundamental part of the proposed 3-D magnetic-bubble model (Figure 2).

5. Light Technology in Neurobiology

Photo-stimulation was first used to stimulate action potentials in the abdominal ganglion cells of the marine mollusk Aplysia California (Fork, 1971). Since then it has been developed three principal technologies based on photon stimulation. The photolysis of caged neurotransmitters that are cleaved with UV light to release the active neurotransmitter at high concentration near neighboring neurons (Kaplan et al., 1978), with very good temporal and spatial resolution (Callaway and Yuste, 1994; Shoham et al., 2005). The second method involves the use of engineered membrane photo-switches that uses synthetic photo-isomerizable nano-compounds to block or open ion channels or receptor proteins (Banghart et al., 2004). Synthetic photo-isomerizable azobenzene-regulated K^+ channel (SPARK) opens with short wavelength light (380–390 nm) triggering a K^+-selective current that hyperpolarizes the membrane potential. Long wavelength light (500–505 nm) accelerates the closure of the channel and turns off the K^+ current, restoring the trans-membrane potential. Expression of this SPARK channel in neurons allows light to reversibly hyperpolarize and therefore silence action potential firing. This K^+ channel protein has been modified to make the pore nonselective to cation permeability. Then, the opening of the channel causes depolarization rather than hyper-polarization of the neuron. Expression of this depolarizing SPARK (D-SPARK) channel causes reversible photo-stimulation, with the same wavelengths that cause photo-silencing of neurons expressing the original hyperpolarizing SPARK (H-SPARK) channel.

The last method is based on the use of natural photo-transduction membrane proteins in two forms: light activated cascades leading to ion channels opening and individual light gated channels. Melanopsin is a G-protein photo-pigment that was recently discovered in a small subset of human retinal ganglion neurons (Foster, 2005), which enable light-evoked depolarization responses (Melyan et al., 2005). Channelrhodopsin-2 (ChR2) is a direct light gated cation channel found in the *Chlamydomonas reinhardtii* algae. It has a fast activation by blue light and a fast deactivation time constant (Boyden et al., 2005). A complementary light sensitive inhibiting hyperpolarization protein NpHR has also been reported recently (Zhang et al., 2007), which is a chloride pump that opens by yellow light (approximately 580 nm) and hyperpolarizes the cells resulting in the inhibition of action potentials. ChR2 and melanopsin have a peak spectral sensitivity in the blue at 470 nm. Besides, it has been reported that a very low power density of 5–12nWμm^{-2} was required to stimulate hippocampal culture cells that expressed ChR2 (Boyden et al., 2005) and recently, Bi and co-workers reported that a power density of only 50pWμm^{-2} was sufficient to stimulate ChR2 expressing mice retinal neuron cells (Bi et al., 2006). In comparison with ChR2, the activation of melanopsin requires a much lower irradiance (0.5-5pWμm^{-2}). This is because the G-protein cascade biochemically amplifies the light-stimulation process.

On the other hand, single- and two-photon un-caging stimulation has been important to demonstrate the Ca^{2+}-dependent release of glio-transmitters by astrocytes in acute brain slices (Fellin et al., 2004; Gordon et al., 2009; Liu et al., 2004; Perea and Araque, 2007) as well as permitting neuronal activation and inhibition in freely moving animals (Aravanis et al., 2007; Gradinaru et al., 2009; Wyart et al., 2009). In conjunction with spatiotemporally resolved photo-stimulation techniques, these photo-sensible tools represent the most promising alternative to electrical stimulation devices to control the activity of specific types of brain cells in time and space with sufficient precision.

Grossman and co-workers have recently developed a special custom-made light-emitting-diode (LED) matrix to stimulate multiple neurons in parallel (Grossman et al., 2010). This micro-LED array is based on Gallium Nitride (GaN) technology. It emits 470nm blue light, which matches the absorption peak of ChR2. Action potentials in rat hippocampal neurons photosensitized with ChR2 were stimulated with LED at intensities of only 50pWμm^{-2} (Poher et al., 2008). The responses from single neurons using a standard patch-clamping technique and the spatiotemporal resolution of the micro-LED array was able to stimulate an arbitrary combination of neurons and a single cell with sub-cellular resolution, showing that single action potentials could be accurately and reliably triggered up to a frequency of 40Hz by light in the visible spectrum. The matrix arrays consist of 64×64 pixels (20μm radius; 50μm pitch) that can be flip-chip bonded to complimentary-metal-oxide-semiconductor (CMOS) controllers. The CMOS allows implement independent oscillator control of the individual pixels rather than raster scanning (Grossman et al., 2010).

Electrophysiological recordings and calcium imaging techniques in acute hippocampal slices have shown that excitation patterns precisely tailored to the shape of multiple neuronal bodies simultaneously excited a group of neurons. Indeed, through holographic photo-stimulation it has been easy to generate action potentials and Ca^{2+} signals on target neurons with a relatively high spatial resolution and low excitation density. In addition, it was demonstrated that fast shaped illumination patterns also induce reliable responses in single glial cells. Taking oligodendrocyte precursor cells expressing the proteoglycan NG2 (Nishiyama et al., 2009) as a cellular model, it was demonstrated that holographic photolysis efficiently elicits glutamatergic currents with fast kinetics and intracellular Ca^{2+} signals in these cells. This means that light can affect Ca^{2+} waves in glial cells changing their electric and magnetic fields. The use of holographic photolysis for the excitation of multiple neurons and glial cells has been developed with low energy corresponding to excitation densities between 0.6 and 33.3 nJ/μm^2 generating shaped illumination patterns that selectively excite the whole cell soma. This approach allowed working at excitation densities well below the photo damage threshold (500 nJ/μm^2), reducing the generation of by-products (Trigo et al., 2009). Besides, this method reduces the axial resolution to around two pyramidal cell layers. This high axial resolution is particularly suitable for photolysis experiments requiring multi-cell excitation since it insures that all neurons located near the focal plane are equally stimulated, even if they lay in slightly different axial planes.

Photo-stimulation in brain slices was able to trigger action potentials in pre-synaptic neurons in order to characterize neuronal circuits by two-photon excitation allowing the excitation of individual neurons (Nikolenko et al., 2007). However, holographic light stimulation is the most suited method for fast and efficient excitation of a group of neurons, with a good axial resolution (Zahid et al., 2010). The versatility of the holographic light stimulation could be of particular interest to study neuronal circuits, but also to study the bidirectional communication between neurons and glia in the neocortex. Indeed, the stimulation patterns can be adjusted according to the target cell type.

The photo-switch approach, the caged neurotransmitter approach, and the natural photo-protein approach provide new opportunities to precisely and remotely control neuronal activity for experimental and potentially medical applications but these technical applications of light are examples that show how Nature can use light for information transmission and transduction. In fact, the natural photo-protein ChR2 is endogenous to parts of the nervous system, playing a key role in the retina photo-transduction. Moreover, these approach work in the visible wavelength spectrum at very low intensities opening the possibility that natural bio-photons generated in neuronal and glial cells could play a physiological function in information processing into the neocortex. These human constructed technologies are examples of how visible light photons at very low intensities may stimulate the simultaneous activities of multiple neurons arranged in a cellular size matrix with micron-spatial and millisecond-temporal resolutions.

6. Principles of Holography

The word holography means complete writing. The concept is that each part of the hologram contains information about the whole. The hologram is a photographic (2-D) emulsion in which the information about an object is recorded in such a way that when is illuminated we can see a three-dimensional representation of the object (Figure 3). Unlike the conventional photographic films, holograms have the property that when they are cut up into small pieces each piece is capable of reconstructing the entire image although with a lesser luminosity and clarity (Gabor, 1946). Then, according to the principle of holography, a detailed three dimensional image of an object can be recorded in a two dimensional photographic film and the image can be reproduced back in a three dimensional space (Figure 4).

The present neurobiological concept is that the generation of action potentials by neurons or a network of neurons triggers a particular memory. In the simplest case the firing of a single cell can trigger a certain memory while on the complex one it would be the near simultaneous firing of a collection of neurons in specific circuits that triggers the retrieval of the memorized events. Then, it would be the integrative emergent response of the other parts of the cortex (including other sensory modalities) that yields the sensation of the retrieval of memories. We think these concepts are fundamentally true but are incomplete because do not explain specific mechanisms of memory storage and retrieval nor how our brain can form or reconstruct such realistic representations that we experiment and recreate in dreams.

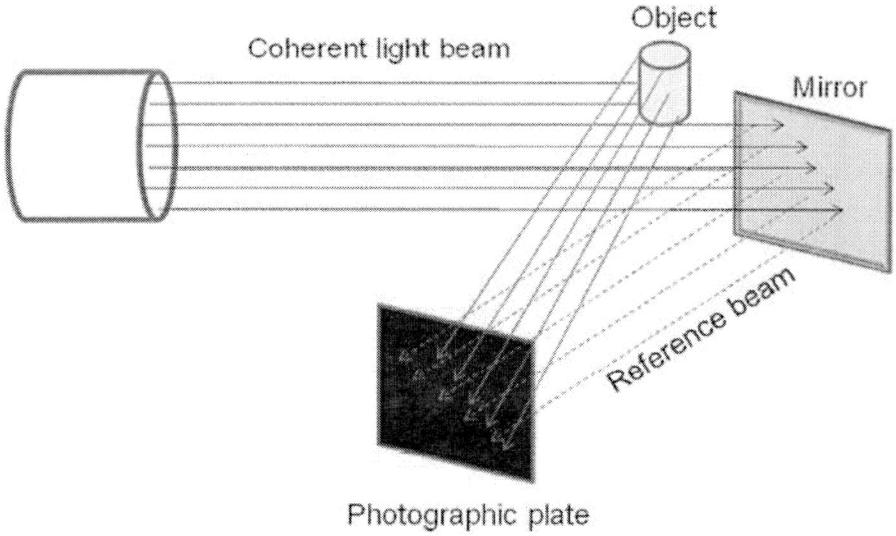

Figure 3. One way to construct a hologram. The hologram plate records an interference pattern between the laser light reflected by a mirror and the scattered laser light reflected by the object. The pattern recorded on the hologram is in the holographic domain. Each part of the hologram plate contains information of the whole object. Light reflected from each point of the object is distributed to every location on the hologram plate.

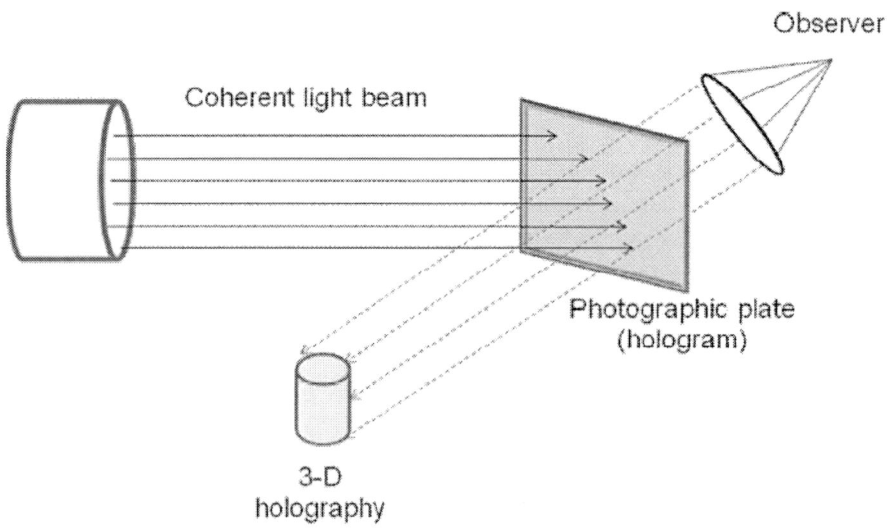

Figure 4. Reconstruction of a 3-D holographic representation. For the reconstruction of a holography, the laser light is shined through the hologram plate (picking up the holographic information from the plate) and becomes incident on the eye which does a transformation (focuses) which forms an image on the retina.

7. Development of Bio-Photonic Representations in the Human Neocortex: The Holographic Model

Photo-stimulation may be an exciting model for explain neocortical functioning at nano-scale size with possible implications in memory retrieval and representations. Triggering neurons and astrocytes with light has many advantages over the classical chemical and electric stimulation in information processing, integration and representation. One important advantage is the potential for multisite stimulation with a high spatial and temporal resolution that seems necessary to explain very complex neuro-cognitive processes. Likewise, the wavelength and irradiance characteristics are sufficient for the use of bio-photons as mediators of complex 3-D holographic representations.

Thar and Kühl (2004) suggested that the real bio-photon intensity within cells can be significantly higher than that measured outside cells. Although photons seems to be coherent light they are strongly scattered and absorbed in tissues suggesting that bio-photonic irradiance may be two orders of magnitude higher than that measured experimentally. As previously mentioned neuronal activity increases bio-photon emission but also and simultaneously produces an associated magnetic field that may be linked to magnetite bio-mineralization. These two synchronous and apparently unrelated effects of neuronal activation may be the basis of the magneto-optical mechanisms that would support holographic representations in the neocortex. Based on the high spatial resolution of the extracellular bio-photons that typically can simultaneously interface with all cells around approximately 100μm; the high selectivity of bio-photons that may preferentially stimulate specific macromolecules; the inherent plasticity of bio-photon-cell interactions and the versatility of different wavelength for stimulation, it is proposed that the generation of bio-photons in neurons and neighboring astrocytes may re-construct physical (optical) representations that under the precise control of the electric and magnetic cellular fields would support short-term, long-term and memory retrieval in the human neocortex (Figure 5).

Magnetite is a spin-polarized Fe^{2+}-Fe^{3+} mixed-valence metal with a DC conductivity at 23°C of about 0.1% that of Cu metal. Its crystals appear black and absorb throughout the UV-visible-IR spectrum. Recent in vitro experiments have shown that superparamagnetic magnetite nano-particles in solution acquire optical properties by self-assembly under magnetic field influences (Kim et al., 2005; Osterloh, 2002). Because of their reduced size, the small aggregates reflected light only weakly but efficiently depolarized the incident light when the magnetic field vector formed a 45° angle with the plane of polarization. Using a setup with two cross-polarized filters, this property allowed the construction of a magnetic light switch. The scattering intensity also strongly depended on the wavelength of the incident light. The observed magnetic birefringence and scattering phenomena were intimately connected with the magnetic properties of the composite. Preliminary magnetization data collected on the magnetite composite with a SQUID revealed its superparamagnetic nature. Tentatively, the authors identified dipolar interactions between adjacent magnetite nano-crystals on the composite sheets as the cause for the observed orientation phenomena of the aggregates in solution. The result of this magnetic anisotropy is a preferential magnetization of the sheets along their planes following external magnetic field force lines, similar to compass needles.

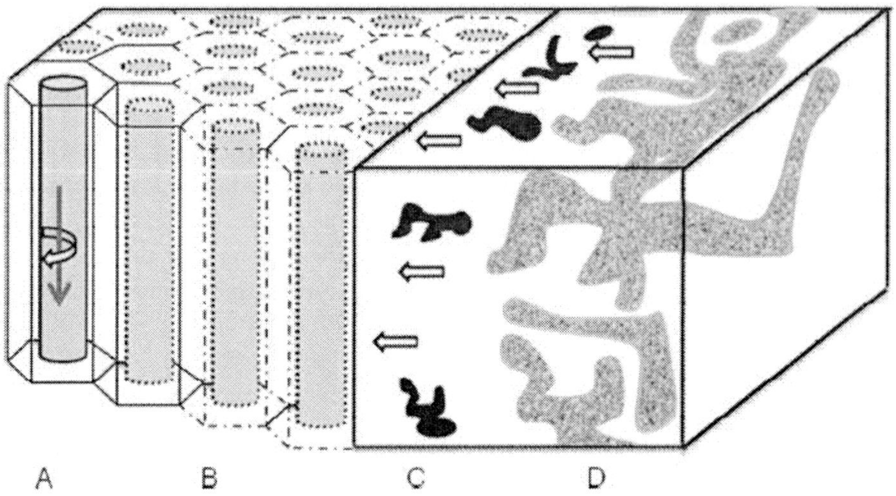

Figure 5. Schematic representation of complex 3-D holographic pictures in neocortex. A) Mini-column associated magnetic fields in the neocortex. B) Magnetite nano-crystal interaction between neuronal and astroglial networks during the processing of information. C) Magnetic bubbles during the retrieval of information. D) Holographic pictures resulting from bio-photon emission and interaction with bio-magnetite in neurons and astrocytes.

Similar magneto-optical properties would be accomplished by biogenic magnetite in agreement with the previously proposed hypothesis about the role of neuronal superparamagnetic magnetite nano-crystals in short-term memory. We have proposed that superparamagnetic magnetite bio-mineralization in mitochondrial and cytoplasmic membranes of neurons may be fundamental for the short-term memory process since NAAMFs would drive and select those neurons electrically more active, allowing the construction of specific arrays of superparamagnetic magnetite nano-crystals in the neocortex. Then, the electric fields generated by action potentials have associated magnetic fields that would drive specific magnetite bio-mineralization in neuronal membranes. This superparamagnetic magnetite linked to specific proteins and phospholipids in the mitochondrial and cytoplasmic membranes would form nano-structures with special magneto-optical properties. These biological compounds would allows the generation of holographic representations using the bio-photons produced by the mitochondrial and cytoplasmic biochemical reactions in working neurons as the source of coherent light (Figure 5). In this way, when specific neuronal minicolumns and layers are activated in response to external stimuli, the synchronized patterns of electric activities produce its associated magnetic fields which may induce changes in superparamagnetic magnetite magnetic moments allowing that bio-photons generated at the same time by the neuronal metabolism would produce specific holographic representations in agreement with the 3-D arrangement of neuronal cyto-architecture. These holographic pictures can be reproduced each time the same pattern of neuronal activity is produced since the hologram has been previously built through the NAAMFs directed bio-mineralization process.

Moreover, NAAMFs would induce and modulate magnetic fields in neighboring astrocytes after time and repetition. These astroglial magnetic fields modulated by NAAMFs depend on Ca^{2+} waves in astrocytes which have been shown to travel through gap-junctions across the astroglial matrix. We have recently conjectured that these Ca^{2+} waves may generate astroglial magnetic bubbles that would drive single-domain magnetite mineralization in neocortical astrocytes supporting long-term memory (Banaclocha and Banaclocha, 2011). The present concept suggests that in the human cerebral cortex there is an electro-magnetic interplay between neurons and astrocytes that allows the generation of innumerable bio-phonic-mediated nano-holograms, which are based on magnetite-compounds associated to neuronal and astroglial membranes.

In the present chapter we have up-dated our previous model for explain memory fixation and retrieval and we have advanced the hypothesis that bio-photons generated by neuronal and astroglial metabolism may produce holographic pictures explaining retrieval of short-term and long-term memories as well as other neuro-cognitive representations such as dreams produced during sleep.

REFERENCES

Adams, DL and Horton, JC. Monocular cells without ocular dominance columns. *Journal Neurophysiology* 2006, 96, 2253-2264.

Aguado, F; Espinosa-Parrilla, J; Carmona, MA and Soriano, E. Neuronal activity regulates correlated network properties of spontaneous calcium transients in astrocytes in situ. *Journal Neurophysiology* 2002, 22, 9430-9444.

Amano, T; Kobayashi, M; Devaraj, B; Usa, M and Inaba, H. Ultraweak biophoton emission imaging of transplanted bladder cancer. *Urology Research* 1995, 23, 315-318.

Amari, S-I. Dynamics of pattern formation in lateral-inhibition type neural fields. *Biology Cybernetics* 1977, 27, 77-87.

Anastassiou, C; Perin, R; Markram, H and Koch, C. Ephaptic coupling of cortical neurons. *Nature Neuroscience* 2011, 14, 217-223.

Arakaki, A; Nakazawa, H; Nemoto, M; Mori, T and Matsunag, T. Formation of magnetite by bacteria and its application. *Journal Royal Society Interface* 2008, 5, 977-999.

Aravanis, AM; Wang, LP; Zhang, F; Meltzer, LA; Mogri, MZ; Schneider, MB and Deisseroth, K. An optical neural interface: in vivo control of rodent motor cortex with integrated fiberoptic and optogenetic technology. *Journal Neural Engineering* 2007, 4, S143-156.

Artem'ev, VV; Goldobin, AS and Gus'kov, LN. Recording of light emission from a nerve. *Biophysics* 1967, 12, 1111-1113.

Banaclocha, MAM. Are neuronal activity-associated magnetic fields the physical base for memory? *Medical Hypotheses* 2002, 59, 555-559.

Banaclocha, MAM. Architectural organization of neuronal activity-associated magnetic fields: a hypothesis for memory. *Medical Hypotheses* 2004, 63, 481-484.

Banaclocha, MAM. Magnetic storage of information in the human cerebral cortex: a hypothesis for memory. *International Journal Neuroscience* 2005, 115, 329-347.

Banaclocha, MAM. Neuromagnetic dialogue between neuronal minicolumns and astroglial network: a new approach for memory and cerebral computation. *Brain Research Bulletin* 2007, 73, 21-27.

Banaclocha, MAM and Banaclocha, H. Spontaneous neocortical activity and cognitive functions: a neuron-astroglial bio-magnetic and self-organized process. *Neuroquantology* 2010, 8, 191-199.

Banaclocha, M.A.M., Bókkon, I., Banaclocha, H., 2010. Long-term memory in brain magnetite. *Med. Hypotheses* 74, 254-257.

Banaclocha, MAM and Banaclocha, H. Magnetite nano-particles in information processing: from the bacteria to the human brain neocortex. In: *Magnetite: Structure, Properties and Applications*. Ed: Angrove, DM. Nova Science Publishers 2011, ISBN: 978-1-61761-839-0.

Banghart, M; Borges, K; Isacoff, E; Trauner, D and Kramer, RH. Light-activated ion channels for remote control of neuronal firing. *Nature Neuroscience* 2004, 7, 1381-1386.

Benninger, RK; Hao, M and Piston, DW. Multi-photon excitation imaging of dynamic processes in living cells and tissues. *Review Physiology Biochemistry Pharmacology* 2008, 160, 71-92.

Bezzi, P and Volterra, A. A neuron-glia signalling network in the active brain. *Current Opinion Neurobiology* 2001, 11, 387-394.

Bi, A; Cui, J; Ma, Y-P; Olshevskaya, E; Pu, M; Dizhoor, AM and Pan, Z-H. Ectopic expression of a microbial-type rhodopsin restores visual responses in mice with photoreceptor degeneration. *Neuron* 2006, 50, 23-33.

Bischof, M. Biophotons- The light in our cells. *Journal Optometric Phototherapy* 2005, 1-5.

Boncheva, M; Andreev, SA; Mahadevan, L; Winkleman, A; Reichman, DR; Prentiss, MG; Whitesides, S and Whitesides, GM. Magnetic self-assembly of three-dimensional surfaces from planar sheets. *Proceeding National Academy Science USA* 2005, 102, 3924-3929.

Bókkon, I; Salari, V; Tuszynski, J and Antal, I. Estimation of the number of biophotons involved in the visual perception of a single object image: Biophoton intensity can be considerably higher inside cells than outside. *Journal Photochemistry Photobiology B: Biology* 2010, 100, 160-166.

Bókkon, I. Visual perception and imagery: a new hypothesis. *Biosystems* 2009, 96, 178-184.

Boyden, ES; Zhang, F; Bamberg, E; Nagel, G and Deisseroth, K. Millisecond-timescale, genetically targeted optical control of neural activity. *Nature* Neuroscience 2005, 8, 1263-1268.

Bradley, JR and Wikswo, JP. The magnetic field of a single axon: a comparison of theory and experiment. *Biophysical Journal* 1985, 48, 93-109.

Brem, F; Tiefenauer, L; Fink, A; Dobson, J and Hirt, A.M. A mixture of ferritin and magnetite nanoparticles mimics the magnetic properties of human brain tissue. *Physical Review* B 2006, 73, 22-227.

Buxhoeveden, DP and Casanova, MF. The minicolumn hypothesis in neuroscience. Brain 2002, 125, 935-951.

Callaway, EM and Yuste, R. Stimulating neurons with light. *Current Opinion Neurobiology* 2002, 12, 587-592.

Cheun, BS; Yi, SH; Baik, KY; Lim, JK; Yoo, JS; Shin, HW and Soh, KS. Biophoton emission of MDCK cell with hydrogen peroxide and 60 Hz AC magnetic field. *Journal Environmental Biology* 2007, 28, 735-740.

Cohen, D. Magnetoencephalography, evidence of magnetic fields produced by alpha-rhythm currents. *Science* 1968, 161, 784-786.

Cohen, D. Magnetoencephalography: detection of brain's electric activity with a superconducting magnetometer. *Science* 1972, 175, 664-666.

Davila, AF; Fleissner, G; Winklhofer, M and Petersen, N. A new model for a magnetoreceptor in homing pigeons based on interacting clusters of superparamagnetic magnetite. *Physical Chemical Earth* 2003, 28, 647-52.

Dedov, VN and Roufogalis, DB. Organisation of mitochondria in living sensory neurons. *FEBS Letters* 1999, 456, 171-174.

DeFelipe, J; Alonso-Nanclares, L and Arellano, JI. Microstructure of the neocortex: comparative aspects. *Journal Neurocytology* 2002, 31, 299-316.

Devaraj, B; Usa, M and Inaba, H. Biophotons: ultraweak light emission from living systems. *Current Opinion Solid State Materials Science* 1997, 2, 188-193.

Dobson, J and Grassi, P. Magnetic properties of human hippocampal tissue: evaluation of artifact and contamination sources. *Brain Research Bulletin* 1996, 39, 255-259.

Estola, K-P and Malmivuo, JA. Air-Core induction coil magnetometer design. *Journal Physics E: Scientist Instruments* 1982, 15, 1110-1113.

Fellin, T; Pascual, O; Gobbo, S; Pozzan, T; Haydon, PG and Carmignoto, G. Neuronal synchrony mediated by astrocytic glutamate through activation of extra synaptic NMDA receptors. *Neuron* 2004, 43, 729-743.

Fleissner, G; Holtkamp-Rotzler, E; Hanzlik, M; Winklhofer, M; Petersen, N. Ultrastructural analysis of a putative magnetoreceptor in the beak of homing pigeons. *Journal Comparative Neurology* 2003, 458, 350-360.

Fork, RL. Laser stimulation of nerve cells in Aplysia. *Science* 1971, 171, 907-908.

Foster, RG. Neurobiology: bright blue times. *Nature* 2005, 433, 698-699.

Gabor, D. Theory of communication. *Journal Institute Electrical Engineers* 1946, 93, 429-441.

Georgiev, D. Electric and magnetic fields inside neurons and their impact upon the cytoskeletal microtubules. *Cogprints Reports*. Cogprints 2003. [http://cogprints.org /3190/].

Gordon, GR; Iremonger, KJ; Kantevari, S; Ellis-Davies, GC; MacVicar, BA and Bains, JS. Astrocyte-mediated distributed plasticity at hypothalamic glutamate synapses. *Neuron* 2009, 64, 391-403.

Gradinaru, V; Mogri, M; Thompson, KR; Henderson, JM and Deisseroth, K. Optical deconstruction of parkinsonian neural circuitry. *Science* 2009, 324, 354-359.

Grossman, N; Poher, V; Grubb, MS; Kennedy, GT; Nikolic, K; McGovern, B; Berlinguer Palmini, R; Gong, Z; Drakakis, EM; Neil, MA; Dawson, MD; Burrone, J; Degenaar, P. Multi-site optical excitation using ChR2 and micro-LED array. *Journal Neural Engineering* 2010, 7 016004 doi: 10.1088/1741-2560/7/1/016004.

Gurwitsch, AG. Das Problem der Zellteilung, physiologisch betrachtet. *Protoplasma* 1926, 1, 473-475.

Gurwitsch, AA. A historical review of the problem of mitogenetic radiation. *Experientia* 1988, 44, 545-550.

Hameroff, SR and Penrose, R. Conscious events as orchestrated space-time selections. *Journal Conscious Studies* 1996, 3, 36-53.

Haydon, PG. Glia: listening and talking to the synapse. *Nature Neuroscience* 2001, 2, 185-193.

Helmstaedter, M; de Kock, CPJ; Feldmeyer, D; Bruno, RM and Sakmann, B. Reconstruction of an average cortical column in silico. *Brain Research Review* 2007, 55, 193-203.

Ho, MW. The Rainbow and the Worm: *The Physics of Organisms*. 2003, 2nd ed.; World Scientific, Singapore.

Horton, JC and Adams, DL. The cortical column: a structure without a function. *Philosophy Transactional Royal Society* B 2005, 360, 837-862.

Hubel, DH and Wiesel, TN. Anatomical demonstration of columns in the monkey striate cortex. *Nature* 1969, 221, 747–750.

Inaba, H; Shimizu, Y; Tsuji, Y and Yamagishi, A. Photon counting spectral analyzing system of extraweak chemi and bioluminescence for biochemical applications. *Photochemistry Photobiology* 1979, 30, 169-175.

Ingber, L. Statistical mechanics of neocortical interactions. Derivation of short-term-memory capacity. *Physical Review A* 1984, 29, 3346-3358.

Ingber, L. Statistical mechanics of neocortical interactions: nonlinear columnar electroencephalography. *Neuroquantology* 2009, 7, 500-529.

Ingber, L. Columnar magnetic vector potential of short-term memory influences on molecular processes: Smoking gun for top-down neocortical information processing. 2011a. www.ingber.com/smni11_stm_potential. pdf.

Ingber, L. Computational algorithms derived from multiple scales of neocortical processing. *Cognitive Computation* 2011b, In press.

Isojima, Y; Isoshima, T; Nagai, K; Kikuchi, K and Nakagawa, H. Ultraweak biochemiluminescence detected from rat hippocampal slices. *Neuroreport* 1995, 6, 658-660.

Kalisman, N; Silberberg, G and Markram, H. The neocortical microcircuit as a tabula rasa. *Proceeding National Academy Science USA* 2005, 102, 880-885.

Kaplan, JH; Forbush, B and Hoffman, JF. Rapid photolytic release of adenosine 5-triphosphate from a protected analogue: utilization by the Na:K pump of human red blood cell ghosts. *Biochemistry* 1978, 17, 1929-1935.

Kataoka, Y; Cui, Y; Yamagata, A; Niigaki, M; Hirohata, T; Oishi, N and Watanabe, Y. Activity-dependent neural tissue oxidation emits intrinsic ultraweak photons. *Biochemical Biophysical Research Communication* 2001, 285, 1007-1011.

Katz, B. *Nerve, Muscle and Synapse*. McGraw-Hilt, New York. 1966.

Kim, JY; Osterloh, FE; Hiramatsu, H; Dumas, RK and Liu K. Synthesis and real-time magnetic manipulation of a biaxial superparamagnetic colloid. *Journal Physics Chemistry* B 2005, 109, 11151-11157.

Kishida, KT and Klann, E. Sources and targets of reactive oxygen species in synaptic plasticity and memory. *Antioxidant Redox Signaling* 2007, 9, 233-244.

Kirschvink, JL. Magnetite biomineralization and geomagnetic sensitivity in higher animals: an update and recommendations for future study. *Bioelectromagnetics* 1989, 10, 239-259.

Kirschvink, JL and Gould, JL. Biogenic magnetite as a basis for magnetic field sensitivity in animals. *Biosystems* 1981, 13, 181-201.

Kirschvink, JL; Kobayashi-Kirschvink, A and Woodford, BJ. Magnetite biomineralization in the human brain. *Proceeding National Academy Science USA* 1992, 89, 7683-7687.

Kobayashi, M; Kikuchi, D and Okamura, H. Imaging of ultraweak spontaneous photon emission from human body displaying diurnal rhythm. *PLoS ONE* 2009, e6256. DOI:10.1371/journal.pone.0006256.

Kobayashi, M; Takeda, M; Ito, K; Kato, H and Inaba, H. Two-dimensional photon counting imaging and spatiotemporal characterization of ultra-weak photon emission from a rat's brain in vivo. *Journal Neuroscience Methods,* 1999a, 93, 163-168.

Kobayashi, M; Takeda, M; Sato,T; Yamazaki, Y; Kaneko, K; Ito, K; Kato, H and Inaba, H. In vivo imaging of spontaneous ultra-weak photon emission from a rat's brain correlated with cerebral energy metabolism and oxidative stress. *Journal Neuroscience Research* 1999b, 34, 103-113.

Liu, QS; Xu, Q; Arcuino, G; Kang, J and Nedergaard, M. Astrocyte-mediated activation of neuronal kainate receptors. *Proceeding National Academy Science USA* 2004, 101, 3172-3177.

Livingstone, MS and Hubel, DH. Specificity of intrinsic connections in primate primary visual cortex. *Journal Neuroscience* 1984, 4, 2830-2835.

Livingstone, MS; Nori, S; Freeman, DC and Hubel, DH. Stereopsis and binocularity in the squirrel monkey. *Vision Research* 1995, 35, 345-354.

Lorente De Nó, R. Cerebral cortex, architecture, intracortical connections, motor projections. In: Fulton JF, editor. *Physiology of the nervous system.* New York: Oxford University Press 1949, 288-330.

Malmivuo, J and Plonsey, R. Theory of biomagnetic measurements. In: *Bioelectromagnetism, principles and applications of bioelectric and biomagnetic fields.* Oxford University Press, New York, 1995, 325-326.

Marin-Padilla, M. Ontogenesis of the pyramidal cell of the mammalian neocortex and developmental cytoarchitectonic: a unifying theory. *Journal Comparative Neurology* 1992, 321, 223-240.

Maxwell, J. *A dynamical theory of the electromagnetic field.* Philosophy Transactional Royal Society London 1865, 155, 459-512.

Melyan, Z; Tarttelin, EE; Bellingham, J; Lucas, RJ and Hankins, MW. Addition of human melanopsin renders mammalian cells photoresponsive. *Nature* 2005, 433, 741-745.

Mountcastle, VB. Modality and topographic properties of single neurons of cat's somatic sensory cortex. *Journal Neurophysiology* 1957, 20, 408-434.

Mugniani, E. Cell junctions of astrocytes, ependyma and related cells in the mammalian central nervous system, with emphasis on the hypothesis of a generalized functional syncytium of supporting cells. In: Ferodoff, S; Vernadakis, A (eds.) Astrocytes: *Development, Morphology, and Regional Specialization of Astrocytes.* London: Academic Press, 1986, 329-371.

Nakano, M. Low-level chemiluminescence during lipid peroxidations and enzymatic reactions. *Journal Biological Chemical Luminescence* 1989, 4, 231-240.

Nedergaard, M; Ransom, B and Goldman, SA. New roles for astrocyte: redefining the functional architecture of the brain. *Trends Neuroscience* 2003, 26, 523-530.

Niggli, HJ. Artificial sunlight irradiation induces ultraweak photon emission in human skin fibroblasts. *Journal Photochemistry Photobiology* B 1993, 18, 281-285.

Nikolenko, V; Poskanzer, KE and Yuste, R. Two-photon photostimulation and imaging of neural circuits. *Nature Methods* 2007, 4, 943-950.

Nishiyama, A; Komitova, M; Suzuki, R and Zhu, X. Polydendrocytes (NG2 cells): multifunctional cells with lineage plasticity. *Nature Review Neuroscience* 2009, 10, 9-22.

Nunez, PL. *Electric fields of the brain: the neurophysics of EEG.* Oxford University Press, London, 1981.

Oberheim, NA; Takano, T; Han, X.; He, W; Lin, JH; Wang, F; Xu, Q; Wyatt, JD; Pilcher, W; Ojemann, JG; Ransom, BR; Goldman, SA and Nedergaard, M. Uniquely hominid features of adult human astrocytes. *Journal Neuroscience* 2009, 29, 3276-3287.

Osterloh, FE. Solution self-assembly of magnetic light modulators from exfoliated perovskite and magnetite nanoparticles. *Journal American Chemical Society* 2002, 124, 6248-6249.

Parpura, V., Basarsky, T.A., Liu, F., Jeftinija, K., Jeftinija, F., Haydon, P.G., 1994. Glutamate-mediated astrocyte-neuron signalling. *Nature* 369, 744–7.

Perea, G and Araque, A. Astrocytes potentiate transmitter release at single hippocampal synapses. *Science* 2007, 317, 1083-1086.

Poher, V; Grossman, N; Kennedy, GT; Nikolic, K; Zhang, HX; Gong, Z; Drakakis, EM; Gu, E; Dawson, MD; French, PMW; Degenaar, P and Neil, MAA. Micro-LED arrays: a tool for two dimensional neuron stimulation. *Journal Physics D: Applied Physics* 2008, 41, 094014 (9pp). stacks.iop. org/JPhysD/41/094014.

Polimeni, JR; Granquist-Fraser, D; Wood, RJ and Schwartz, EL. Physical limits to spatial resolution of optical recording: clarifying the spatial structure of cortical hypercolumns. *Proceeding National Academy Science USA* 2005, 102, 4158-4163.

Popp, FA. Coherent photon storage of biological systems. In: Electromagnetic bio-information. Popp, FA; Becker, G; Koenig, HL and Peschka, W (eds). *Urban and Schwarzenberg,* Munchen, 1979, 123-149.

Popp, FA; Chang, JJ; Herzog, A; Yan Z and Yan, Y. Evidence of nonclassical (squeezed) light in biological systems. *Physics Letters* A 2002, 293, 98-102.

Popp, FA; Nagl, W; Li, K; Ssholz, W; Weingartner, O and Wolf, R. Biophoton emission. New evidence for coherence and DNA as source. *Cell Biophysics* 1984, 6, 33-52.

Popp, FA and Yan, Y. Delayed luminescence of biological systems in terms of coherent states. *Physics Letters A* 2002, 293, 93-97.

Rahnama, M; Bokkon, I; Tuszynski, J; Cifra, M; Sardar, P and Salari, V. Emission of Biophotons and Neural Activity of the Brain. *Neuroscience Research* 2010, 1-18. arXiv:1012.3371 [physics.

Rakic, P. Radial versus tangential migration of neuronal clones in the developing cerebral cortex. *Proceeding National Academy Science USA* 1995, 92, 11323-11327.

Ramon y Cajal, S. *Histology of the nervous system of man and vertebrates*, 1897. Reprint (Swanson N, Swanson LW, translator). Oxford: Oxford University Press, 1995.

Reisin, HD and Colombo, JA. Considerations on the astroglial architecture and the columnar organization of the cerebral cortex. *Cellular Molecular Neurobiology* 2002, 22, 634-644.

Santello, M and Volterra, A. Astrocytes as aide-mémoires. *Nature* 2010, 463, 169-170.

Shaner, NC; Steinbach, PA and Tsien, RY. A guide to choosing fluorescent proteins. *Nature Methods* 2005, 2, 905-909.

Shcherbakov, VP and Winklhofer, M. The osmotic magnetometer: a new model for magnetite-based magnetoreceptors in animals. *European Biophysical Journal* 1999, 28, 380-392.

Shoham, S; O'Connor, DH; Sarkisov, DV and Wang, SS. Rapid neurotransmitter uncaging in spatially defined patterns. *Nature Methods* 2005, 2, 837-843.

Shu, X; Royant, A; Lin, MZ; Aguilera, TA; Lev-Ram, V; Steinbach PA and Tsien, RY. Mammalian expression of infrared fluorescent proteins engineered from a bacterial phytochrome. *Science* 2009, 324, 804-807.

Skulachev, VP. Mitochondrial filaments and clusters as intracellular power-transmitting cables. *Trends Biochemical Sciences* 2001, 26, 23-29.

Slawinski, J; Ezzahir, A; Godlewski, M; Kwiecinska, T; Rajfur, Z; Sitko D and Wierzuchowska, D. Stress-induced photon emission from perturbed organisms. *Experientia* 1992, 48, 1041-1058.

Sonnier, H and Marino, AA. Sensory transduction as a proposed model for biological detection of electromagnetic fields. *Electrobiology and Magnetobiology* 2010, 20, 153-175.

Spacek, J and Harris, KM. Three-dimensional organisation of cell adhesion junctions at synapses and dendritic spines in area CA1 of the rat hippocampus. *Journal Comparative Neurology* 1998, 393, 58-68.

Stringer, SM; Rolls, ET; Trappenberg, TP and de Araujo, IET. Self-organising continuous attractor networks and motor function. *Neural Networks* 2003, 16, 161-182.

Stringer, SM; Rolls, ET and Trappenberg, T.P. Self-organising continuous attractor networks with multiple activity packets, and the representation of space. *Neural Networks* 2004, 17, 5-27.

Sun, Y; Wang, C; andDai, J. Biophotons as neural communication signals demonstrated by in situ biophoton autography. *Photochemical Photobiological Sciences* 2010, DOI: 10.1039/b9pp00125e.

Taylor, JG. Perception by neural networks. *Neural Networks* 1997, 4, 363-395.

Taylor, JG. Neural 'bubble' dynamics in two dimensions: foundations. *Biological Cybernetics* 2000, 80, 393-409.

Taylor, JG. Bubbles in the brain? *Trends Cognitive Science* 2003, 7, 429-431.

Tilbury, RN. The effect of stress factors on the spontaneous photon emission from microorganisms. *Experientia* 1992, 48, 1030-1041.

Thar, R and Kühl, M: Propagation of electromagnetic radiation in mitochondria? *Journal Theoretical Biology* 2004, 230, 261-270.

Trigo, FF; Corrie, JE and Ogden, D. Laser photolysis of caged compounds at 405 nm: photochemical advantages, localisation, phototoxicity and methods for calibration. *Journal Neuroscience Methods* 2009, 180, 9-21.

Tuszynski, JA and Dixon, JM. Quantitative analysis of the frequency spectrum of the radiation emitted by cytochrome oxidase enzymes. *Physical Review* E 2001, 64 051915.

Van Hooser, SD. Similarity and diversity in visual cortex: is there a unifying theory of cortical computation? *Neuroscientist* 2007, 13, 639-656.

Van Wijk, EP; Ackerman, J and Van Wijk, R. Effect of meditation on hand and forehead ultraweak photon emission. *Forsch Komplementärmed Klass Naturheilkd* 2005, 12, 107-112.

Van Wijk, R; Bosman, S; Ackerman, J and Van Wijk, EP. Correlation between fluctuations in human ultra-weak photon emission and EEG alpha rhythm. *Neuroquantology* 2008, 6, 452-463.

Van Wijk, R. Bio-photons and bio-communication. *Journal Scientific Exploration* 2001, 15, 183-197.

Volterra, A; Trotti, D; Tromba, C; Floridi, S and Racagni, G. Glutamate uptake inhibition by oxygen free radicals in rat cortical astrocytes. *Journal Neuroscience* 1994, 14, 2924-2932

Wang, X and Liang, L. Effects of static magnetic fields on magnetosome formation and expression of mama, mms13, mms6 and magA in Magnetospirillum magneticum AMB-1. *Bioelectromagnetics* 2009, 30, 313-321.

Wang, Ch; Bókkon, I; Dai, J and Antal, I. Spontaneous and visible light-induced ultraweak photon emission from rat eyes. *Brain Research* 2010 DOI: 10.1016 /j.brainres.2010.10.077.

Wikswo, JP; Barach, JP and Freeman, JA. Magnetic field of a nerve impulse: first measurements. *Science* 1980, 208, 53-55.

Wininger, FA; Schei, JL and Rector, MD. Complete optical neurophysiology: toward optical stimulation and recording of neural tissue. *Applied Optics* 2009, 48, D218-D224.

Wyart, C; Del Bene, F; Warp, E; Scott, EK; Trauner, D; Baier, H and Isacoff, EY. Optogenetic dissection of a behavioural module in the vertebrate spinal cord. *Nature* 2009, 461, 407-410.

Yoon, YZ; Kim, J; Lee, BC; Kim, YU; Lee, SK and Soh, KS. Changes in ultraweak photon emission and heart rate variability of epinephrine-injected rats. *Genetic Physiology Biophysics* 2005, 24, 147-159.

Zahid, M; Vélez-Fort, M; Papagiakoumou, E; Ventalon, C; Angulo, MC and Emiliani, V. Holographic photolysis for multiple cell stimulation in mouse hippocampal slices. *PLoS ONE* 2010, 5, e9431. doi:10.1371/journal.pone. 0009431.

Zhang, F; Wang, LP; Brauner, M; Liewald, JF; Kay, K; Watzke, N; Wood, PG; Bamberg, E; Nagel, G; Gottschalk, A and Deisseroth, K. Multimodal fast optical interrogation of neural circuitry. *Nature* 2007, 446, 633-639.

Zhang, HX; Gu, E; Jeon, CW; Gong, Z; Dawson, MD; Neil, MAA and French, PMW. Microstripe-array jn GaN light-emitting diodes with individually addressable elements. *IEEE Photonics Technology Letters* 2006, 18, 1681-1683.

Zhang, F; Wang, LP; Boyden, ES and Deisseroth, K. Channel rhodopsin-2 and optical control of excitable cells. *Nature Methods* 2006, 3, 785-792.

In: Short-Term Memory: New Research
Editors: Garifallia Kalivas and Sappho F. Petralia
ISBN: 978-1-62100-860-6

Chapter 5

VISUAL SHORT-TERM MEMORY AND THE BILATERAL FIELD ADVANTAGE

Jean-Francois Delvenne
Institute of Psychological Sciences, University of Leeds, UK

ABSTRACT

Past research has demonstrated superior visual processing when the information is distributed across the left and right visual fields rather than within the same single hemifield. This effect is known as the *bilateral field advantage* (BFA). Recent studies have recently begun to investigate whether a BFA also arises in visual short-term memory (VSTM), with a direct effect on its storage capacity. In other words, the question is whether it is possible to remember more visual objects when they are distributed between the two hemifields than when they are all located within a single one.

The goal of this chapter is to provide a synthesis of the current data regarding the possible existence of a BFA in VSTM. Those data reveal that a BFA can be found in spatial short-term memory, namely when the task requires holding spatial information. However, no BFA has been found in object short-term memory (i.e., when the task is to hold detailed visual properties of the objects), unless attentional selective processes are dominantly engaged in the task, suggesting that the BFA is a general feature of selective attention.

1. INTRODUCTION

In everyday life, the transfer of sensory input to the visual system is often interrupted by events such as eye blinks and saccades, or by full or partial occlusions from irrelevant information. To maintain and integrate relevant visual information across those interruptions, and to draw on this information to guide behaviours, we need a temporary buffer known as *visual short-term memory* (VSTM) (Philips, 1974), or *visual working memory* (Baddeley and Hitch, 1974). VSTM is vital for nearly all cognitive activities. For example, when driving a car, we must incessantly look at our surroundings and remember relevant information, such as the location of the other vehicles on the road to avoid collisions, or the traffic signs to guide driving behaviours. When reading comic strips, we must look at and remember one drawing at a time while we read the short text that relates to it. In any social contacts, such as team sports, conversations, or simply walking in town with our mates for instance, we must encode and remember the identities and the whereabouts of the people around us to properly interact.

Intuitively, we may assume that we can encode and remember a large proportion of information that is presented in our visual field. However, the last decades of research have shown that only a small amount of information can actually reach visual awareness and be stored in VSTM at any one time. Probably the first compelling demonstration of this limitation was provided by Luck and Vogel (1997). In their seminal study, Luck and Vogel used the change detection paradigm (Philips, 1974) in which participants were required to detect a change between two successive visual displays. More specifically, participants were first briefly presented with a memory array containing a number of "objects" (e.g., simple coloured squares or oriented bars). The memory array was then followed by a brief blank screen and finally by the test array. In half of the trials, the objects in the test array were similar as the ones in the memory array, whereas in the other half of the trials, one object was different. Luck and Vogel observed that in average change detection performance was near perfect on array sizes containing up to four objects but dropped dramatically and systematically with larger set sizes. For the last 15 years, those findings have been repeatedly replicated and it is now fairly established that the capacity of VSTM is around 3-4 objects (e.g., Cowan, 2001; Sperling, 1960, Pashler, 1990; Vogel, Woodman, and Luck, 2001; see also the review by Brady, Konkle, and Alvarez, 2011).

The discovery of this capacity limit is not only a laboratory curio. The severe limitation of our VSTM capacity can also be observed in, and has an impact on, our everyday life. For instance, research has shown that gross changes between two seemingly similar visual scenes can often be undetected, a phenomenon known as "change blindness" (e.g., Rensink, O'Regan, and Clark, 1997; Simons and Levin, 1997, 1998). Because the detection of a change requires a comparison of the visual input to a previous representation of the information held in memory, the limitation of VSTM capacity is thought to be at least to a certain extent accountable for this phenomenon. Furthermore, the failure to store in memory more than just a few objects at one time may also explain many human errors that occur in a variety of situations where a large amount of visual information needs to be processed simultaneously. For instance, the capacity limit has been suggested to be linked with road crash risk (e.g., Langham, Hole, Edwards, and O'Neill, 2002).

Since the publication of Luck and Vogel (1997)'s paper, the majority of the research on VSTM has tried to identify the factors that may influence its capacity. Indeed, determining the factors that may improve our processing capacities, such as our mnemonic capacities, has become crucial if one wish to cope effectively with the information-rich environment in which we all live nowadays. Among those factors, there is object complexity (i.e., VSTM capacity decreases as function of object complexity - Alvarez and Cavanagh, 2004), the nature of the features (i.e., VSTM capacity increases when the to-be-remembered features belong to distinct dimensions, such as colour, shape, orientation, texture, etc., as compared to when they belong to the same dimension – Wheeler and Treisman, 2002; Xu, 2002a, Delvenne and Bruyer, 2004), the perceptual integration (i.e., VSTM capacity increases when the to-be-remembered features are bound into a smaller number of objects as compared to when the features are all separated– Delvenne and Bruyer, 2004; Luck and Vogel, 1997, Olson and Jiang, 2002; Vogel, Woodman, and Luck, 2001; Wheeler and Treisman, 2002), the spatial arrangement of object parts (i.e., VSTM capacity increases when the features belong to the same object parts as compared to different parts - Delvenne and Bruyer, 2004; Xu, 2002b), the configural organisation of the objects within the display (i.e., the encoding of the spatial relationships between the objects benefits VSTM capacity – Delvenne, Braithwaite, Riddoch and Humphreys, 2002; Delvenne and Bruyer, 2006, Jiang, Olson, and Chun, 2000), the third dimension (i.e., VSTM capacity increases when objects are placed in a 3-D space as compared to a 2D space– Xu and Nakayama, 2007), and perceptual expertise (i.e., VSTM capacity increases as function of visual expertise – Curby, Glazek, and Gauthier, 2009; Jackson and Raymond, 2008).

In our visual world, objects can be located at the centre of our visual field, namely within the small region of space that we fix at a particular moment. However, in most cases other objects will also be presented elsewhere within our visual field, specifically to the left or right sides of fixation. Because of the crossing of the neural projections from the retina to the striate cortex, visual information that occurs in one half of the visual field is predominantly processed and represented in the contralateral cerebral hemisphere (see Bullier, 2004; Eviatar and Zaidel, 1994; Manson and Kandel, 1991). Only visual stimuli along the vertical meridian are projected to both hemispheres (Chiang, Walsh, and Lavidor, 2004; Lavidor and Walsh, 2004). As we will see in Section 2, one major effect of this contralateral organization of the visual system is that it allows us to process more effectively the visual inputs when the information is distributed across the left and right hemifields, thus projected to two hemispheres, as compared to when the same information is presented within one hemifield only, therefore projected to a single hemisphere. This phenomenon is known as the *Bilateral Field Advantage* (BFA).

In the VSTM domain, very little is known about how the contralateral organisation of the visual system may influence its storage capacity. In particular, it is not clear whether VSTM capacity is fixed regardless of whether the to-be-remembered objects share the same or different hemifields or whether VSTM capacity may be modulated by the spatial distribution of the objects across the two half visual fields. If the latter were true, it would grant us with a better appreciation of what determines VSTM capacity. It may also help us find ways to improve VSTM capacity, and thus behavioural performance that relies on it in real environments.

The goal of this chapter is to provide a synthesis of the current data regarding the possible existence of a BFA in VSTM. I will first review the evidence showing the BFA in visual information processing (section 2). Then, I will review the recent studies that have directly investigated the possible existence of a BFA in VSTM (section 3).

2. Bilateral Field Advantage in Visual Information Processing

The bilateral field advantage (BFA) in visual information processing refers to the fact that visual tasks are processed more quickly and/or more accurately when the visual inputs are distributed across the vertical meridian than when they are all presented within the same single hemifield[1]. Because of the contralateral organisation of the visual system, the general interpretation of this phenomenon is that the two cerebral hemispheres possess some degree of processing resources independence.

Probably one of the first demonstrations of a BFA was provided 40 years ago by Dimond and Beaumont (1971). The authors used the divided visual field technique in which participants had to report pairs of digits that were briefly presented for 250ms either within the same hemifield or across the two hemifields. The authors observed that a significant higher number of pairs of digits were correctly reported when the stimuli were displayed to both hemifields as compared to only one hemifield. Dimond and Beaumont later confirmed the performance improvement in visual processing capacity for bilateral presentations in a task that employed non-verbal information (Dimond and Beaumont, 1972). In this study, the authors found faster reaction times when participants had to match two complex visuo-spatial figures that occurred in separate hemifields as compared to within the same single hemifield. The two studies of Dimond and Beaumont mentioned here constitute a good illustration of the two main categories of visual tasks that have been used over the years to demonstrate the BFA. Specifically, some tasks have been designed to investigate whether independent processing capacities exist in the left and right hemispheres (section 2.1.). Other tasks have been used to investigate the efficiency of inter-hemispheric interaction (2.2.).

2.1. Bilateral Field Advantage as an Index of Hemispheric Independence

In some studies, the BFA suggests the existence of some degree of independence in visual processing capacity in the left and right hemispheres. Those studies use visual tasks that simply require processing each stimulus independently, in parallel, without the need of processing the information about their relationship to one another. For example, they may be designed to investigate whether a larger number of stimuli can be processed in bilateral arrays as compared to unilateral arrays. The digits report task used by Dimond and Beaumont (1971), in which two stimuli are briefly presented to a single hemifield or one each to a different hemifield, falls into that category. Typically, results reveal the best performance when each stimulus is presented to a different hemifield (i.e., the BFA). The effect has been observed in several studies and holds true whether the task involves identifying digits or letters (Awh and Pashler, 2000; Chakravarthi and Cavanagh, 2006; Scalf, Banich, Kramer, Narechania, and Simon, 2007), detecting simple targets (Castiello and Umilta, 1992; Reardon, Kelly, and Matthews, 2009), searching for a target amongst distracters (Alvarez and Cavanagh, 2006), detecting and discriminating orientations (Chakravarthi and Cavanagh, 2006; Reardon et al., 2009), or even encoding and remembering spatial information (Delvenne, 2005; Umemoto, Drew, Ester, and Awh, 2010 – see section 3).

Probably the most compelling demonstration of a BFA in this category of visual tasks was provided by Alvarez and Cavanagh (2005). Alvarez and Cavanagh used a Multiple Object Tracking task (Pylyshyn and Storm, 1988), in which participants were required to attentionally track a number of moving targets presented amongst moving distracters. When

[1] In some studies, the term *bilateral field advantage* has also been used to refer to a distinct phenomenon whereby presenting similar stimuli to both visual fields produces better performance than presenting a single stimulus to either hemifield alone (Baird and Burton, 2008; Miniussi, Girelli, and Marzi, 1998). A phenomenon also called *bilateral redundancy gain*.

all the targets were presented within the same hemifield, participants could accurately track two targets, but performance dramatically decreased when four targets had to be tracked. By contrast, participants could track four targets as well as two targets if they were distributed in separate hemifields. This shows that in some tasks it is even possible to process twice more objects when they are split between the two half fields, a result rendering possible only if one assume some kinds of hemispheric independence in visual processing.

This notion of hemispheric independence is strengthen by studies of split-brain patients (Gazzaniga and Young, 1967; Holtzman and Gazzaniga, 1985; Luck, Hillyard, Mangun, and Gazzaniga, 1989, 1994). Split-brain patients have their corpus callosum seriously damaged or sectioned after a surgical operation usually undertaken at the last resort for the control of intractable epilepsy. As a result, the two cerebral hemispheres in those patients are unable to exchange visual information and the stimuli presented in one visual field are exclusively processed by the contralateral hemisphere (see Eviatar and Zaidel, 1994). Studies have shown that split-brain patients can either perform better than normal healthy subjects if the visual inputs are distributed between the left and right visual fields (Luck et al., 1989), or exhibit a BFA in their performance while control subjects do not (Luck et al., 1994). For example, using a visual search task, Luck and colleagues (1994) discovered that split-brain patients can scan bilateral stimulus arrays at a much faster rate (twice as fast in some cases) than unilateral arrays. This BFA observed with split-brain patients, however, was not found in normal control subjects, suggesting that the hemispheric independence in processing capacities can sometimes be erased when the two hemispheres are able to exchange information via the corpus callosum. However, as we will see in section 2.2., the unavoidable cost in inter-hemispheric interaction is often too small to erase entirely the benefit of parallel processing by the two hemispheres.

2.2. Bilateral Field Advantage as an Index of Inter-Hemispheric Interaction

In everyday life, most visual tasks entail the information from one hemifield to be integrated or compared with the information from the other hemifield. For example, when we enumerate a set of objects placed in our visual field, objects from our left and right hemifields need to be combined in order to obtain a single quantity. This means that at higher levels, the two hemispheres need to exchange information via the corpus callosum (see Bullier, 2004), and this is inevitably accompanied with some costs in processing times or efficiency. In some studies, the BFA particularly refers to the fact that the initial benefits of parallel processing by the two hemispheres outweigh the cost of inter-hemispheric interaction. Those studies use visual tasks that not only involve processing each stimulus individually, but require also the integration or comparison of information presented within or across hemifields. The complex figures matching task used by Dimond and Beaumont (1972), for example, in which two stimuli presented either unilaterally or bilaterally had to be compared, falls into this category. The matching task, as a way to reveal a BFA, has been extensively used in the literature (Banich and Belger, 1990; Belger and Banich, 1992, 1998; Berger, 1988; Brown, Jeeves, Dietrich, and Burnison, 1999; Collin, McMullen, and Seguin, 2009; Compton, 2002; Davis and Schmit, 1971; Koivisto, 2000; Kraft, Muller, Hagendorf, Schira, Dick, Fendrich, and Brandt, 2005; Kraft, Pape, Hagendorf, Schmidt, Naito, and Brandt, 2007; Liederman, Merola, and Martinez, 1985; Ludwig, Jeeves, Norman, and DeWitt, 1993; Muller, Malinowski,

Gruber, and Hillyard, 2003; Norman, Jeeves, Milne, and Ludwig, 1992; Reuter-Lorenz, Stanczak, and Miller, 1999; Sereno and Kosslyn, 1991; Weissman and Banich, 2000; Weissman, Banich, and Puente, 2000; Zhang and Feng, 1999). Other studies have also observed the same phenomenon using different types of tasks that also require integration of information presented at different locations within the visual field, therefore involving, in the case of bilateral presentations, inter-hemispheric interaction. For example, Hatta and Tuji (1993) used a task in which participants were required to add numbers. In the same vein, with my colleagues (Delvenne, Castronovo, Demeyere, and Humphreys, 2011a), we have recently found a BFA in a visual enumeration task in which participants were required to enumerate simple dots that appeared briefly on the computer screen.

The BFA appears to be contingent on the complexity or difficulty of the task. Many studies have revealed that the BFA increases, or simply becomes apparent, as the difficulty of the task increases (Banich and Belger, 1990; Belger and Banich, 1992, 1998; Delvenne et al., 2011a; Merola and Liederman, 1990; Norman et al., 1992; Reuter-Lorenz et al., 1999; Weissman and Banich, 2000; Weisman et al., 2000; Zhang and Feng, 1999). For example, in our visual enumeration task, the BFA was only observed when more than four dots had to be enumerated (Delvenne et al., 2011a). Moreover, when the task is relatively simple and does not require many processing resources, a *unilateral field advantage* can sometimes occur (Banich and Belger, 1990; Butcher and Cavanagh, 2008; Hayes, Swallow, and Jiang, 2010; Weisman et al., 2000). For instance, using a letter-matching task, Banich and Belger (1990) observed that when the two letters to be-matched were perceptually identical (e.g., A and A), performance was better for unilateral than bilateral arrays. By contrast, when the letters were perceptually dissimilar (A and a), or when the number of letters displayed on the screen was increased to five (Belger and Banich, 1992), the task difficulty increased and performance was better for bilateral than unilateral arrays. Consistent with these findings, neuroimaging studies have demonstrated that computationally complex tasks often produce more bilateral activities than do simpler tasks (e.g., Awh, Smith, and Jonides, 1995; Klingberg, O'Sullivan, and Roland, 1997; Pollman, Zaidel, and von Cramon, 2003).

In sum, a large body of research, especially over the last two decades, has shown that (1) the two cerebral hemispheres have, at least to some extent, their own independent resources for processing visual information; (2) the independent, parallel processing provides a gain in efficiency if the task is sufficiently demanding and if it recruits both cerebral hemispheres; (3) in most visual tasks, the benefits of this initial hemispheric independence outweigh the cost of exchanging and integrating information between the hemispheres.

3. Bilateral Field Advantage in Visual Short-Term Memory

The capacity of VSTM typically refers to the maximum number of items that can be encoded and held in memory simultaneously. However, research suggests that the capacity may not be only defined by the number of memory representations, but also by their precision or resolution. (Alvarez and Cavanagh, 2004; Xu and Chun, 2006; Zhang and Luck, 2008). The number and resolution of memory representations may even represent distinct and independent aspect of VSTM. For example, Xu and Chun (2006) found that the neural regions that are sensitive to the number of memory items (i.e., inferior intraparietal sulcus) are distinct from those that are sensitive to the complexity of the stored items (i.e., superior parietal and lateral occipital cortex). Therefore, a BFA in VSTM implies that the distribution of visual information across both hemifields increases the maximum number of items that can be encoded and held in memory simultaneously, and/or improves the resolution of their representations compared to when the items occupied the same single hemifield.

While the existence of a BFA in visual processing is pretty much well established nowadays (see section 2), the question of whether the BFA extends to memory only started to be directly addressed a couple of years ago and, as we will see, reveals conflicting findings. Yet, reasons as to why a BFA can be expected in VSTM are to be found in the close relationship between VSTM (the 'off-line' processing) and perception (the 'online' processing). A growing body of neuroimaging (Awh and Jonides, 2001; Harrison and Tong, 2009; Postle, 2006; Serences, Ester, Vogel and Awh, 2009) and single-unit studies (Miller, Erickson, and Desimone, 1996; Supèr, Spekreijse, and Lamme, 2001) suggests that the early cortical regions recruited to encode sensory information are also sustainably activated during VSTM storage. Thus, visual objects are represented in brain areas where object processing occurs. In the same vein, it has been proposed that the contralateral organization of the visual system extends in VSTM, where information presented in one hemifield is maintained by sustained activity in the contralateral visual cortex (see Gratton, 1998; Gratton, Corballis, and Jain, 1997). Much evidence comes from recent event-related potentials studies that have identified a specific contralateral electrophysiological correlate of the contents of VSTM (e.g., Delvenne, Kaddour, and Castronovo, 2011b; Eimer and Kiss, 2009; Jolicoeur, Sessa, Dell'Acqua, and Robitaille, 2006a, 2006b; Klaver, Talsma, Wijers, Heinze, and Mulder, 1999; McCollough, Machizawa and Vogel, 2007; Vogel and Machizawa, 2004; Vogel, McCollough, and Machizawa, 2005). In those studies, participants are presented with a number of visual items to both sides of fixation and are required to memorize the items of either the left or right side. A sustained posterior negative wave is observed throughout the memory retention period, which is larger over the contralateral side of the brain (with respect to the position of the memory items in the visual field) relative to the ipsilateral side. Importantly, the amplitude of this contralateral delay activity (CDA – also called SPCN, for sustained posterior contralateral negativity) increases progressively with the number of items to be remembered, reaching an asymptotic limit at around 3-4 items. The contralateral organization of visual memories raises logically the possibility that each hemisphere has its own capacity of storage.

In addition, as mentioned in section 2.1., the clearest demonstration of a BFA in visual processing was provided in an attentional tracking task (Alvarez and Cavanagh, 2005), where the overall tracking capacity (i.e., around 4 objects) was equal to the sum of two independent tracking capacities, one in each hemisphere (i.e., around 2 objects). For the last ten years, numerous behavioural and neuroimaging studies have found a functional overlap between attentional tracking and VSTM. Not only do they share the same overall capacity limit of approximately 3-4 objects (Alvarez and Cavanagh, 2005; Luck and Vogel, 1997; Oksama and Hyönä, 2004; Pashler, 1988; Pylyshyn and Storm, 1988), but they also correlate in an individual's performance (Oksama and Hyönä, 2004) and interfere each other when participants have to simultaneously attentionally track and remember objects in VSTM (Fougnie and Marois, 2006). Functional MRI studies have also identified similar brain regions (i.e., intraparietal sulcus and frontal eye fields) activated during both tracking and

VSTM tasks (Culham, Cavanagh, and Kanwisher, 2001; Todd and Marois, 2004; 2005; Xu and Chun, 2006) and event-related potentials studies have found similar waveforms (i.e., the CDA) (Drew and Vogel, 2008; Vogel and Machizawa, 2004).

3.1. Empirical Evidence

3.1.1. Evidence Supporting the Bilateral Field Advantage in Visual Short-Term Memory

In 2001, Gratton and colleagues (Gratton, Fabiani, and Corballis, 2001) briefly reported unpublished data in which they found a BFA in a VSTM task. Specifically, the authors used a recognition task where a number of patterns of randomly oriented lines were sequentially presented on a computer screen for 200 ms each and separated by an 800 ms interval. Following the memory set (that consisted of 5 stimuli), a test stimulus was presented at the centre of the screen and the task was to decide whether the stimulus belonged to the memory set. The results showed that the participants were faster at recognizing the test stimulus as being part of the memory set when the memory set stimuli were distributed across the left and right hemifields as when they were presented unilaterally.

However, to the best of my knowledge, there are currently only two published studies in humans that have provided a clear demonstration of a BFA in VSTM. The first study that directly investigated this question was the one I conducted a couple of years ago (Delvenne, 2005). I used a standard change detection task in which a number of squares were simultaneously and briefly presented for 200 ms either within the same hemifield (*unilateral condition*) or across both hemifields (*bilateral condition*). Following a short retention interval of 1000 ms, the stimuli reappeared and the participants had to detect a change in the spatial location of one of the items. The results revealed better performance when the items were spread across the two hemifields as compared to when they occupied a single hemifield (Figure 1). Note that the amplitude of the BFA also increased with the number of locations to be remembered (absent with 4 items, $p < 0.01$ with 6 items, and $p<0.005$ with 8 items), supporting the notion that the BFA emerges only when the task is sufficiently complex (Banich and Belger, 1990; Belger and Banich, 1992, 1998; Delvenne et al., 2011a; Merola and Liederman, 1990; Norman et al., 1992; Reuter-Lorenz et al., 1999; Weissman and Banich, 2000; Weisman et al., 2000; Zhang and Feng, 1999).

The second demonstration of a BFA in VSTM was recently provided by Umemoto and colleagues (2010). The authors used an orientation recall task in which teardrop stimuli or simple lines presented in various orientations were displayed unilaterally or bilaterally for 150 ms. Following a retention interval of 1000 ms, a randomly oriented test stimulus was presented and the task was to adjust its orientation with the computer mouse to match the orientation of the stimulus that occupied the same location in the memory array. The results showed fewer errors in the bilateral condition compared to the unilateral condition (Figure 2), replicated therefore the main results I observed a couple of year ago (Delvenne, 2005).

However, the study of Umemoto and colleagues also revealed two additional new findings. Firstly, they demonstrated the existence of a BFA in VSTM even when the stimuli were sequentially presented one at a time within the memory array.

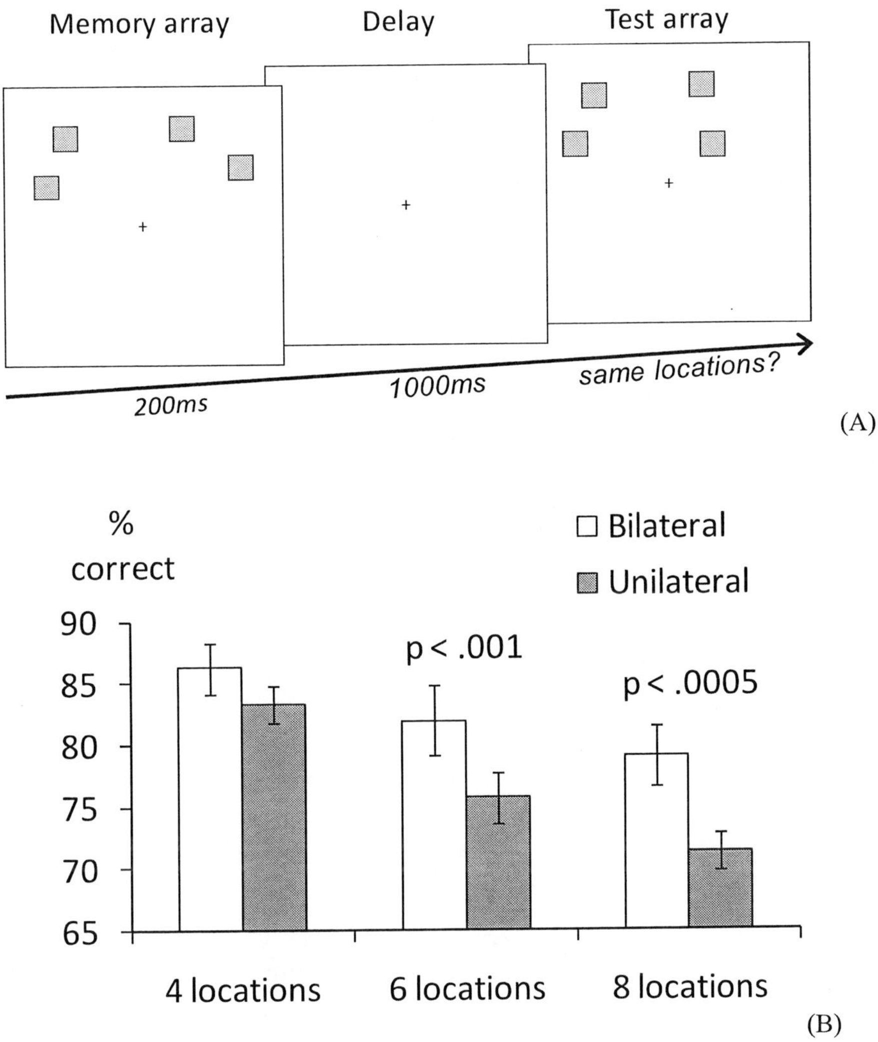

Figure 1. (A) Trial sequence (from the bilateral '4 locations' condition) used in the location VSTM study of Delvenne (2005). (B) Results of the experiment. Error bars represent standard errors of the means. (Adapted from Delvenne, 2005.).

This suggests that the BFA in VSTM cannot be, at least exclusively, explained by a difference in the encoding quality between unilaterally and bilaterally presented stimuli.

Secondly, using an analytic approach developed by Zhang and Luck (2008)[2], the authors found that the bilateral distribution of information affected the number of items that can be held in VSTM, but not their resolution.

---

[2] In order to provide independent estimates of the number and resolution of the memory representations, Zhang and Luck (2008) used a recall paradigm in which participants had to memorize several colours, and following a brief retention interval, were asked to recall the colour of a probe item by selecting it on a colour wheel. The rational is that if the colour was stored in memory, the selected colour will be near to the original colour. By contrast, if the colour was not stored in memory, the selected colour should be random. The distance between the selected colour and the original one provided some information about the resolution of the memory representations (see Zhang and Luck, 2008, for further details about this approach).

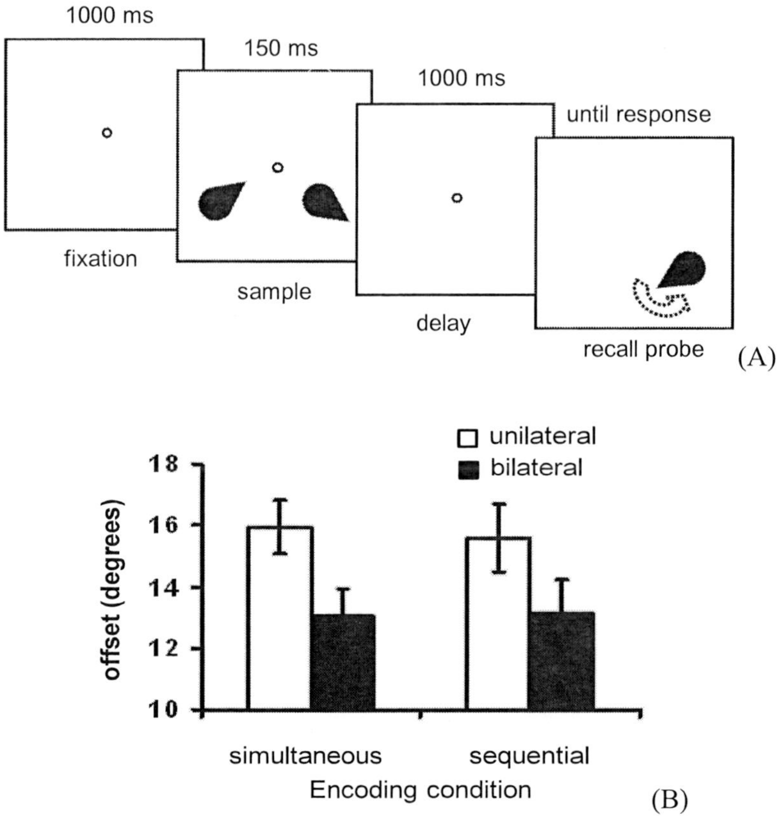

Figure 2. (A) Trial sequence and (B) results of the spatial orientation VSTM study of Umemoto et al. (2010). Error bars represent 95% confidence interval. (Adapted from Umemoto et al., 2010.).

To sum-up, current findings have revealed a BFA in VSTM when the task involves detecting a location (Delvenne, 2005) or orientation (Gratton et al., 2001; Umemoto et al., 2010) change between two successive visual displays.

3.1.2. Evidence against the Bilateral Field Advantage in Visual Short-Term Memory

There are also studies that have failed to find a BFA in VSTM as well as others that have indirectly suggested that the capacity of VSTM does not dependent on the spatial layout of information in the visual field. If the overall capacity of VSTM is the sum of independent capacities in each hemifield, VSTM capacity in one hemifield should be smaller than the overall average capacity in humans, typically estimated at around four items. However, electrophysiological studies that have used the contralateral method (McCollough et al., 2007; Vogel and Machizawa, 2004; Vogel et al., 2005), in which only items in one hemifield had to be stored in memory, have found that the amplitude of the CDA, the electrophysiological marker of VSTM capacity in one hemifield, reached an asymptotic limit at around four items. This limit is similar to the estimated overall average VSTM capacity, indirectly suggesting a similar capacity within and across hemifields.

In the study I conducted in 2005 (Delvenne, 2005), although a BFA was found when the task entailed remembering spatial locations (see previous section), no BFA was observed if the task implied remembering colour information. Specifically, I used a standard change detection task in which a number of coloured squares were briefly presented for 200 ms either within the same hemifield (unilateral condition) or split between both hemifields (bilateral condition). Following a retention interval of 1000 ms, the colours reappeared and the participants had to detect a change in the colour of one of the items. Performance was found to be similar for unilaterally and bilaterally presented stimuli, suggesting no BFA for colour VSTM (Figure 3).

These findings are supported by two recent change detection studies. Xu and Nakayama (2007) presented participants with two sets of three colours that needed to be encoded and held in memory. The two sets were presented sequentially either in the same single hemifield or one set on the left hemifield and one set on the right hemifield. Xu and Nakayama observed no difference in change detection performance between those two conditions. Likewise, Mance and colleagues (Mance, Becker, and Liu, 2011) asked participants to encode and maintain two colours that appeared either within the same hemifield or in opposite hemifields. The two colours appeared also either simultaneously or sequentially. Again, the results revealed no BFA, be it in the simultaneous or sequential mode of presentation.

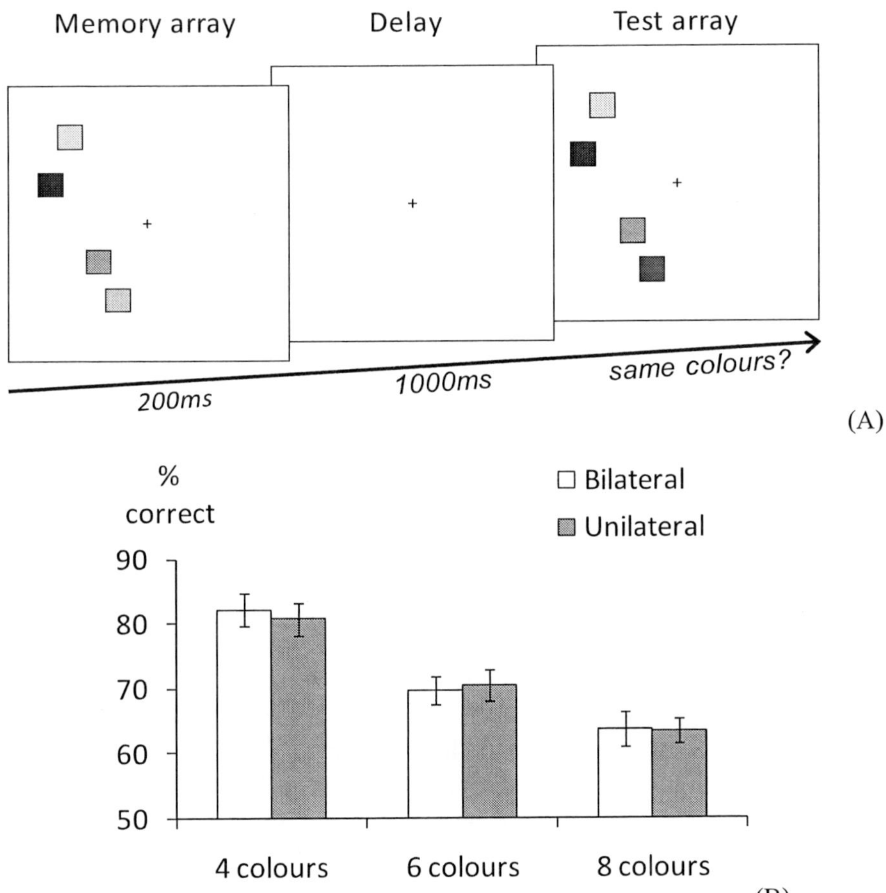

Figure 3. (A) Trial sequence (from the unilateral '4 colours' condition) used in the colour VSTM study of Delvenne (2005). The different grey levels represent different colours. (B) Results of the experiment. Error bars represent standard errors of the means. (Adapted from Delvenne, 2005.).

It may be argued that the change detection paradigm may not be totally appropriate and sensitive enough to reveal a BFA as it is not a direct measure of VSTM capacity. Since a comparison process between a visual input (i.e., the test array) and a memory representation (i.e., the memory array) is required in a change detection task, performance reflects what remains available in memory after the onset of the test array and during the comparison process. For example, it has been shown that a failure in the comparison process can occur despite the successful encoding and storage of the to-be-compared item (Mitroff, Simons, and Levin, 2004).

As a result, the change detection paradigm may lead to underestimation of the maximum number of items that can actually be held in VSTM (Awh, Barton, and Vogel, 2007; Delvenne, Cleeremans, and Laloyaux, 2010; Hollingsworth, 2003; Landman, Spekreijse, and Lamme, 2003). It is therefore possible that this paradigm obscures the effects of the bilateral presentation. This speculation falls in line with the findings from Umemoto and colleagues (2010) showing a consistent BFA for orientation information using recall procedures, namely when the test array and the comparison process stage were removed from the task, but less constant BFA for the same stimuli when using the change detection paradigm.

However, evidence suggests that the failure to find a BFA in the colour memory task (Delvenne, 2005) cannot be explained by the lack of sensibility of the change detection paradigm. Firstly, Umemoto and colleagues (2010) reported having found no BFA with colour information, even in a recall paradigm (p. 78). Secondly, we recently provided evidence for the absence of a BFA in colour VSTM in an electrophysiological study (Delvenne et al., 2011b). The great benefit of using electrophysiological measures is that it allows us to track the on-line maintenance of visual information in memory, prior the onset of the test array. Here, the dependent variable was not the change detection accuracy, but rather the amplitude of the CDA during memory maintenance. Participants were required to maintain multiple colours either from one hemifield (unilateral condition) or from both hemifields (bilateral condition). Consistent with previous research (McCollough et al., 2007; Vogel and Machizawa, 2004), the CDA amplitude increased as function of set size but ceased getting larger for arrays of four colours in the unilateral condition. In the bilateral condition, however, this contralateral activity already reached its asymptotic limit for arrays of two colours per side (i.e., four colours across both hemifields) (Figure 4). This shows that despite the contralateral nature of the CDA, this activity is modulated by the overall number of items presented in both hemifields, supporting the notion that VSTM capacity is insensitive to the spatial distribution of information across hemifields.

The absence of a BFA in VSTM is also supported, although indirectly, by the neuropsychological investigation carried out by Duncan and colleagues in patients with unilateral (right) parietal lobe lesions and showing signs of spatial neglect (Duncan, Bundesen, Olson, Humphreys, Chavda, and Shibuya, 1999). The patients were asked to report letters (one to five) that briefly appeared in the left or right visual field. If independent capacities exist in the left and right hemispheres for VSTM, one might expect performance in those patients to be impaired when the to-be-remembered items are presented to the contralateral side of the lesion (i.e., the left hemifield), but not when the items are presented to the ipsilateral side (i.e., the right hemifield). Against this hypothesis, the results revealed that VSTM capacity was equally impaired on the two sides in those patients.

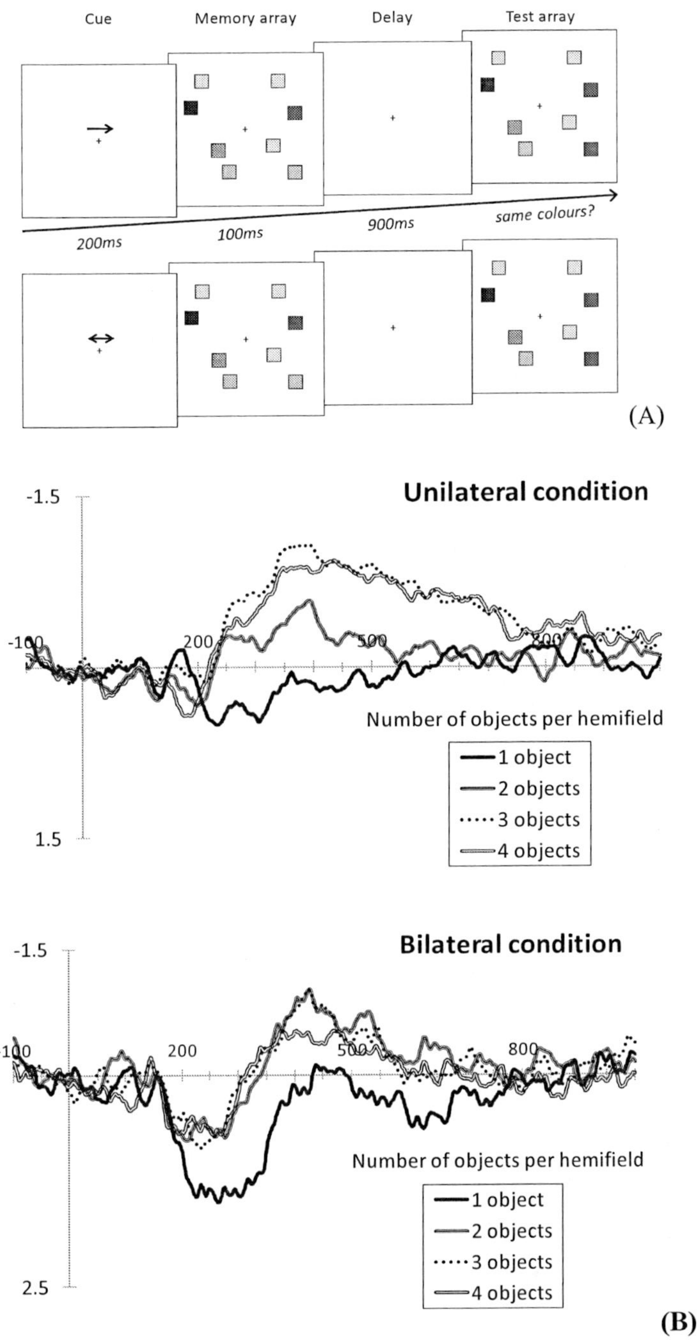

Figure 4. (A) Trial sequences (from the unilateral and bilateral '4 objects' conditions) used in the EEG study of Delvenne et al. (2011b). The different grey levels represent different colours. (B) CDAs (ipsilateral activity subtracted from contralateral activity) at posterior electrode sites for arrays of one, two, three, and four objects per hemifield obtained in the unilateral and bilateral conditions. (Adapted from Delvenne et al., 2011b.).

In summary, current evidence have revealed the absence of a BFA in VSTM when the task involves detecting a colour change between two successive visual displays (Delvenne,

2005; Delvenne et al., 2011b; Mance et al., 2011; Umemoto et al., 2011; Xu and Nakayama, 2007) or when it implies reporting previously presented letters (Duncan et al, 1999).

3.2. Review of Possible Accounts

3.2.1. Task Complexity

Why have past studies yielded inconsistent evidence for a BFA in VSTM? Although clearly further research is needed to fully understand the BFA and its effect on memory, one possibility is that the BFA is contingent on task complexity. Indeed, past research using non-mnemonic visual tasks, such as matching (Banich and Belger, 1990; Belger and Banich, 1992, 1998; Merola and Liederman, 1990; Norman et al., 1992; Reuter-Lorenz et al., 1999; Weissman and Banich, 2000; Weisman et al., 2000; Zhang and Feng, 1999) or enumerating visual items (Delvenne et al., 2011a) for instance, has shown that the BFA happens to emerge only when the task is sufficiently complex and attentionally demanding. Albeit the memory studies reviewed here seem rather alike in terms of task and procedure that they used (i.e., they mainly used the change detection paradigm), none of them were exactly similar and some tasks may have been logically more complex than others. It is therefore sensible to examine whether the inconsistency in finding a BFA in VSTM could be explain by a difference in the complexity of the tasks used in those studies.

The complexity undeniably plays an important role on the emergence of the BFA. If the task is too easy – and this applies for any sorts of task, not only memory tasks – it will be difficult to find some factors that can increase the level of already-high performance. To observe a benefit of splitting the information between both hemifields, performance should not be already at ceiling or nearly flawless when information is presented in only one hemifield. The need of a minimum of complexity can be witnessed in Delvenne (2005)'s study, for example, in which the BFA in the spatial location short-term memory task occurred only in the most complex conditions. In particular, the BFA was observed in larger set sizes (i.e., when four or six locations had to be remembered), but not in the smallest set size (i.e., when two locations had to be held in memory) (see Figure 1).

However, a closer examination of the performance across experiments and studies does not seem to suggest a direct cause-effect relationship between task complexity and the emergence of the BFA in VSTM. For example, in Delvenne (2005)'s study, the same participants performed both the spatial and colour short-term memory tasks. In average, performance was the lowest in the colour memory task, suggesting that this task was more complex than the spatial task. Nonetheless, the BFA was only observed in the spatial memory task (i.e., the less difficult task), and not in the colour memory task. Thus, although the memory task must be sufficiently complex for a BFA to emerge, complexity itself cannot explain the inconsistency of past research, nor forecast whether or not a BFA will occur.

3.2.2. Spatial/Object Short-Term Memory Dissociation

The most obvious disparity that can be found between studies that have revealed a BFA in VSTM and those that have not is the type of information that participants were required to encode and hold in memory. Studies that have found a BFA in VSTM had examined memory for spatial information, particularly spatial locations (Delvenne, 2005) and orientations

(Gratton et al., 2001; Umemoto et al., 2010). By contrast, studies that have failed to observe it had examined memory for identity information, in particular colour information (Delvenne, 2005; Delvenne et al., 2011b; Mance et al., 2011; Umemoto et al., 2011; Xu and Nakayama, 2007) and letters (Duncan et al, 1999). In view of this distinction, one possibility is that the spatial distribution of visual inputs in the left and right visual fields affects memory for spatial information, and not memory for object identity.

In vision, it is widely acknowledged that processing the location of an object requires some distinct brain regions from those involved in processing the identity of the object (Goodale and Milner, 1992; Ungerleider and Mishkin, 1982). Spatial locations is processed in the occipito-parietal regions (also known as the "dorsal stream" or "where pathway") and object identification involves the occipito-temporal regions ("ventral stream" or "what pathway"). A number of behavioural (Darling, Della Sala, and Logie, 2009; Tresch, Sinnamon, and Seamon, 1993; Woodman and Luck, 2004; Woodman, Vogel, and Luck, 2001), neuropsychological (Darling, Della Sala, Logie, and Cantagallo, 2006; Della Sala, Gray, Baddeley, Allamano, and Wilson, 1999; De Renzi and Nichelli, 1975; Hanley, Young, and Person, 1991) and neuroimaging studies (Courtney, Ungerleider, Keil, and Haxby, 1996; Courtney, Petit, Maisog, Ungerleider, and Haxby, 1998; Fuster and Jervey, 1981; McCarthy, Puce, Constable, Krystal, Gore, and Goldman-Rakic, 1996; Smith and Jonides, 1997; Ungerleider, Courtney, and Haxby, 1998; Ventre-Dominey, Bailly, Lavenne, LeBars, Mollion, Costes, and Dominey, 2005; Xu, 2009; Xu and Chun, 2006) have suggested that the division between spatial and object processing extends to short-term memory. For example, using positron emission tomography (PET), Ventre-Dominey and colleagues (2005) found that spatial short-term memory (STM) tasks activated dorsal circuits mainly in the occipito-parietal cortex and the dorsal region of the prefrontal cortex, whereas object STM tasks recruited ventral circuits in the occipito-temporal regions, the ventral area of the prefrontal cortex, and the striatum.

The idea that the bilateral field presentation of visual inputs affects memory for dorsal stream visual properties, but not memory for ventral stream visual properties, implies that the contralateral organisation of the visual system extends to the parietal cortex, but not to the temporal cortex. In support to this assumption, it has been shown that the parietal cortex, including the intra-parietal sulcus (IPS), contains a map of retinotopically-coded neurons that represent spatial locations (Kusonoki and Goldberg, 2003; Sereno, Pitzalis, and Martinez, 2001). In addition, damage to the left or right parietal lobe can result in denying awareness of information in the contralateral visual field, a syndrome known as *unilateral neglect* (Brain, 1941). Furthermore, although recent electrophysiological studies have demonstrated the existence of the contralateral organization of visual memories by revealing the CDA (McCollough et al., 2007; Vogel and Machizawa, 2004), the potential candidate source localization of this activity has been proposed to be the parietal cortex, in particular the intra-parietal sulcus (IPS). Indeed, like the CDA, the neural activity in the IPS has been found to be strongly modulated by the number of items held in memory and to reach also an asymptotic limit of approximately 4 items (Todd and Marois, 2004; Xu, 2009; Xu and Chun, 2006). The dorsal scalp topography of the CDA suggests that the contralateral organization of visual memories finds its source in the parietal cortex, mainly involved in spatial processing. By contrast, the preservation of the contralateral organisation in the temporal cortex is less clear. Some data seem to suggest that such organisation is retained in the inferior regions of the temporal cortex (Chelazzi, Miller, Duncan, and Desimone, 1993) while neuropsychological data suggest that the temporal cortex represents information from both sides. For instance, damage to either temporal lobe can result in difficulty in identifying and recognizing visual objects presented to either hemifield, a syndrome called *agnosia* (Lissauer, 1890).

If processing spatial information is, to some extent, independent in the left and right hemifields, it is plausible to suggest that the bilateral field presentation of visual information would benefit spatial processing, including spatial STM. By contrast, if processing non-spatial object information in one hemifield involves neural activity in both temporal lobes, one may assume that the bilateral field presentation of visual information would not benefit object processing, including object STM. In support to this, and as mentioned in previous sections, the clearest and strongest BFA found in a high-level visual task was demonstrated in a MOT task, in which spatial locations needed to be continually monitored (Alvarez and Cavanagh, 2005). MOT and spatial STM are closely related as they both recruit dorsal circuits. Importantly, spatial STM but not visual STM has been found to be impaired by a concurrent MOT task (Zhang, Xuan, Fu, and Pylyshyn, 2010). Together, those findings suggest that the source of the BFA in VSTM might be spatial processing.

3.2.3. Attentional Selection

Although the spatial/object processing dissociation account appears to be a good candidate to explain the BFA in VSTM, it might encounter some difficulties at explaining a number of past BFA demonstrations in visual non-mnemonic tasks. Specifically, if the BFA is a signature of spatial processing, how can this effect occur in tasks involving the identification of targets (Awh and Pashler, 2000; Chakravarthi and Cavanagh, 2006; Reardon et al., 2009; Scalf et al., 2007) or the search for a target in a visual display (Alvarez and Cavanagh, 2006)? Because those tasks are dominated by the identification process rather than by spatial processing, they should not exhibit a BFA according to the spatial/object processing dissociation account. However, a close examination of those studies reveals that the BFA emerged only when the targets had to be selected to the exclusion of distracters. In the absence of distracters, the BFA failed to emerge. For example, in Reardon and colleagues (2009)'s study, participants were required to detect peripheral Gabor targets with Gabor distracters present in half of the trials. The stimuli were either presented in one hemifield or divided across the left and right hemifield. Detection performance exhibited a BFA only when distracters were present, thus when attentional requirements were high.

If the process of attentional selection is particularly sensitive to bilateral presentations, would we then observe a BFA in an object STM task provided that the to-be-remembered objects had to be selected to the exclusion of distracters? The answer seems to be "yes". We have recently examined this idea in a colour change detection task (Holt and Delvenne, *submitted for publication*). We contrasted three conditions: in the *2 targets* and *4 targets conditions*, two and four coloured circles were presented, respectively, whereas in the *distracters condition*, two coloured circles together with two coloured crosses were displayed. The stimuli were presented either bilaterally or unilaterally, and all those conditions were randomly mixed. Participants were asked to ignore the colours of the crosses and to make their change detection judgment on the colours of the circles only. The results revealed a BFA in the *distracters condition* only, indicating a major role of attentional selection in the emergence of the BFA (Figure 5). Those findings also suggest that it might not be the nature of the to-be-remembered features (i.e., spatial/object) per se that determines whether a BFA would emerge.

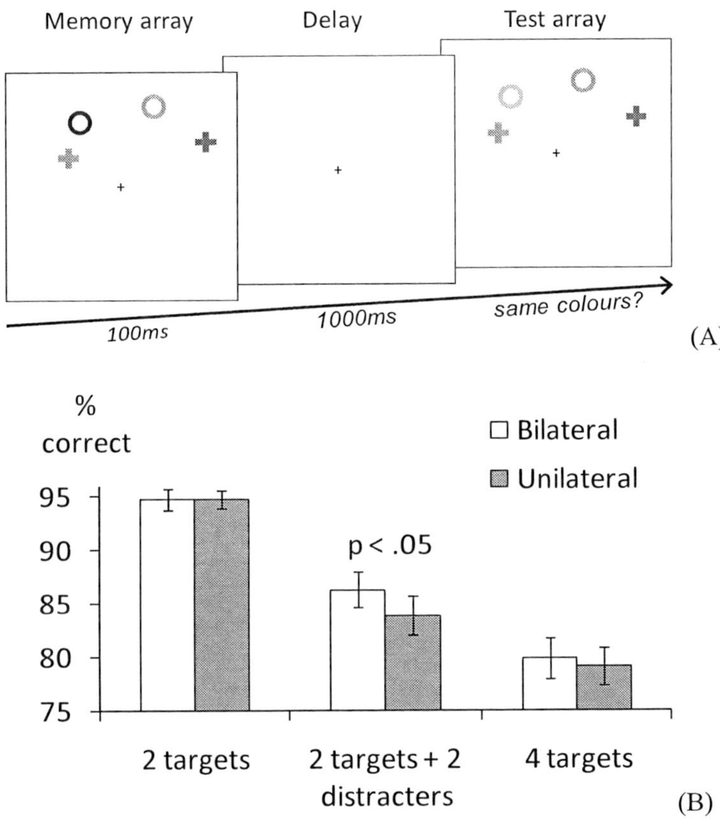

Figure 5. (A) Trial sequence (from the bilateral, distracter condition) used in the study of Holt and Delvenne (*submitted for publication*). The different grey levels represent different colours. (B) Results of the experiment. Error bars represent standard errors of the means. (Adapted from Holt and Delvenne, *submitted for publication*).

If attentional selection is the source of the BFA, why does spatial STM show a BFA even when no distracters are present in the visual display (Delvenne, 2005; Gratton et al., 2001; Umemoto et al., 2010)? Although no definitive explanation can be given at present, one possibility is that, by definition, a spatial STM task is already dominated by the attentional selection stage. This hypothesis makes sense if we assume that VSTM is a sequence of capacity-limited processes, beginning with the selection of the to-be-remembered objects through their spatial locations (i.e., object individuation – Xu and Chun, 2006) and then proceeding to higher-level operations such as the encoding of objects details (i.e., object identification – Xu and Chun, 2006), and finally the maintenance in memory (i.e., object storage). For example, using the functional Magnetic Resonance Imaging (fMRI) technique, Xu and colleagues (Xu, 2009; Xu and Chun, 2006) have recently provided clear evidence for separate neural mechanisms underlying object individuation and object identification. Specifically, Xu and colleagues found that the inferior intra-parietal sulcus (IPS) selects a fixed number of approximately four objects via their spatial locations (object individuation) and the superior IPS and the lateral occipital complex (LOC) process a subset of the objects selected and encode their detailed visual properties (object identification). Perhaps, the bilateral field presentation of visual inputs affects the object individuation process rather than the object identification process.

As Xu and Chun (2006) suggested, the selection of information by object individuation mechanisms may not only determine which objects can be held in VSTM, but also which ones can be enumerated or attentionally tracked. Evidence for a BFA in both visual enumeration (Delvenne et al., 2011a) and object tracking (Alvarez and Cavanagh, 2005) strongly supports the idea that the BFA takes its source at the object individuation stage.

Furthermore, because the objects need to be selected before they can be identified, the object individuation-identification theory suggests that object individuation precedes object identification. This asymmetry between spatial processing and object processing is also supported by Jiang and colleagues (2000), who found in a change detection study that altering the shape or colour of the items had no effects on memory for their locations, whereas changing the location of the items affected memory for their colour or shape. In that context, we may assume that spatial STM mainly involves two stages. Firstly, the objects are selected via their spatial locations (object individuation). Secondly, those locations are held in memory (object storage). Because there is no need to encode the detailed properties of the objects (object identification) in a spatial STM task, it is plausible to suggest that such a task is dominated by the object individuation stage, in which the attentional selection process plays a major role. If the BFA is a signature of attentional selection, then there is a great chance this effect will emerge in a spatial STM task, as shown in recent studies (Delvenne, 2005; Gratton et al., 2001; Umemoto et al., 2010). By contrast, an object STM task requires the additional stage of object individuation. First, the objects are selected (object individuation), then their detailed visual properties are processed and encoded (object identification), and finally those object details are maintained in memory (object storage). An object STM task may be particularly dominated by the object identification stage since this stage is subsequent to the object individuation stage. This may result in obscuring the initial BFA, as demonstrated in previous studies (Delvenne, 2005; Delvenne et al., 2011b; Mance et al., 2011; Umemoto et al., 2010; Xu and Nakayama, 2007). As shown by our recent findings (Holt and Delvenne, *submitted for publication*), a BFA can emerge in an object STM task, but only when the demand of attentional resources onto the object individuation stage is particularly high (e.g., selecting targets amongst distracters).

The process of target selection is not limited to the encoding stage but can also operate within memory representations. A large body of recent research has found that once objects are transferred into VSTM, they can still be selectively accessed by attentional mechanisms (Delvenne et al., 2010; Griffin and Nobre, 2003; Landman et al., 2003; Makovski and Jiang, 2007; Makovski, Sussman, and Jiang, 2008; Matsukura, Luck, and Vecera, 2007; Nobre, Coull, Maquet, Frith, Vandenberghe, and Mesulam, 2004). Those studies used the retro-cuing paradigm, in which an attentional spatial cue (e.g., an arrow) that pointed to the location previously occupied by an object was presented during the retention interval of the memory task. It was found that memory for the cued object was significantly better than memory for the uncued objects. Importantly, the process of selecting a subset of objects held in memory appears to also exhibit a BFA. In a retro-cuing study, we have recently observed that selecting two memory objects that were presented in separate hemifields within the memory array is more efficient than selecting two objects from within the same hemifield (Delvenne and Holt, *submitted for publication*). Such a benefit of splitting attention across the two sides of internal representations may account for the BFA observed when the items were sequentially presented within the memory array (Gratton et al., 2001; Umemoto et al., 2010). In a sequential presentation, the selection of information at the encoding stage is controlled in that all the items are selected in the same way, be it in a bilateral or unilateral condition. But because attention can still operate beyond the phase of perceptual encoding, namely on internal representations, the BFA in a sequential presentation may still reflect the better ability to split attentional selection mechanisms across both hemifields as compared to within a single one.

CONCLUSION

The study of VSTM has become a very active area of research over the past 15 years and has largely focused on its storage capacity. Albeit highly limited, the capacity of this system has been found to be modulated by a number of factors, such as object complexity (Alvarez and Cavanagh, 2004), the nature of the features (Delvenne and Bruyer, 2004) or perceptual integration (Luck and Vogel, 1997), among others. Determining what may influence the number of visual objects that can be simultaneously held in memory is crucial as it may help us to develop ways to improve VSTM capacity, and thus daily behavioural performance that depends on it (Xu and Nakayama, 2007).

This chapter was focused on a newly discovered factor, namely the spatial distribution of the to-be-remembered objects across the left and right visual fields. Despite few published reports, current data seem to suggest that the capacity of VSTM can benefit from the division of visual inputs across both hemifields, thanks to independent (or at least semi-independent) attentional resources in the left and right hemifields. A BFA can therefore be observed in VSTM when the task is dominated by the spatial selective attention stage, such as VSTM for spatial information (Delvenne, 2005; Gratton et al., 2001; Umemoto et al., 2010) or VSTM for a subset of targets that have to be selected to the exclusion of distracters (Holt and Delvenne, *submitted for publication*).

More research is needed to elucidate the source of the BFA in VSTM. Nonetheless, in view of these recent discoveries, it is clear that to further understand VSTM, it will be critical to take into account the existence of the contralateral organisation of the visual space at early stages of visual processing and the possible existence of independent attentional resources in the left and right hemifields. If determining the factors that influence VSTM capacity may be essential to understand why VTSM is limited in the first place, understanding the BFA may be critical to answering an even broader question about the human brain, specifically why it is divided into two cerebral hemispheres.

REFERENCES

Alvarez, G. A. and Cavanagh, P. (2004). The capacity of visual short-term memory is set both by visual information load and by number of objects. *Psychological Science, 15*, 106–111.

Alvarez, G. A, and Cavanagh, P. (2005). Independent resources for attentional tracking in the left and right visual hemifield. *Psychological Science, 16*, 637–643.

Alvarez, G. A. and Cavanagh, P. (2006). Hemifield independence is a signature of location-based attentional filtering. *Journal of Vision*, *6*(6), 943a.

Awh, E., Barton, B., Vogel, E. K. (2007). Visual working memory represents a fixed number of items, regardless of complexity. *Psychological Science, 18(7)*, 622-628.

Awh, E. and Jonides, J. (2001). Overlapping mechanisms of attention and working memory. *Trends in Cognitive Sciences, 5(3)*, 119-126.

Awh, E. and Pashler, H. (2000). Evidence for split attentional foci. *Journal of Experimental Psychology: Human Perception and Performance, 26*, 834–846.

Awh, E., Smith, E. E., and Jonides, J. (1995). Human rehearsal processes and the frontal lobes: PET evidence. In J. Grafman, K. Holyoak, and F. Boller (Eds.) *Structure and functions of the human prefrontal cortex Annals of the New York Academy of Sciences., vol. 769*, 97-119. New York, NY:, New York Academy of Sciences.

Baddeley, A. D. and Hitch, G. J. (1974). Working memory. In G.A. Bower (ed.), *Recent Advances in Learning and Motivation*, Vol. 8 (pp. 47–89). New York: Academic Press.

Baird, L. M. and Burton, A. M. (2008). The bilateral advantage for famous faces: Interhemispheric communication or competition? *Neuropsychologia, 46(5),* 1581-1587.

Banich, M. T. and Belger, A. (1990). Interhemispheric interaction: How do the hemispheres divide and conquer a task? *Cortex, 26*, 77-94.

Belger, A. and Banich, M. T. (1992). Interhemispheric interactions affected by computational complexity. *Neuropsychologia, 30*, 923-929.

Belger, A. and Banich, M. T. (1998). Costs and benefits of integrating information between the hemispheres: a computational perspective. *Neuropsychology, 12,* 380-398.

Berger, J. M. (1988). Interhemispheric cooperation and activation in integration of verbal information. *Behavioural Brain Research, 29*, 193-200.

Brady, T. F., Konkle, T., and Alvarez, G. A. (2011). A review of visual memory capacity: Beyond individual items and toward structured representations. *Journal of Vision, 11(5)*, 1-4.

Brain, R. W. (1941). Visual disorientation with special reference to lesion of the right brain hemisphere. *Brain, 64,* 244-272.

Brown, W. S., Jeeves, M. A., Dietrich, R., and Burnison, D. S. (1999). Bilateral field advantage and evoked potential interhemispheric transmission in commissurotomy and callosal agenesis. *Neuropsychologia, 37*, 1154-1180.

Bullier, J. (2004). Communications between cortical areas of the visual system. In L.M. Chalupa and J.S. Werner (Eds.), *The visual neurosciences* (pp. 522–540). Cambridge, MA: MIT Press.

Butcher, S. and Cavanagh, P. (2008). Unilateral field advantage for detecting repeated elements. *Perception and Psychophysics, 70*, 714-724.

Castiello, U., and Umilta, C. (1992). Splitting focal attention. *Journal of Experimental Psychology: Human Perception and Performance, 18(3)*, 837–848.

Chakravarthi, R. and Cavanagh, P. (2009). Bilateral field advantage in visual crowding. *Vision Research, 49*, 1638-1646.

Chelazzi, L., Miller, E. K., Duncan, J., and Desimone, R. (1993). A neural basis for visual search in inferior temporal (IT) cortex. *Nature, 363*, 345-347.

Chiang, T. C., Walsh, V., and Lavidor, M. (2004). The cortical representation of foveal stimuli: evidence from quadrantanopia and TMS-induced suppression. *Brain Research. Cognitive Brain Research, 21*, 309–316.

Collin, C. A., McMullen, P. A., and Seguin, J.-A. (2009). A significant bilateral field advantage for shapes defined by static and motion cues. *Perception, 38*, 1132-1143.

Compton, R. J. (2002). Inter-hemispheric interaction facilitates face processing. *Neuropsychologia, 40*, 2409–2419.

Courtney, S. M., Petit, L., Maisog, J. M., Ungerleider, L. G., and Haxby, J. V. (1998). An area specialized for spatial working memory in human frontal cortex. *Science, 279,* 1347–1351.

Courtney, S. M., Ungerleider, L. M., Keil, K., and Haxby, J. V. (1996). Object and spatial visual working memory activate separate neural systems in human cortex. *Cerebral Cortex, 6*, 39–49.

Cowan, N. (2001). The magical number 4 in short-term memory: A reconsideration of mental storage capacity. *Behavioral and Brain Sciences, 24*, 87-114.

Culham, J., Cavanagh, P., and Kanwisher, N. (2001). Attention Response Functions: Characterizing Brain Areas Using fMRI Activation during Parametric Variations of Attentional Load. *Neuron, 32,* 737-745.

Curby, K. M., Glazek, K., and Gauthier. I. (2009). A visual short-term memory advantage for objects of expertise. *Journal of Experimental Psychology: Human Perception and Performance, 35*, 94 - 107.

Darling, S., Della Sala, S., Logie, R.H. (2009). Dissociation between appearance and location within visuo-spatial working memory. *Quarterly Journal of Experimental Psychology, 62,* 417-425.

Darling, S., Della Sala, S., Logie, R. H., and Cantagallo, A. (2006). Neuropsychological evidence for separating components of visuo-spatial working memory. *Journal of Neurology, 253*, 176–180.

Davis, R. and Schmit, V. (1971). Timing the transfer of information between the hemispheres in man. *Acta Psychologica, 36*, 335-346.

Della Sala, S., Gray, C., Baddeley, A. D., Allamano, N., and Wilson, L. (1999). Pattern span: A tool for unwelding visuo-spatial memory. *Neuropsychologia, 37*, 1189–1199.

Delvenne, J.-F. (2005). The capacity of visual short-term memory within and between hemifields. Cognition, 96, B79–B88.

Delvenne, J.-F., Braithwaite, J. J., Riddoch, M. J., and Humphreys, G. W. (2002). Capacity limits in Visual Short-Term Memory for local orientations. *Current Psychology of Cognition, 21(6),* 681-690.

Delvenne, J.-F. and Bruyer, R. (2004). Does visual short-term memory store bound features? *Visual Cognition, 11(1)*, 1-27.

Delvenne, J.-F. and Bruyer, R. (2006). A configural effect in visual short-term memory for features from different parts of an object. *The Quarterly Journal of Experimental Psychology, 59(9)*, 1567-1580.

Delvenne, J.-F., Castronovo, J., Demeyere, N., and Humphreys, G. W. (2011a). Bilateral field advantage in visual enumeration. *PLoSONE 6(3)*: e17743.

Delvenne, J.-F., Cleeremans, A., and Laloyaux, C. (2010). Feature bindings are maintained in visual short-term memory without sustained focused attention. *Experimental Psychology, 57(2)*, 108-116.

Delvenne, J.-F. and Holt, J. L. (*submitted for publication*). Splitting attention across the two visual fields in visual short-term memory.

Delvenne, J.-F., Kaddour, L., and Castronovo, J. (2011b). An electrophysiological measure of visual short-term memory capacity within and across hemispheres. *Psychophysiology, 48*, 333-336.

De Renzi, E. and Nichelli, P. (1975). Verbal and non-verbal short-term memory impairment following hemispheric damage. *Cortex, 11*, 341-354.

Dimond, S. J. and Beaumont, J. G. (1971). Use of two cerebral hemispheres to increase brain capacity. *Nature, 232*, 270-271.

Dimond, S. J. and Beaumont, J. G. (1972). Processing in perceptual integration between and within the cerebral hemispheres. *British Journal of Psychology, 63(4)*, 509-517.

Drew, T. and Vogel, E. K. (2008). Neural measures of individual differences in selecting and tracking multiple moving objects. *Journal of Neuroscience, 28*, 4183–4191.

Duncan, J., Bundesen, C., Olson, A., Humphreys, G. W., Chavda, S., and Shibuya, H. (1999). Systematic analysis of deficits in visual attention. *Journal of Experimental Psychology: General, 128*, 450–478.

Eimer, M. and Kiss, M. (2010). An electrophysiological measure of access to representations in visual working memory. *Psychophysiology, 47*, 197-200.

Eviatar, Z. and Zaidel, E. (1994). Letter matching within and between the disconnected hemispheres. *Brain and Cognition, 25*, 128-137.

Fougnie, D. and Marois, R. (2006). Distinct capacity limits for attention and working memory: Evidence from attentive tracking and visual working memory paradigms. *Psychological Science, 17*(6), 526-534.

Fuster, J. M. and Jervey, J. P. (1981). Inferotemporal neurons distinguish and retain behaviorally relevant features of visual stimuli. *Science, 212,* 952-955.

Gazzaniga, M. S. and Young, E. D. (1967). Effects of commissurotomy on the processing of visual information. *Experimental Brain Research,* 3, 368-371.

Goodale, M. A. and Milner, A. D. (1992). Separate visual pathways for perception and action. *Trends in Neuroscience, 15*(1), 20-25.

Gratton, G. (1998). The contralateral organization of visual memory: A theoretical concept and a research tool. *Psychophysiology, 35*, 638-647.

Gratton, G., Corballis, P. M., and Jain, S. (1997). Hemispheric organization of visual memories. *Journal of Cognitive Neuroscience, 9*, 92-104.

Gratton, G., Fabiani, M., and Corballis, P. M. (2001).Working memory capacity and the hemispheric organization of the brain: A commentary to Cowan, 2001. *Behavioral and Brain Sciences, 24(1)*, 121-122.

Griffin, I. C. and Nobre, A. C. (2003). Orienting attention to locations in internal representations. *Journal of Cognitive Neuroscience, 15*, 1176-1194.

Hanley, J. R., Young, A. W., and Pearson, N. A. (1991). Impairment of the visuo-spatial sketch pad. *Quarterly Journal of Experimental Psychology: Human Experimental Psychology, 43A(1),* 101-125.

Harrison, S. A. and Tong, F. (2009). Decoding reveals the contents of visual working memory in early visual areas. *Nature, 458*, 632–635.

Hatta, T. and Tuji, S. (1993). Interhemispheric integration of number stimuli: comparison of Arabic with kanji numerals. *Cortex, 29*, 359–364.

Hayes, M. T., Swallow, K. M., and Jiang, Y. V. (2010). The unilateral field advantage in repetition detection: Effects of perceptual grouping and task demands. *Attention, Perception, and Psychophysics*, *72 (3),* 583-590.

Hollingworth, A. (2003). Failures of retrieval and comparison constrain change detection in natural scenes. *Journal of Experimental Psychology: Human Perception and Performance, 29*, 388-403.

Holt, J. L., and Delvenne, J.-F. (*Submitted for publication*). A bilateral field advantage in controlling access to visual short-term memory.

Holtzman, J. D. and Gazzaniga, M. S. (1985). Enhanced dual task performance following callosal commissurotomy in humans. *Neuropsychologia, 23*, 315-321.

Jackson, M. C. and Raymond, J. E. (2008). Familiarity enhances visual working memory for faces. *Journal of Experimental Psychology: Human Perception and Performance, 34*(3), 556-568.

Jiang, Y., Olson, I. R., and Chun, M. M. (2000). Organization of visual short-term memory. *Journal of Experimental Psychology: Learning, Memory, and Cognition*, *26*, 683-702.

Jolicoeur, P., Sessa, P., Dell�Acqua, R., and Robitaille, N. (2006a). Attentional control and capture in the attentional blink paradigm: Evidence from human electrophysiology. *European Journal of Cognitive Psychology, 18*, 560–578.

Jolicoeur, P., Sessa, P., Dell�Acqua, R., and Robitaille, N. (2006b). On the control of visual spatial attention: Evidence from human electrophysiology. *Psychological Research, 70*, 414–424.

Klingberg, T., O'Sullivan, B. T., and Roland, P. E. (1997). Bilateral activation of fronto-parietal networks by incrementing demand in a working memory task. *Cerebral Cortex, 7,* 465–471.

Klaver, P., Talsma, D., Wijers, A. A., Heinze, H. J., and Mulder, G. (1999). An event-related brain potential correlate of visual short-term memory. *Neuroreport, 10*, 2001–2005.

Koivisto, M. (2000). Interhemispheric interaction in semantic categorization of pictures. *Cognitive Brain Research, 9*, 45-51.

Kraft, A., Muller, N. G., Hagendorf, H., Schira, M. M., Dick, S., Fendrich, R. M., and Brandt, S. A. (2005). Interactions between task difficulty and hemispheric distribution of attended locations: Implications for the splitting attention debate. *Cognitive Brain Research, 24(1),* 19–32.

Kraft, A., Pape, N., Hagendorf, H., Schmidt, S., Naito, A., and Brandt, S. A. (2007). What determines sustained visual attention? The impact of distracter positions, task difficulty and visual fields compared. *Brain Research, 1133(1),* 123–135.

Kusonoki, M. and Goldberg, M. E. (2003). The time course of perisaccadic receptive field shifts in the lateral intraparietal area of the monkey. *Journal of Neurophysiololy, 89(3),* 1519-27.

Landman, R., Spekreijse, H., and Lamme, V. A. F. (2003). Large capacity of storage of integrated objects before change blindness. *Vision Research, 43*, 149-164.

Langham, M., Hole, G., Edwards, J., and O'Neill, C. (2002). An analysis of 'looked but failed to see' accidents involving parked police cars. *Ergonomics, 45*, 167–185.

Lavidor, M. and Walsh, V. (2004). The nature of foveal representation. *Nature Reviews Neuroscience*, *5*, 729–735.

Liederman, J., Merola, J. and Martinez, S. (1985). Interhemispheric Collaboration in Response to Simultaneous Bilateral Input. *Neuropsychologia, 23,* 673-683.

Lissauer, H. (1890). Ein Fall von Seelenblindheit nebst einem beitrage zur Theorie derselben. *Archiv für Psychiatrie und Nervenkrankheiten*, *21*, 22–270. English translation by Jackson, M. (1988). Lissauer on agnosia. *Cognitive Neuropsychology*, *5*, 155–192.

Luck, S. J., Hillyard, S. A., Mangun, G. R., and Gazzaniga, M. S. (1989). Independent hemispheric attentional systems mediate visual search in split-brain patients. *Nature, 342*, 543–545.

Luck, S. J., Hillyard, S. A., Mangun, G. R., and Gazzaniga, M. S. (1994). Independent attentional scanning in the separated hemispheres of split-brain patients. *Journal of Cognitive Neuroscience*, *6*, 84-91.

Luck, S. J. and Vogel, E. K. (1997). The capacity of visual working memory for features and conjunctions. *Nature, 390*, 279–281.

Ludwig, T. E., Jeeves, M. A., Norman, W. D., and DeWitt, R. (1993). The bilateral field advantage on a letter-matching task. *Cortex, 29*, 691-713.

Makovski, T. and Jiang Y. V. (2007). Distributing versus focusing attention in visual short-term memory. *Psychonomic Bulletin and Review, 14(6),* 1072-1078.

Makovski, T., Sussman, R., and Jiang, Y. V. (2008). Orienting attention in visual working memory reduces interference from memory probes. *Journal of Experimental Psychology: Learning, Memory, and Cognition, 34(2),* 369-380.

Mance, I., Becker, M. W., and Liu, T (2011, May 30). Parallel consolidation of simple features into visual short-term memory. *Journal of Experimental Psychology: Human Perception and Performance.* Advance online publication. doi: 10.1037/a0023925.

Mason, C. and Kandel, E. R. (1991). Central visual pathways. In E. R. Kandel, J. H. Schwarz, and T. M. Jessell (Eds.), *Principles of neural science* (3rd ed., pp. 420–439). Norwalk, Connecticut: Appleton and Lange.

Matsukura, M., Luck, S. J., and Vecera, S. P. (2007). Attention effects during visual short-term memory maintenance: Protection or prioritization? *Perception and Psychophysics, 69*, 1422-1434.

McCarthy, G., Puce, A., Constable, R. T., Krystal, J. H., Gore, J. C., and Goldman-Rakic, P. (1996). Activation of human prefrontal cortex during spatial and nonspatial working memory tasks measured by functional MRI. *Cerebral Cortex, 6,* 600–611.

McCollough, A. W., Machizawa, M. G., and Vogel, E. K. (2007). Electrophysiological measures of maintaining representations in visual working memory. *Cortex, 43*(1), 77-94.

Merola, J. L. and Liederman, J. (1990). The effect of task difficulty upon the extent to which performance benefits from between-hemisphere division of inputs. *International Journal of Neuroscience, 51,* 35–44.

Miller, E. K, Erickson, C. A, Desimone, R. (1996). Neural mechanisms of visual working memory in prefrontal cortex of the macaque. *Journal of Neuroscience, 16*, 5154 –5167.

Miniussi, C., Girelli, M., and Marzi, C. A. (1998). Neural site of the redundant target effect: electrophysiological evidence. *Journal of Cognitive Neuroscience, 10*, 2, 216-230.

Mitroff, S. R., Simons, D. J., and Levin, D. T. (2004). Nothing compares 2 views: Change blindness can occur despite preserved access to the changed information. *Perception and Psychophysics, 66,* 1268-1281.

Muller, M. M., Malinowski, P., Gruber, T., and Hillyard, S. A. (2003). Sustained division of the attentional spotlight. *Nature, 424*, 309–312.

Nobre, A. C., Coull, J. T., Maquet, P., Frith, C. D., Vandenberghe, R., and Mesulam, M. M. (2004). Orienting Attention to Locations in Perceptual Versus Mental Representations. *Journal of Cognitive Neuroscience, 16,* 363-373.

Norman, W. D., Jeeves, M. A., Milne, A., and Ludwig, T. E. (1992). Hemispheric interactions: The bilateral advantage and task difficulty. *Cortex* , *28* , 623-642.

Oksama, L. and Hyönä, J. (2004). Is multiple object tracking carried out automatically by an early vision mechanism independent of higher order cognition? An individual difference approach. *Visual Cognition, 11*, 631–671.

Olson, I. R. and Jiang, Y. (2002). Is visual short-term memory object based? Rejection of the "strong-object" hypothesis. *Perception and Psychophysics, 64*, 1055–1067.

Pashler, H. (1988). Familiarity and visual change detection. *Perception and Psychophysics, 44*, 369-378.

Phillips, W. A. (1974). On the distinction between sensory storage and short-term visual memory. *Perception and Psychophysics, 16*, 283-290.

Pollman, S., Zaidel, E., and von Cramon, D. Y. (2003). The neural basis of the bilateral distribution advantage. *Experimental Brain Research, 221,* 322–333.

Postle, B. R. (2006). Working memory as an emergent property of the mind and brain. *Neuroscience, 139*, 23-38.

Pylyshyn, Z. W. and Storm, R. W. (1988). Tracking multiple independent targets: evidence for a parallel tracking mechanism. *Spatial Vision, 3(3*), 1-19.

Reardon, K. M., Kelly, J. G., and Matthews, N. (2009). Bilateral Attentional Advantage on Elementary Visual Tasks. *Vision Research, 49(7)*, 692-702.

Rensink, R. A., O'Regan, J. K., and Clark, J. J. (1997). To see or not to see: The need for attention to perceive changes in scenes. *Psychological Science, 8*, 368–373.

Reuter-Lorenz, P. A., Stanczak, L., and Miller, A. (1999). Neural recruitment and cognitive aging: Two hemispheres are better than one especially as you age. *Psychological Science 10*, 494-500.

Scalf, P., Banich, M. T., Kramer, A. F., Narechania, K., and Simon, C. D. (2007). Double take: Parallel processing by the cerebral hemispheres reduces the attentional blink. *Journal of Experimental Psychology: Human Perception and Performance, 33*, 298–329.

Serences, J., Ester, E., Vogel, E. K., and Awh, E. (2009). Stimulus-specific delay activity in human primary visual cortex. *Psychological Science, 20(2)*, 207-214.

Sereno, A. B. and Kosslyn, S. M. (1991). Discrimination within and between hemifields: A new constraint on theories of attention. *Neuropsychologia, 29*, 659-675.

Sereno, M. I., Pitzalis, S., and Martinez, A. (2001). Mapping of contralateral space in retinotopic coordinates by a parietal cortical area in humans. *Science, 294,* 1350-1354.

Simons, D. J. and Levin, D. T. (1997). Change Blindness. *Trends in Cognitive Science, 1*, 261–267.

Simons, D. J. and Levin, D. T. (1998). Failure to detect changes to people in a real-world interaction. *Psychonomic Bulletin and Review, 5(4),* 644–649.

Smith, E. E. and Jonides, J. (1997). Working memory: A view from neuroimaging. *Cognitive Psychology, 33*, 5-42.

Sperling, G. (1960). The information available in brief visual presentations. *Psychological Monographs: General and Applied, 74*, 1-29.

Supèr, H., Spekreijse, H., and Lamme, V. A. F. (2001). A neural correlate of working memory in the monkey primary visual cortex. *Science, 293,* 120 –124.

Todd, J. J. and Marois, R. (2004). Capacity limit of visual short-term memory in human posterior parietal cortex. *Nature, 428*, 751-754.

Todd, J. J. and Marois, R. (2005). Posterior parietal cortex activity predicts individual differences in visual short-term memory capacity. *Cognitive, Affective, and Behavioral Neuroscience, 5*(2), 144-155.

Tresch, M. C., Sinnamon, H. M., and Seamon, J. G. (1993). Double dissociation of spatial and object visual memory: Evidence from selective interference in intact human subjects. *Neuropsychologia, 31*, 211–219.

Umemoto, A., Drew, T., Ester, E. F., and Awh, E. (2010). A Bilateral Advantage for Storage in Visual Working Memory. *Cognition, 117,* 69-79.

Ungerleider, L. G., Courtney, S. M., and Haxby, J. V. (1998). A neural system for human visual working memory. *Proceedings of the National Academy of Sciences, U.S.A., 95,* 883–890.

Ungerleider, L. G. and Mishkin, M. (1982). Two cortical visual systems. In D. J. Ingle, M. A. Goodale, and R. J. W. Mansfield (Eds.), *Analysis of visual behavior* (pp. 549–586). Cambridge, MA: MIT Press.

Ventre-Dominey, J., Bailly, A., Lavenne, F., Lebars, D., Mollion, H., Costes, N., and Dominey, P. F. (2005). Double dissociation in neural correlates of visual working memory: a PET study. *Cognitive Brain Research, 25(3)*, 747-59.

Vogel, E. K. and Machizawa, M. G. (2004). Neural activity predicts individual differences in visual working memory capacity. *Nature, 428*, 748-751.

Vogel, E. K., McCollough, A. W., and Machizawa, M. G. (2005). Neural measures reveal individual differences in controlling access to working memory. *Nature, 438*, 500-503.

Vogel, E. K., Woodman, G. F., and Luck, S. J. (2001). Storage of features, conjunctions, and objects in visual working memory. *Journal of Experimental Psychology: Human Perception and Performance*, 27, 92-114.

Weissman, D. H. and Banich, M. T. (2000). Cooperation between the cerebral hemispheres underlies the performance of complex but not simple tasks. *Neuropsychology, 14,* 41-59.

Weissman, D. H., Banich, M. T., and Puente, E. I. (2000). An unbalanced distribution of inputs across the hemispheres facilitates interhemispheric interaction. *Journal of International Neuropsychological Society, 6(3),* 313-321.

Wheeler, M. E. and Treisman, A. M. (2002). Binding in short-term visual memory. *Journal of Experimental Psychology: General*, *131*, 48-64.

Woodman, G. F. and Luck, S. J. (2004). Visual search is slowed when visuospatial working memory is occupied. *Psychonomic Bulletin and Review*, *11*, 269-274.

Woodman, G. F., Vogel, E. K., and Luck, S. J. (2001). Visual search remains efficient when visual working memory is full. *Psychological Science*, *12*, 219-224.

Xu, Y. (2002a). Limitations in object-based feature encoding in visual short-term memory. *Journal of Experimental Psychology: Human Perception and Performance, 28,* 458–468.

Xu, Y. (2002b). Integrating color and shape in visual short-term memory for objects with parts. *Perception and Psychophysics, 64*, 1260–1280.

Xu, Y. (2009). Distinctive neural mechanisms supporting visual object individuation and identification. *Journal of Cognitive Neuroscience, 21*, 511–518.

Xu, Y. and Chun, M.M. (2006). Dissociable neural mechanism supporting visual short-term memory for objects. *Nature, 440*, 91–95.

Xu, Y. and Nakayama, K. (2007). Visual short-term memory benefit for objects on different 3D surfaces. *Journal of Experimental Psychology: General, 136,* 653-662.

Zhang, H., Xuan, Y., Fu, X., and Pylyshyn, Z. W. (2010). Do objects in working memory compete with objects in perception? *Visual Cognition*, *18*(4), 617-640.

Zhang, W. and Feng, L. (1999). Interhemispheric interaction affected by identification of Chinese characters. *Brain and Cognition, 39,* 93–99.

Zhang, W. and Luck, S. J. (2008). Discrete fixed-resolution representations in visual working memory. *Nature, 452*, 233–235.

In: Short-Term Memory: New Research
Editors: Garifallia Kalivas and Sappho F. Petralia
ISBN: 978-1-62100-860-6

Chapter 6

Mechanisms of Short-term Working Memory Deficit

***N. M. Dubrovskaya*[1,*], *N. N. Nalivaeva*[1,2], *D. S. Vasilev*[1], *D. I. Bagrova*[1] and *I. A. Zhuravin*[1]**

[1]I.M. Sechenov Institute of Evolutionary Physiology and Biochemistry, Russian Academy of Sciences, St. Petersburg, Russia

[2]Institute of Molecular and Cellular Biology, Faculty of Biological Sciences, University of Leeds, Leeds, United Kingdom

Abstract

Short-term working memory provides a basis for performance of current behavioral and cognitive tasks. It is based on repeated circulation of impulses in a circuit of neurons in the cortical and subcortical structures through which the perception of this information, its analysis and storage is carried out. Disruption of short-term working memory (and in particular of its spatial form) is observed in ageing and, to a greater extent, in Alzheimer's disease patients. Prenatal stress also leads to disruption of short-term memory in later life and according to our data one of the reasons of short-term memory deficit after prenatal hypoxia lies in a decrease in the number of synaptopodin-positive labile spines and the levels of activity and expression of a metallopeptidase neprilysin (NEP) which is involved in metabolism of some neuropeptides and, in particular, in amyloid β peptide degradation. As such, we postulate that there is a link between the decrease of the amyloid-degrading enzymes activity, in particular of NEP and a reduced number of labile interneuronal contacts which might be one of the reasons of short-term working memory decline caused by early development pathology, normal ageing or neurodegenerative deceases. This decline can be compensated by up-regulation of NEP expression and activity.

* Corresponding author: Dr Nadezhda M Dubrovskaya, PhD. Senior Research Fellow, I.M. Institute of Evolutionary Physiology and Biochemistry, 44 M Thorez avenue, 194223 St. Petersburg, Russia. Tel: 007 812 5523166; FAX: 007 812 4423112. E-mail: ndub@iephb.ru

INTRODUCTION

Short-term working memory is a brief retention of conscious information which provides a basis for performance of current behavioral and cognitive tasks via storage and processing of incoming information from the sensory organs and long-term memory storage circuits. One of the important conditions for transition of information from perceptive (sensory) memory to short-term memory is "working" with this information, i.e. focusing attention on it [1]. Memory capacity, duration and reliability as well as the ability of the brain to process complex signals and form reflexes increase during evolution. These brain properties develop along with the increase in the number of brain neurones and the complexity of the brain. There is an opinion that working memory specifically underlies the qualitative differences between the cognitive capacities of humans and primates [2]. It also determines the variability of intellectual abilities between humans [3-5].

NEURONAL MECHANISMS OF SHORT-TERM MEMORY

There is an opinion that short- and long-term memory represents subsequent stages of the same process although some authors suggest their parallel processing [6, 7]. We are inclined to support the first opinion. The difference between short-term working and long-term memory lies in the processes of memory coding at the molecular level. While working memory retains the incoming information mostly by means of the electrical activity, long-term memory depends on formation of new peptide bonds and proteins [8]. Information from short-term memory not always is transferred into the long-term memory. The transition phase when short-term memory is being transformed into long-term memory requires consolidation of memory imprints and is sometimes considered as a separate entity, the intermediate memory. This phase increases the capacity of short-term memory and prolongs its duration up to minutes and hours [9, 10]. The intermediate-term memory involves conformation changes in structural proteins and enzymes as well as the changes in concentration and distribution of neuromediators (Figure 1).

The concept that repeated circulation of impulses within the circuits of neuronal cells underlies short-term memory was originally proposed by Hebb [11]. It is based on the histological evidence of existence of numerous recurrent fiber connections in the cerebral cortex [12]. The circuits can also be formed within the same neurone by returning impulses from the terminal (or lateral) branches of the same axon on the dendrites of the same neurone. As the result of the repeated impulses in neuronal circuits the latter undergo steady modifications which provide the basis of long-term memory. These circuits can involve not only excitatory but also inhibitory neurones [13]. The reverberation hypothesis of short-term memory suggests that neuronal circuits transmitting the excitatory impulses can be formed either within the cortex or between the cortex and subcortical structures containing both sensory and associative neurones [14-16]. Intracortical and thalamocortical reverberation circuits as the neurophysiological basis of short-term memory are formed by cortical pyramidal cells from the V-VI layers in the frontal and parietal areas of the neocortex. Participation of the hippocampus and the limbic system of the brain in the short-term memory underlies the ability of these brain structures to recognise the novelty of the signals and perception of the afferent information received by the awake brain [17, 18].

LTP as a Basis of Memory

Despite the differences between various hypotheses and theories about the nature of short-term memory, all of them base it on the transient reversible changes in the physico-chemical properties of cell membranes and dynamics of mediators in the synapses. Indeed, changes in the ion currents together with short-term metabolic shifts induced by various stimuli during activation of the synapses lead to alterations of the efficacy of the synaptic transmission which last for several seconds. The results of some electrophysiological studies have suggested that short-term memory is based on posttetanic potentiation caused by reverberating incoming impulses which results in an increase in the number of modifiable synapses after rhythmic stimulation of presynaptic fibers [19].

The long-term potentiation (LTP) following posttetanic potentiation underlies memory and can be divided into two phases - early (up to 4 hours) and late (more than 4 hours) phases [20, 21]. LTP duration is critically dependent on the expression of genes and protein synthesis since inhibition of these processes or physical isolation of neuronal cell bodies from the synapses result in LTP decay within 1-4 hours. Thus, LTP requires appearance in the synapses of new proteins or increased synthesis of existing proteins which testifies to structural transformation of synapses during LTP [22].

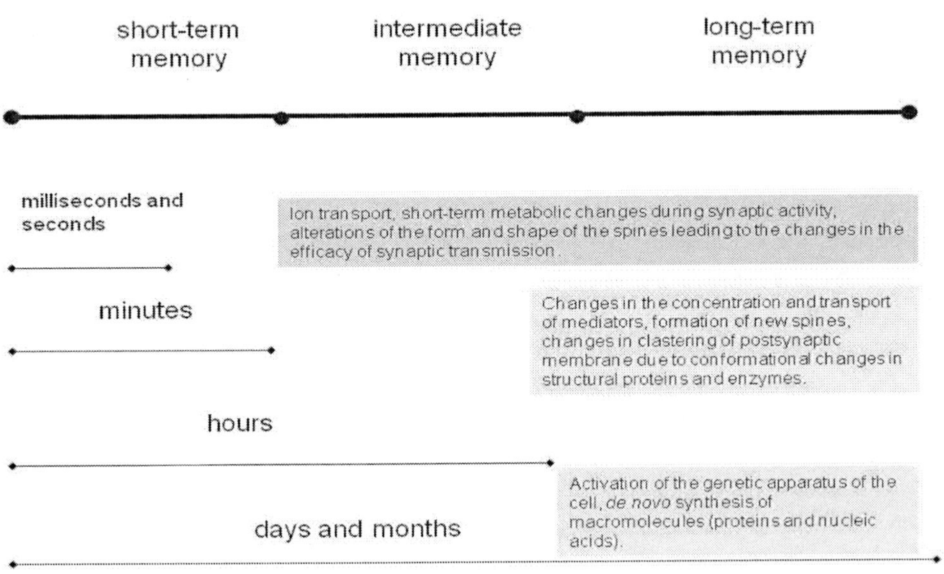

Figure 1. Duration and types of memory. Schematic representation of the molecular processes involved in memory and their duration.

During the first minutes of LTP changes in the synaptic plasticity mainly involve functional alterations of receptors for neuromediators [23] suggesting that this might be the physical substrate of short-term memory at the early stage of LTP. Numerous attempts to elucidate whether LTP involves changes in the number and/or in morphology of synapses revealed that at the early phase of LTP there are changes in the size and form of dendritic spines. They can also disappear or reappear. At the same time, alterations of such important components of the synapses as the postsynaptic density take place during LTP. However, the results of the studies on synapse morphology performed even by similar techniques are quite different [24-27]. For example it was shown that in the dentate gyrus during the first 1-2 hours of LTP there were only changes in the form of the synaptic components rather than changes in the number of synapses [25-27].

As described in the previous section, various types of memory can be classified from the point of view of the duration of the processes underlying them (Figure 1). The most persistent processes involved in memory are linked with formation of new interneuronal contacts in the reverberating circuits. Newly formed dendritic spines can rather quickly establish synaptic contacts and become active within several hours [28]. Duration of the processes involving alteration of the form and volume of the spine, modification of postsynaptic membrane, clustering of its active elements and changes in the receptor composition is determined by the process of transcription (several hours), translation (within 1-3 hours) and posttranslational modifications of proteins (minutes). The synapse itself is the place of rather fast (seconds to minutes) plastic rearrangements which affect the efficacy of signal transduction [29, 30]. It is most likely that formation of memory traces involves both fast modulation of synaptic activity and more slow processes of structural reorganisation required for prolonged storage of memory imprints [31]. However, the precise molecular mechanisms of memory and mechanisms of LTP underlying it are still far from understood.

The most studied is the NMDAR-dependent mechanism of LTP initiation [32] which is mediated by voltage-gated L-type calcium channels [33]. The cascade of reaction underlying LTP requires release of Ca^{2+} from its intracellular depot which involves the endoplasmic reticulum of the dendrite and the spine apparatus [34]. On the other hand, the most important condition for LTP initiation and maintenance is appearance in the synapses of completely new or additional amounts of the same proteins required for their structural transformation [22]. At present the processes of local protein synthesis in the dendritic spines and adjacent compartment of the dendrite is under active investigation [35, 36]. It has been suggested that in the process of long-term structural and functional changes of synapses, the cascade of reactions leading to activation of gene expression is initiated by the transcription factor CREB, since CREB-dependent activation of gene expression was observed both during direct stimulation of neurones and in learning paradigms [37, 38]. In its active form CREB initiates transcription of numerous genes including the immediate-early genes c-fos and c-jun [39]. On the other hand, CREB is involved in numerous cellular processes and signalling pathways which suggests that there should be some, still not discovered, mechanisms, directing CREB-dependent pathways towards the synthesis of structural and functional proteins specific for LTP.

Finally, there are the data on the role of NMDAR- and Ca^{2+}-independent LTP [40] demonstrating the variety of molecular mechanisms underlying LTP initiation which makes the search for a universal mechanism of memory retention and acquisition rather challenging. Moreover, all alterations at the structural and molecular levels involved in the mechanisms of memory *in vivo* are continuous and interlinked which suggests that the precise boundaries between different types of memory are rather artificial [41].

Dendritic Spines as One a Major Substrate of Neuronal Plasticity

In axon-spine synapses the spine apparatus is involved in the local process of protein synthesis, posttranslational modifications and transport of numerous synapse-associated proteins [42]. The presence of the spine apparatus with its precise organisation seems to be the main factor determining that the mushroom shaped dendritic spines with developed spine apparatus are the most labile and capable of fast changes of their form and size (Figure 2). On the contrary, thin and filopodia-like spines without the spine apparatus and small spines do not undergo structural changes [43]. The first, probably, possess the most complex system of functional regulation and are of particular importance for studying the processes of formation of temporal neuronal contacts during animal training. In the process of ontogenesis the inactive thin filopodia-like spines seem to serve as the precursors of larger functionally active spines and their transformation into active spines requires formation of the synaptic contacts [44]. Despite the importance of filopodia-like spines as the precursors of new synaptic contacts their role in the adult brain is not yet clarified [45] although it is accepted that formation of new spines and stabilization of axon-spine contacts represent the basis of memory consolidation [46]. This also supported by the fact that an enriched environment and associative learning in rodents and primates lead to an increase of dendritic spine density [47] and changes in their morphology [46]. These animals also demonstrated higher ability to learn new experimental tasks [48]. On the other hand, sensory deprivation has the opposite effects [49]. Functional properties of the spines to a great extent are determined by their morphology and internal structure. There is also a correlation between spine morphology and its functional load and the larger is a spine, the higher is the current amplitude in the cell body [50]. Changes of the size and shape of the spine appear in parallel with an increase or decrease of synaptic transmission [51]. Some authors suggest that large mushroom-like spines are responsible for long-term memory while the small ones with induction of LTP [52]. However, it is still not clear what mostly affects the strength of synaptic transmission: the shape and size of its head [43, 53] or the length and width of its neck [54]. Nevertheless, all researchers agree that there is a correlation between synaptic conductivity of the spine and its volume [50]. However, in the literature there are no data evaluating the role of labile and stable axon-spine synapses in memory or evaluating their ratio in the nervous system of naпve and trained animals at various stages of ontogenesis under normal or pathological conditions.

Dendritic spines are not only highly variable in size and shape but in various brain structures their density and location also vary to a great extent. Within the brain, the axon-spine synapses are mostly represented in the cortical areas of the brain but their characteristic features in individual cortical layers are different. This determines regional functional properties of neuronal circuits including their plasticity and adaptive potential. The highest density of the spines can be found in the hippocampus [55]. In the neocortex, spine density increases from the internal to the external cortical layers being the highest in the layers I-III. And exactly these areas of the brain are considered as principal for memory consolidation.

One of the specific proteins of the spine apparatus is synaptopodin. In particular, this actin-associated protein is regarded as a specific marker of labile spines involved in neuronal network rearrangement during the learning processes. A short form of this protein (characteristic for neurones) in the spine apparatus is linked to α-actin and participates in stabilisation of actin components of the cytoskeleton in the neck of the spine [56]. Synaptopodin is essential for organisation of the spine apparatus and remodelling of its cytoskeleton during transformations of the size and shape of the spines [57, 58]. In the hippocampus of synaptopodin knock-out mice the dendritic spines lack the spine apparatus and these animals have impaired LTP and short-term memory [57]. On the other hand, over-expression of synaptopodin does not affect the size and number of dendritic spines. Moreover, LTP itself can up-regulate expression of synaptopodin. Thus Okubo-Suzuki and colleagues [59] demonstrated that high-frequency stimulation of the dentate gyrus of the hippocampus resulted in an increased expression of the short form of synaptopodin which stabilised the early and late phases of LTP (E- and L-LTP). These findings suggests that synaptopodin is essential for maintenance of neuronal plasticity due to its role in reorganisation and redistribution of labile axon-spine inter-neuronal contacts [42] and that it plays an important role in memory consolidation since it is involved in LTP [58]. It is also reasonable to suggest that synaptopodin-positive spines with the spine apparatus are involved in learning and memory and the density of their distribution can correlate with the changes in short-term memory caused both by various pathogenic impacts and normal ageing.

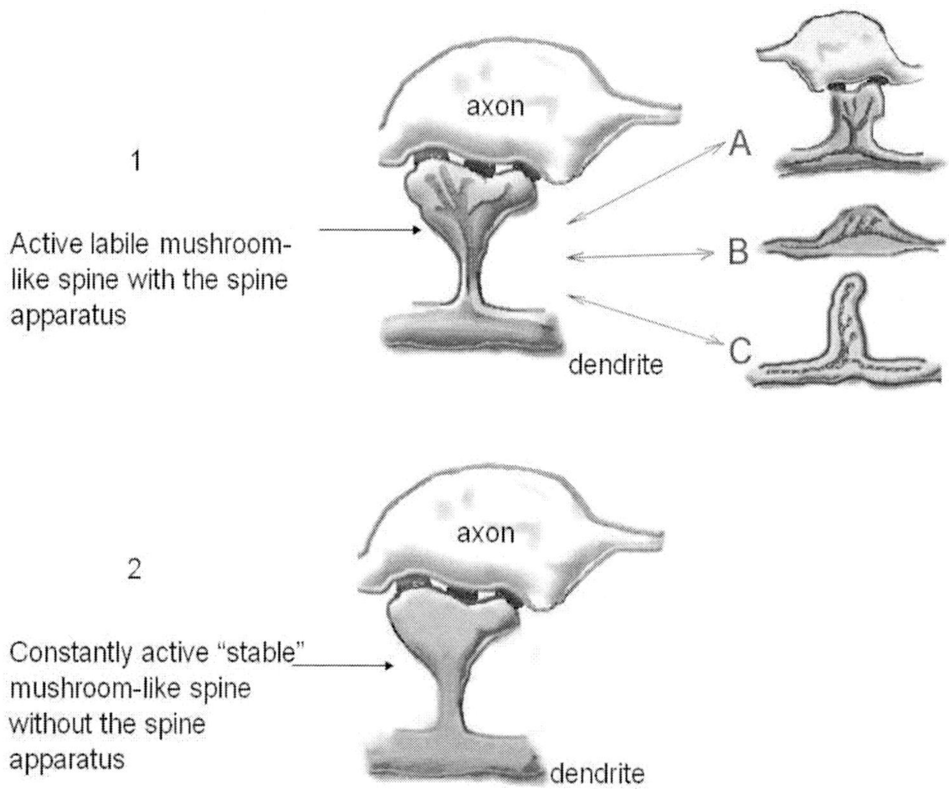

Figure 2. Schematic difference between labile and "stable" dendrite spines. The labile spines (1), unlike the stable spines (2), possess the spine apparatus and due to this are capable of fast (seconds, minutes) changes of the form and size of their head (see A, B and C) and the area of postsynaptic membrane (e.g. in A) as an additional way of regulation of synaptic transmission. The scheme represents our current model based on the data of literature discussed in the chapter.

Factors Underlying Neurodegeneration and Memory Loss

Ageing

In the process of ageing, normally functioning brain undergoes numerous changes of morphological and biochemical characteristics of its major structures which result in alteration of its functioning. For example, the density of dendritic spines decreases [60] with parallel reduction in the plasticity of the CNS and increase in vulnerability of the brain to the harmful effects of internal and external factors which underlie development of various age-related pathologies [31]. In recent years the decrease of adaptive properties of the brain and, in particular, of its synaptic plasticity and ability to establish new inter-neuronal contacts, is being considered as one of the reasons of memory deterioration and age-related dementia [31]. Ageing is also one of the main factors determining development of the sporadic form of Alzheimer's disease (AD, or senile dementia of Alzheimer's type).

At the molecular level it has been demonstrated that in the hippocampus of old rats the number of functionally active synapses, their NMDAR-dependent response and expression of several genes involved in synaptic plasticity are significantly reduced leading to impairment of LTP [61, 62]. In our studies we have found that there is also an age-related decrease in the number of labile synaptopodin-positive spines in the hippocampus and neocortex of rats [63, 64]. Age-related neuronal death and impairment of neuronal circuits in animals lead to deterioration of their short-term memory tested by various paradigms and also to declined learning abilities. These changes are also characteristic of ageing humans who first suffer from short-term memory deficit and inability to acquire new skills [65].

Neurodegenerative disorders and cognitive decline are linked with various metabolic changes in the nervous tissue. In particular, increased lipid peroxidation can lead to reorganisation of cellular membranes (their phospho- and glycolipid composition, fluidity and ion permeability) resulting in impaired calcium balance, functioning of enzymes and receptors, disruption of mirochondrial processes and energy homeostasis [66, 67].

Another important age-related process leading to various pathologies is modification of proteins, e.g. of their proteolytic processing and posttranslation modifications which result in formation of non-functional structural proteins and enzymes. For example AD is accompanied by disruption of the processes of production and clearance of amyloid β peptide (Aβ) and accumulation of hyperphosphorylated tau proteins which lead to neuronal death and cognitive decline (for review see [68]). One of the proteins undergoing age-related changes is a metallopeptidase neprilysin (NEP) which is currently considered as a major Aβ-degrading enzyme. Levels of NEP expression reduce with age in the cortex and hippocampus [69, 70] and it is also undergoes oxidative changes resulting in formation of an inactive 4-hydroxynonenal (HNE)-modified product [71]. Reduced age-related NEP expression in the cortex and hippocampus, but not in the striatum (where amyloid deposits usually are not formed), testify to its important role in amyloid clearance [69, 72]. Levels of NEP expression and activity are also reduced in AD brains [73, 74]. Expression of other amyloid-degrading enzymes, e.g. of insulin-degrading enzyme, also decreases with age, especially in the hippocampus [76].

Thus, age-related cognitive deficit can be underlined by a variety of changes in the metabolism of neuronal cells which in the long term cause their death. Some of these changes take place when neuronal cell death is still at its normal physiological rate and neurodegenerative changes are still not pronounced but neuronal plasticity of the brain is already reduced and slight changes in memory can already be revealed by behavioural tests. This early stage of neurodegenerative processes can be related to some changes in metabolism of structural proteins and enzymes, e.g. to a decrease in expression and activity of amyloid-degrading enzymes, which at a later stage will result in development of characteristic morphological and behavioural features of neurodegeneration.

As was shown in numerous studies, amyloid precursor protein (APP) metabolism undergoes significant changes in the ageing brain which results in a decreased formation of its neuroprotective soluble form sAPPα [77] and increased production of toxic forms of Aβ [78]. These changes might not only be linked with the alterations in expression of APP itself but also with the process of its intracellular modifications and transport and also with the changes in expression of the main proteolytic enzymes metabolising APP, namely α-secretase (ADAM10 and ADAM17) and β-secretase (BACE1) [79-82]. Impaired APP metabolism in ageing brain can also be linked to the changes in membrane clustering and alteration of composition of lipid rafts where APP is being mostly processed by β and γ-secretases [83-84].

Ageing is also accompanied by alteration in cerebral vasculature which reduces perivascular drainage of brain metabolites including Aβ and results in accumulation of Aβ deposits around brain vessels. Hardening of brain vessels also leads to reduced oxygen supply which is one of the main reasons for development of brain ischemia and cerebral angiopathy [85, 86].

Hypoxia

Hypoxia and ischemia are the major factors predisposing to development of various brain pathologies including memory deficit. Thus, in patients suffering from stroke the frequency of diagnosed AD and Parkinson's disease is much higher compared to other age-matched groups [87-89]. There is also a correlation between development of cognitive impairments and AD in patients with obstructive lung diseases [90]. It has been shown that hypoxia/ischemia results in metabolic changes in the brain characteristic of AD pathology [91-93]. For example, Ca^{2+} homeostasis, mitochondrial dysfunctions, production of reactive oxygen species, changes of DNA structure, accumulation of hyperphosphorylated tau and immunoreactive Aβ products were recorded in the ischemic/hypoxic brains [94-96]. Moreover, hypoxia can also increase expression and content of APP and affect various stages of its proteolytic processing, including decrease of non-amyloidogenic α-secretase [69, 97], increase of BACE activity leading to Aβ production [96, 98, 99] and reduction in amyloid-degrading enzymes [100].

Presence of a variety of amyloid-degrading enzymes in the brain capable to control concentration of Aβ inside neuronal cells, along axon and dendrites, in the synapses and in the extracellular medium suggests that there is a rather well developed defense system against accumulation of toxic concentrations of Aβ [101]. However, starting from the embryonic period and in later life the brain is exposed to various damaging factors, including hypoxia, which can disturb normal functioning of this defence system leading to the disturbance of brain metabolism and accumulation of harmful molecular species including Aβ [102, 103].

There are data demonstrating cellular response of such amyloid-degrading enzymes as NEP and endothelin-converting enzyme (ECE-1) to reduced oxygen content in the environment [99, 103]. Moreover, NEP plays an important role in functioning of the carotid body determining physiological levels of its substrate, substance P, which participates in transduction of hypoxic stimulus in this organ. As such NEP participates in modification of ventilator response to hypoxia [105-107]. On the other hand expression of ECE-1, controlling blood pressure via its substrate endothelin, was shown to be altered in the aorta of animals subjected to hypoxic episodes [108]. In the brain of rats subjected to prenatal hypoxia we also observed reduced levels of NEP and ECE-1 [69].

To conclude, accumulation of Aβ in the brain leading to AD can be either a result of an increased expression of APP and activation of β- and/or γ-secretases or a deficit of α-secretase and /or amyloid-degrading enzymes. These changes in Aβ metabolism indeed take place during normal ageing and are accelerated after hypoxia.

MECHANISMS INVOLVED IN SHORT-TERM WORKING MEMORY DEFICIT

At present it is becoming more and more evident that the oligomeric forms of Aβ are the most toxic species for neuronal cells leading to inhibition of neuronal plasticity and cell death [109]. In the brain of a transgenic mouse model of AD a decrease in expression of proteins participating in synaptic transmission, including synaptopodin, was detected in the areas with the highest Aβ content and amyloid deposits (the cortex and hippocampus) [110]. As such we hypothesized that any decrease in synaptopodin or other important pre- and postsynaptic proteins content could result in impaired neuronal plasticity and that there is a link between synaptopodin and Aβ metabolism in the affected brain areas. In our experiments with Wistar males rats we have observed a positive correlation (by Spearman Runk Order Correlation, $p < 0,05$) between the number of correct runs in a radial maze and the number of synaptopodin-positive spines in their hippocampus. There was also a positive correlation between the number of correct runs and NEP activity in the hippocampus. To further investigate possible mechanisms of short-term memory deficit we have performed a correlative analysis of rat working memory in the radial maze, in the new object recognition test, the number of synaptopodin-positive spines and NEP activity in the cortical structures of rats under various experimental paradigms (prenatal hypoxia, normal aging, administration of pharmacological compounds).

The data of this study demonstrated that prenatal hypoxia (E14, 7% O_2, 3 hours) resulted in impaired short-term memory in the radial maze and new-recognition test as well as in a decreased number of synaptopodin-positive spines in the molecular layer of the cortex and in the hippocampus [64, 111]. These changes have been accompanied by a decrease in NEP activity in the same brain areas [63, 111].

As we have found, normal ageing also resulted in impaired short-term memory tested in the two-level maze, a decreased number of synaptopodin-positive spines and reduced NEP activity in the parietal cortex and hippocampus of rats older than 12 months. To elucidate the effects of NEP activity on short-term memory, we have performed injections into rat brain cortex of various drugs capable of changing NEP expression and activity.

First, we have analysed the effect of an NEP inhibitor phosphoramidon ($2x10^{-3}$ M, via osmotic minipumps, rate 0.25 μl per hour during 28 days) into the cortex of intact adult rats. Second, we have injected rats with an anticonvulsant drug valproic acid (VA, 200 mg/kg, during 24 days, daily) which was shown to increase expression of NEP in neuronal cells [112]. VA is histone deacetylase (HDAC) inhibitor which was shown to compete with a transcription factor AICD, derived from APP cleavage by β- and γ-secretase, for binding to the *NEP* promoter causing up-regulation of the *NEP* gene expression [113]. Another class of biologically active compounds capable of increasing NEP expression and activity are antioxidants of green tea which were shown to have neuroprotective effects in various neurodegenerative disorders [114, 115]. As demonstrated previously, green tea extracts EFLA85942 and epigallocatechin gallate (EGCG) increase NEP expression and activity in human neuroblastoma cells SH-SY5Y, SK-N-SH and NB7 ([116]; our own unpublished data). Taking into account the effects of green tea compounds we have also analysed the effect of EGCG administration to rats ($2x10^{-3}$ M, via osmotic minipumps, 0.25 μl per hour, during 28 days). These experiments demonstrated that chronic (within 28 days) *i.c.* administration of phosphoramidon to adult rats resulted in impaired short-term memory tested in the radial maze. It also led to a reduction of the number of synaptopodin-positive spines in the molecular layer of the cortex. These data agree with our previous observations [111] obtained in experiments with multiple injections (6-8 times with one day interval) of the NEP inhibitors phosphoramidon and thiorphan.

With the aim to restore brain NEP activity in adult rats subjected to prenatal hypoxia, we performed two series of experiments with *i.p.* injections of VA and *i.c.* administration of EGCG to adult rats subjected to prenatal hypoxia. Usually after prenatal hypoxia NEP activity in the brain cortex was reduced by 40% while VA or EGCG administration led to a statistically significant ($p<0.05$) increase of NEP activity up to the levels recorded in control age-matched animals. In rats subjected to prenatal hypoxia and administration of VA or EGCG we have also observed an improved performance in the radial maze and improvement of short-term and long-term memory in the novel object recognition test. Animals treated with VA also had an increased number of synaptopodin-positive dendritic spines in the cortex while EGCG injections resulted in an increase of spines in the hippocampus compared to the age-matched rats subjected to prenatal hypoxia [63].

CONCLUDING REMARKS

The results of our studies summarized in the Table 1 allow us to suggest that one of the reasons of impaired brain functions after prenatal hypoxia and normal ageing is reduced neuronal plasticity of the brain which is linked with the alterations in the activity of the enzymes participating in Aβ catabolism, in particular of NEP. It is also linked with a decrease in the number of synaptopodin-positive dendritic spines resulting in deterioration of short-term working memory. However, these brain properties can be restored by administration of such pharmacologically active compounds as VA and EGCG which testifies to their therapeutic value in treatment of diseases which are accompanied by memory impairment.

Table 1. Effects of various experimental conditions on memory, number of synaptopodin-positive spines and neprilysin activity in rat

Conditions	Short-term working memory		Number of synapotopodin-positive spines		Neprilysin activity	
	Testing in a radial maze	Testing by the new object recognition test for 10 min	Parietal cortex	Hippocampus	Parietal cortex	Hippocampus
Prenatal hypoxia	Deterioration compared to control	Deterioration compared to control	Decreased compared to control	Decreased compared to control	Decreased compared to control	Decreased compared to control
Ageing	Deterioration compared to 3-4-month old rats	No statistically significant changes	Decreased compared to 3-4-month old rats	Decreased compared to 3-4-month old rats	Decreased compared to 3-4-month old rats	Decreased compared to 3-4-month old rats
Administration of phosphoramidon to adult control rats	Deterioration compared to control	No statistically significant changes	Decreased compared to control	No statistically significant changes	Decreased compared to control	Decreased compared to control
Injections of sodium valproate to adult rats, subjected to prenatal hypoxia on E14	Improvement compared to rats subjected to prenatal hypoxia	Improvement compared to rats subjected to prenatal hypoxia	Increased compared to rats subjected to prenatal hypoxia	No statistically significant changes	Increased compared to rats subjected to prenatal hypoxia	Increased compared to rats subjected to prenatal hypoxia
Injections of EGCG to adult rats subjected to prenatal hypoxia on E14	Improvement compared to rats subjected to prenatal hypoxia	Improvement compared to rats subjected to prenatal hypoxia	No statistically significant changes	Increased compared to rats subjected to prenatal hypoxia	Increased compared to rats subjected to prenatal hypoxia	Increased compared to rats subjected to prenatal hypoxia

Further investigation of neuronal network properties *in vivo* using various structural proteins as specific markers of labile inter-neuronal contacts might be of particular interest for further elucidation of the mechanisms of brain plasticity and it role in memory. Besides this, such approaches employed along with various models of developmental pathology are of importance for the analysis of the adaptive potential and compensative mechanisms of the brain.

ACKNOWLEDGMENTS

Supported by the RFBR 10-04-01156, the Medical Research Council, UK and Russian Academy of Science Programme "Fundamental Sciences to Medicine".

REFERENCES

[1] Velichkovsky, B. M.; Challis, B. H.; Pomplun, M., Working memory and work with memory: visual-spatial and further components of processing. *Z Exp Psychol* 1995, 42, (4), 672-701.
[2] Read, D.; van der Leeuw, S., Biology is only part of the story ... *Philos Trans R Soc Lond B Biol Sci* 2008, 363, (1499), 1959-68.
[3] Kyllonen, P. C.; Christal, R. E., Reasoning ability is (little more than) working-memory capacity?! *Intelligence* 1990, 14, 389-433.
[4] SuB, H. M.; Oberauer, K.; Wittmann, W. W.; Wilhelm, O.; Schulze, R., Working-memory capacity explains reasoning a bility – and a little bit more. *Intelligence* 2002, 20, 261-88.
[5] Unsworth, N.; Redick, T. S.; Spillers, G. J.; Brewer, G. A., Variation in working memory capacity and cognitive control: Goal maintenance and microadjustments of control. *Q J Exp Psychol (Colchester).* 2011 Aug 15. [Epub ahead of print]
[6] McGaugh, J., Memory – a century of consolidation. *Science* 2000, 287, 248-51.
[7] McGaugh, J. L., Time-dependent processes in memory storage. *Science* 1966, 153, (742), 1351-8.
[8] Klingberg, T., *The overflowing brain: information overload and the limits of working memory*. New York, Oxford University Press, 2009, p. 202.
[9] Hawkins, R. D.; Kandel, E.R.; Bailey, C.H., Molecular mechanisms of memory storage in Aplysia. *Biol Bull* 2006, 210, (3), 174-91.
[10] Crow, T., Xue-Bian, J. J., Proteomic analysis of short- and intermediate-term memory in Hermissenda. *Neuroscience* 2011, 192, 102-11.
[11] Hebb, D.O., The Organization of Behavior. John Wiley and Sons, New York, 1949.
[12] Lorente de No, R., Cerebral cortex*: Architecture, intracortical connections, motor projections.* In: Fulton, J. Ed., Physiology of the Nervous System. University Press, New York, 1949, 288-315.
[13] Frost, W. N.; Clark, G. A.; Kandel, E. R., Parallel processing of short-term memory for sensitization in Aplysia. *J Neurobiol* 1988, 19, (4), 297-334.

[14] Batuev, A.S., Two neuronal systems involved in short-term spatial memory in monkeys.*Acta Neurobiol Exp (Wars).* 1994, 54, (4), 335-44.

[15] Eccles, J.C., The modular operation of the cerebral neocortex considered as the material basis of mental events. *Neuroscience* 1981, 6, 1839–56.

[16] Fuster, J.M. Cortical dynamics of memory. *International Journal of Psychophysiology* 2000, 35, 155-164.

[17] Borisyuk, R.; Denham, M.; Hoppensteadt, F.; Kazanovich, Y.; Vinogradova. O., An oscillatory neural network model of sparse distributed memory and novelty detection. *Biosystems* 2000, 58, (1-3), 265-72.

[18] Vinogradova, O. S., Hippocampus as comparator: role of the two input and two output systems of the hippocampus in selection and registration of information. *Hippocampus.* 2001, 11, (5), 578-98.

[19] Sil'kis, I. G.; Rapoport, S. Sh.; Veber, N. V., Long-term posttetantic changes in the reaction of neighboring neurons in microsegments of the cat motor cortex. *Neurosci Behav Physiol* 1995, 25, (1), 15-24.

[20] Abraham, W. C., How long will long-term potentiation last? *Philos Trans R Soc Lond B Biol Sci* 2003, 358, (1432), 735-44.

[21] Lynch, M. A., Long-Term Potentiation and Memory. *Physiol Rev* 2004, 84, 87-136.

[22] Adams, J. P.; Dudek, S. M., Late-phase long-term potentiation: getting to the nucleus. *Nat Rev Neurosci* 2005, 6, (9), 737-43.

[23] Malenka, R. C., Nicoll, R. A. Long-term potentiation--a decade of progress? *Science* 1999, 285, (5435), 1870-4.

[24] Yuste, R.; Bonhoeffer, T., Morphological changes in dendritic spines associated with long-term synaptic plasticity. *Annu Rev Neurosci* 2001, 24, 1071-89.

[25] Buchs, P. A.; Muller, D., Induction of long-term potentiation is associated with major ultrastructural changes of activated synapses. *Proc Natl Acad Sci U S A* 1996, 93, (15), 8040-5.

[26] Desmond, N. L.; Levy, W. B., Changes in the numerical density of synaptic contacts with long-term potentiation in the hippocampal dentate gyrus. *J Comp Neurol* 1986, 253, (4), 466-75.

[27] Desmond, N. L.; Levy, W. B., Anatomy of Associative Long-Term Synaptic Modification. *Long-Term Potentiation: From Biophysics to Behavior*; edited by Landfield P.W. and Deadwyler S.A. Alan R. Liss Inc., 1988, 265-305.

[28] Zito, K.; Scheuss, V.; Knott, G.; Hill, T.; Svoboda, K., Rapid functional maturation of nascent dendritic spines. *Neuron* 2009, 61, (2), 247-58.

[29] Martin, K. C.; Barad, M.; Kandel, E. R., Local protein synthesis and its role in synapse-specific plasticity. *Currr Opin Neurobiol* 2000, 10, (5), 587-92.

[30] Prescott, S. A.; Chase, R., Sites of plasticity in the neural circuit mediating tentacle withdrawal in the snail Helix aspersa: implications for behavioral change and learning kinetics. *Learn Mem* 1999, 6, (4), 363-80.

[31] Arendt, T., Synaptic plasticity and cell cycle activation in neurons are alternative effector pathways: the 'Dr. Jekyll and Mr. Hyde concept' of Alzheimer's disease or the yin and yang of neuroplasticity. *Progress in Neurobiology* 2003, 71, 83-248.

[32] Fortin, D. A.; Davare, M. A.; Srivastava, T.; Brady, J.D.; Nygaard, S.; Derkach, V.A.; Soderling, T.R. Long-term potentiation-dependent spine enlargement requires synaptic

Ca2+-permeable AMPA receptors recruited by CaM-kinase I. *J Neurosci* 2010, 30, (35), 11565-75.

[33] Weisskopf, M. G.; Bauer, E. P.; LeDoux, J. E., L-type voltage-gated calcium channels mediate NMDA-independent associative long-term potentiation at thalamic input synapses to the amygdala. *J Neurosci* 1999, 19, (23), 10512-19.

[34] Jedlicka, P.; Vlachos, A.; Schwarzacher, S.W.; Deller, T., A role for the spine apparatus in LTP and spatial learning. *J. Behavioural Brain Research* 2008, 192, 12–9.

[35] Govindarajan, A.; Kelleher, R. J.; Tonegawa, S., A clustered plasticity model of long-term memory engrams. *Nat Rev Neurosci* 2006, 7, (7), 575-83.

[36] Govindarajan, A.; Israely, I.; Huang, S. Y.; Tonegawa, S., The dendritic branch is the preferred integrative unit for protein synthesis-dependent LTP. *Neuron* 2011, 69, (1), 132-46.

[37] Bozon B.; Kelly A.; Josselyn S.A.; Silva A.J.; Davis S.; Laroche S., MAPK, CREB and zif268 are all required for the consolidation of recognition memory. *Philos Trans R Soc Lond Biol Sci* 2003, 358, (1432), 805-14.

[38] Kang, H.; Sun, L.D.; Atkins, C.M.; Soderling, T.R.; Wilson, M.A.; Tonegawa, S., An important role of neural activity-dependent CaMKIV signaling in the consolidation of long-term memory. *Cell* 2001, 106, (6), 771-83.

[39] Plбtenнk, J.; Kuramoto, N.; Yoneda, Y., Molecular mechanisms associated with long-term consolidation of the NMDA signals. *Life Sci* 2000, 67, (4), 335-64.

[40] Mellor, J.; Nicoll, R. A., Hippocampal mossy fiber LTP is independent of postsynaptic calcium. *Nat Neurosci* 2001, 4, (2), 125-6.

[41] Rose, S., *The Making Of Memory: From Molecules to Mind*. Vintage, 2003; p 432.

[42] Segal, M., Dendritic spines, synaptic plasticity and neuronal survival: activity shapes dendritic spines to enhance neuronal viability. *Eur J Neurosci* 2010, 31, (12), 2178-84.

[43] Holtmaat, A.; De Paola, V.; Wilbrecht, L.; Knott, G. W., Imaging of experience-dependent structural plasticity in the mouse neocortex in vivo. *Behavioural Brain Research* 2008, 192, 20–5.

[44] Fiala, J. C; Feinberg, M.; Popov, V.; Harris, K. M., Synaptogenesis via dendritic filopodia in developing hippocampal area CA1. *J Neurosci* 1998, 18, (21), 8900-11.

[45] Arellano, J. I.; Benavides-Piccione, R.; Defelipe, J.; Yuste R., Ultrastructure of dendritic spines: correlation between synaptic and spine morphologies. *Front Neurosci* 2007, 1, 131-43

[46] Bourne, J. N., Harris, K. M., Balancing structure and function at hippocampal dendritic spines. *Annu. Rev. Neurosci* 2008, 31, 47–67.

[47] Engert, F; Bonhoeffer, T., Dendritic spine changes associated with hippocampal long-term synaptic plasticity. *Nature* 1999, 399, (6731), 66-70

[48] von Bohlen Und Halbach, O. Structure and function of dendritic spines within the hippocampus. *J. Ann. Anat* 2009, 191, 518-31.

[49] Zuo, Y.; Yang, G.; Kwon, E.; Gan, W. B., Long-term sensory deprivation prevents dendritic spine loss in primary somatosensory cortex. *Nature* 2005, 436, 261–5.

[50] Zito, K.; Scheuss, V.; Knott, G.; Hill, T.; Svoboda, K., Rapid functional maturation of nascent dendritic spines. *Neuron* 2009, 61, (2), 247-58.

[51] Zhou, Q.; Homma, K. J.; Poo, M. M., Shrinkage of dendritic spines associated with long-term depression of hippocampal synapses. *Neuron* 2004, 44, 749-75.

[52] Matsuzaki, M.; Ellis-Davies, G. C.; Nemoto, T.; Miyashita, Y.; Iino, M.; Kasai, H., Dendritic spine geometry is critical for AMPA receptor expression in hippocampal CA1 pyramidal neurons. *Nat. Neurosci* 2001, 4, 1086-92.

[53] Kasai, H.; Hayama, T.; Ishikawa, M.; Watanabe, S.; Yagishita, S.; Noguchi, J., Learning rules and persistence of dendritic spines. *Eur J Neurosci.* 2010, 32, (2), 241-9.

[54] Araya, R.; Jiang, J.; Eisenthal, K. B.; Yuste, R., The spine neck filters membrane potentials. *Proc Natl Acad Sci U S A* 2006, 103, 17961-66.

[55] Konur, S.; Rabinowitz, D.; Fenstermaker, V.; Yuste, R., Systematic regulation of spine head diameters and densities in pyramidal neurons from juvenile mice. *J. Neurobiol* 2003, 56, 95-112.

[56] Mundel P., Heid H.W., Mundel T.M., Kruger M., Reiser J., Kriz W. Synaptopodin: an actin-associated protein in telencephalic dendrites and renal podocytes. J Cell Biol 1997, 139, 193-204.

[57] Asanuma, K.; Kim, K.; Oh, J.; Giardino, L.; Chabanis, S.; Faul, C.; Reiser, J.; Mundel, P., Synaptopodin regulates the actin-bundling activity of α-actinin in an isoform-specific manner. *J Clin Invest* 2005, 115, (5), 1188-98.

[58] Deller, T.; Korte, M.; Chabanis, S.; Drakew, A.; Schwegler, H.; Stefanie, G.G.; Zuniga, A.; Schwarz, K.; Bonhoeffer, T.; Zeller, F.; Frotscher, M.; Mundel, P., Synaptopodin-deficient mice lack a spine apparatus and show deficits in synaptic plasticity. *Proc Natl Acad Sci U S A* 2003, 100, (18), 10494-99.

[59] Okubo-Suzuki, R.; Okada, D.; Sekiguchi, M.; Inokuchi, K., Synaptopodin maintains the neural activity-dependent enlargement of dendritic spines in hippocampal neurons. *J Mol Cell Neurosci.* 2008, 38, (2), 266-76.

[60] Duan, H.; Wearne, S. L.; Rocher, A.B.; Macedo, A.; Morrison, J. H.; Hof, P. R., Age-related dendritic and spine changes in corticocortically projecting neurons in macaque monkeys. *Cereb Cortex* 2003, 13, (9), 950-61.

[61] Burke, S. N.; Barnes, C. A., Neural plasticity in the ageing brain. *Nat Rev Neurosci* 2006, 7, (1), 30–40.

[62] Rosenzweig, E. S.; Barnes, C. A., Impact of aging on hippocampal function: plasticity, network dynamics, and cognition. *Prog Neurobiol* 2003, 69, (3), 143–79.

[63] Nalivaeva, N. N.; Dubrovskaya, N. M.; Vasiliev, D. S.; Tumanova, N. L.; Kochkina, E. G.; Plesneva, S. A.; Turner, A. J.; Zhuravin, I. A., Changes in the activity of amyloid-degrading enzymes might affect cognitive functions in rats via alteration of synaptopodin-positive dendritic network. *Molecular mechanisms of neurological and psychiatric disorders*. 2011, 1, 244-52.

[64] Zhuravin, I. A.; Tumanova, N. L.; Vasilyev, D. S., Changes in the mechanisms of brain adaption during postnatal ontogeny of rats exposed to prenatal hypoxia. *Doklady Biological Sciences*, 2009, 425, (1), 91-3.

[65] Britton, G. B.; Rao, K. S., Cognitive aging and early diagnosis challenges in Alzheimer's disease. *J Alzheimers Dis* 2011, 24 Suppl 2, 153-9.

[66] Hoyer, S.; Lannert, H.; Latteier, E.; Meisel, T., Relationship between cerebral energy metabolism in parietotemporal cortex and hippocampus and mental activity during aging in rats. *J Neural Transm* 2004, 111, (5), 575-89.

[67] Toescu, E. C.; Verkhratsky, A., Ca2+ and mitochondria as substrates for deficits in synaptic plasticity in normal brain ageing. *J Cell Mol Med* 2004, 8, (2), 181-90.

[68] Turner, A. J.; Fisk, L.; Nalivaeva, N. N., Targeting amyloid-degrading enzymes as therapeutic strategies in neurodegeneration. *Ann N Y Acad Sci* 2004, 1035, 1-20.

[69] Nalivaeva, N. N.; Fisk, L.; Canet Aviles, R. M.; Plesneva, S. A.; Zhuravin, I. A.; Turner, A. J., Effect of prenatal hypoxia on expression of amyloid precursor protein and metallopeptidases in the rat brain. *Lett. Peptide Sci* 2004, 10, 455-62

[70] Nalivaeva, N. N.; Belyaev, N. D.; Lewis, D I.; Pickles, A. R.; Makova, N. Z.; Bagrova D. I.; Dubrovskaya, N. M.; Plesneva, S A.; Zhuravin, I. A.; Turner, A. J., Effect of Sodium Valproate Administration on Brain Neprilysin Expression and Memory in Rats *J Mol Neurosci* 2011, Sep 20. [Epub ahead of print].

[71] Wang, D. S.; Iwata, N.; Hama, E.; Saido, T. C.; Dickson, D. W., Oxidized neprilysin in aging and Alzheimer's disease brains. *Biochem Biophys Res Commun* 2003, 310, (1), 236-41.

[72] Iwata, N.; Takaki, Y.; Fukami, S.; Tsubuki, S.; Saido T. C., Region-specific reduction of Aβ-degrading endopeptidase, neprilysin, in mouse hippocampus upon aging *Neurosci Res* 2002, 70, 493–500.

[73] Russo, R.; Borghi, R.; Markesbery, W.; Tabaton, M.; Piccini, A., Neurobiol Aging. Neprylisin decreases uniformly in Alzheimer's disease and in normal aging. *FEBS Lett* 2005, 579, (27), 6027-30.

[74] Hellstrцm-Lindahl, E.; Ravid, R.; Nordberg, A., Age-dependent decline of neprilysin in Alzheimer's disease and normal brain: inverse correlation with A beta levels. *Neurobiol Aging* 2008, 29, (2), 210-21.

[75] Iwata, N.; Takaki, Y.; Fukami, S.; Tsubuki, S.; Saido, T. C., Region-specific reduction of Aβ-degrading endopeptidase, neprilysin, in mouse hippocampus upon aging. *J Neurosci Res* 2002, 70, 493–500.

[76] Caccamo, A.; Oddo, S.; Sugarman, M. C.; Akbari, Y.; LaFerla, F. M., Age- and region-dependent alterations in Abeta-degrading enzymes: implications for Abeta-induced disorders. *Neurobiol Aging* 2005, 26, (5), 645-54.

[77] Kern, A.; Roempp, B.; Prager, K.; Walter, J.; Behl, C., Down-regulation of endogenous amyloid precursor protein processing due to cellular aging. *J Biol Chem* 2006, 281, (5), 2405-13.

[78] Cai, Y.; Xiong, K.; Zhang, X. M.; Cai, H.; Luo, X. G.; Feng, J. C.; Clough, R. W.; Struble, R. G.; Patrylo, P. R.; Chu, Y.; Kordower, J. H.; Yan, X. X., β-Secretase-1 elevation in aged monkey and Alzheimer's disease human cerebral cortex occurs around the vasculature in partnership with multisystem axon terminal pathogenesis and β-amyloid accumulation. *Eur J Neurosci* 2010, 32, (7), 1223-38.

[79] Jeong, S. J.; Kim, K.; Suh, Y.H,. Age-related changes in the expression of Alzheimer's beta APP in the brain of senescence accelerated mouse (SAM)-P/10. *Neuroreport* 1997, 8, (7), 1733-37.

[80] Schmitt, H. P., εGlycation, APP and Aβ in ageing and Alzheimer disease: a hypothesis. *Med Hypotheses* 2006, 66, (5), 898-906.

[81] Bernstein, H. G.; Stricker, R.; Lendeckel, U.; Bertram, I.; Dobrowolny, H.; Steiner, J.; Bogerts, B.; Reiser, G., Reduced neuronal co-localisation of nardilysin and the putative alpha-secretases ADAM10 and ADAM17 in Alzheimer's disease and Down syndrome brains. *Age (Dordr)* 2009, 31, (1), 11-25.

[82] Fukumoto, H.; Cheung, B. S.; Hyman, B. T.; Irizarry, M. C., β-secretase protein and activity are increased in the neocortex in Alzheimer disease. *Arch Neurol* 2002, 59, (9), 1381-9

[83] Head, B. P.; Peart, J. N.; Panneerselvam, M.; Yokoyama, T.; Pearn, M. L.; Niesman, I. R.; Bonds, J. A.; Schilling, J. M.; Miyanohara, A.; Headrick, J.; Ali, S. S.; Roth, D. M.; Patel, P. M.; Patel, H. H., Loss of caveolin-1 accelerates neurodegeneration and aging. *PLoS One* 2010, 5, (12), e15697.

[84] Kang, M. J.; Chung, Y. H.; Hwang, C. I.; Murata, M.; Fujimoto, T.; Mook-Jung, I. H.; Cha, C. I.; Park, W. Y., Caveolin-1 upregulation in senescent neurons alters amyloid precursor protein processing. *Exp Mol Med* 2006, 38, (2), 126-33.

[85] Hawkes, C. H.; Chawda, S.; Derakshani, S.; Muhammed, N.; Visentin, E.; Boniface, D., MRI and visual-evoked potentials in partners of multiple sclerosis patients. *Acta Neurol Scand* 2011, Aug 25. doi: 10.1111/j.1600-0404.2011.01586.x. [Epub ahead of print].

[86] Weller, R. O; Preston, S. D., The spectrum of vascular disease in dementia. From ischaemia to amyloid angiopathy. *Adv Exp Med Biol* 2001, 487, 111-22.

[87] Di Legge, S.; Hachinski, V., Prospects for prevention and treatment of vascular cognitive impairment. *Curr Opin Invest Drugs* 2003, 4, 1082-7.

[88] Egashira, N.; Iwasaki, K.; Ishibashi, M.; Hatip-Al-Khatib, I.; Wolozin, B.; Mishima, K.; Irie, K.; Fujiwara, M., Hypoxia enhances β-amyloid-induced apoptosis in rat cultured hippocampal neurons. *Jpn J Pharmacol* 2002, 90, 321-7.

[89] Swaminath, P. V.; Ragothaman, M.; Muthane, U. B.; Udupa, S. A. H.; Rao, S. L.; Govindappa, S. S., Parkinsonism and Personality Changes Following an Acute Hypoxic Insult During Mountaineering. *Movement Disorders* 2006, 21, (8), 1296-7.

[90] Antonelli, I. R.; Marra, C.; Giordano, A.; Calcagni, M. L.; Cappa, A.; Basso, S.; Pagliari, G.; Fuso, L., Cognitive impairment in chronic abstructive pulmonary disease – a neuropsychological and spect study. *J Neurol* 2003, 250, (3), 325-32.

[91] Blass, J. P., Brain metabolism and brain desease: is metabolic deficiency the proximate cause of Alzheimer dementia? *J Neurosci Res* 2001, 66, (5), 851-6.

[92] Jendorska, K.; Poewe, W.; Daniel, S.E.; Pluess, J.; Iwerssen-Sschmidt, H.; Paulsen, J.; Barthel, S.; Schelosky, L.; Cervos-Navarro, J.; DeArmond, S. J., Ischemic stress induces deposition of amyloid beta immunoreactivity in human brain. *Acta Neuropat* 1995, 90, (5), 461-6.

[93] Peers, C.; Smith, I. F.; Boyle, J. P.; Pearson, H. A., Remodeling of Ca^{2+} homeostasis in type I cortical astocytes by hypoxia: evidance for association with Alzheimer's desease. *Biol Chem* 2004, 385, (3-4), 285-9.

[94] Bazan, N. G.; Palacios-Pelaez, R.; Lukiw, E. J., Hypoxia signaling to genes: significance Alzheimer's desease. *Mol. Neurobiol* 2002, 26, (2-3), 283-98.

[95] Chen G. J.; Xu J.; Lahousse S. A.; Caggiano N. L.; de la Monte S. M., Transient hypoxia causes Alzheimer-type molecular and biochemical abnormalities in cortical neurons: potential strategies for neuroprotection *J Alzh Dis* 2003, 5, (3), 209-228.

[96] Wen, Y.; Onyewuchi, O.; Yang, Sh.; Lliu, R.; Simpkins, J. W., Increased β-secretase activity and expression in rats following transient cerebral ischemia. *Brain Res* 2004, 1009, 1-8.

[97] Lichtenthaler, S. F.; Haass, C., Amyloid at the cutting edge: activation of α-secretase prevents amyloidogenesis in an Alzheimer disease mouse model. *J Clin Invest* 2004, 113, 1384-7.

[98] Mattson, M. P., Cellular action of β-amyloid precursor protein and soluble and fibrillogenic derivatives. *Physiol Rev* 1999, 77, 1081-132.

[99] Vassar, R.; Citron, M., Aβ-generation enzymes: recent advances in β- and γ-secretases research. *Neuron* 2000, 27, 419-22.

[100] Fisk, L.; Nalivaeva, N. N.; Boyle, J. P.; Peers, C. S.; Turner, A. J., Effects of hypoxia and oxidative stress on expression of neprilysin in human neuroblastoma cells and rat cortical neurones and astrocytes. *Neurochem Res* 2007, 32, (10), 1741-8.

[101] Nalivaeva, N. N.; Fisk, L. R.; Belyaev, N. D.; Turner, A. J., Amyloid-degrading enzymes as therapeutic targets in Alzheimer's disease. *Curr Alzheimer Res* 2008, 5, (2), 212-24.

[102] Turner, A. J.; Nalivaeva, N. N., New insights into the roles of metalloproteinases in neurodegeneration and neuroprotection. *Int Rev Neurobiol* 2007, 82,113-35.

[103] Aliev, G.; Smith, M. A.; Seyidov, D.; Neal, M. L.; Lamb, B. T.; Nunomura, A.; Gasimov, E. K.; Vinters, H. V.; Perry, G.; LaManna, J. C.; Friedland, R. P., The role of oxidative stress in the pathophysiology of cerebrovascular lesions in Alzheimer's disease. *Brain Pathol* 2002, 12, (1), 21-35.

[104] Fisk, L.; Nalivaeva, N. N.; Turner, A. J., Regulation of endothelin-converting enzyme-1 expression in human neuroblastoma cells. *Exp Biol Med (Maywood)* 2006, 231, (6), 1048-53.

[105] Graseman, H.; Lu, B.; Jiao, A.; Boudreau, J.; Gerard, N. P., Targeted deletion of the neutral endopeptidase gene alters ventilatory responses to acute hypoxia in mice. *Appl Phusiol* 1999, 87, 1266-71.

[106] Kumar, G. K., Peptidases of the peripheral chemoreceptors: biochemical, immunological, in vitro hydrolytic studies and electron microscopic analysis of neutral endopeptidase-like activity of the carotid body. *Brain Res* 1997. 748, (1-2), 39-50.

[107] Kumar, V. B.; Farr, S. A.; Flood, J. F.; Kamlesh, V.; Franko, M.; Banks, W. A.; Morley, J. E., Site-directed antisense oligonucleotide decreases the expression of amyloid precursor protein and reverses deficits in learning and memory in aged SAMP8 mice. *Peptides* 2000, 21, 1769-75.

[108] Doi Y.; Kudo H.; Nischino T.; Yamamoto O.; Nagata T.; Nara S.; Morta M.; Fujimoto S., Enhanced expression of endothelin-1 and endothelin-converting enzyme-1 in acute hypoxic rat aorta. *Histol Histopathol* 2002, 17, 97-105.

[109] Huang, S. M.; Mouri, A.; Kokubo, H.; Nakajima, R.; Suemoto, T.; Higuchi, M.; Staufenbiel, M.; Noda, Y.; Yamaguchi, H.; Nabeshima, T.; Saido, T. C.; Iwata, N., Neprilysin-sensitive synapse-associated amyloid-β peptide oligomers impair neuronal plasticity and cognitive function. *J Biol Chem* 2006, 281, 17941-51.

[110] Dickey, C. A.; Loring, J. F.; Montgomery, J.; Gordon, M. N.; Eastman, P. S.; Morgan, D., Selectively reduced expression of synaptic plasticity-related genes in amyloid precursor protein + presenilin-1 transgenic mice. *J Neurosci* 2003, 23, 5219 –26.

[111] Dubrovskaya, N. M., Nalivaeva, N. N., Plesneva, S. A., Feponova, A. A., Turner, A. J., Zhuravin, I. A. Changes in the activity of amyloid-degrading metallopeptidases leads to disruption of memory in rars. *Neurosci and Behavioral Physiol* 2010, 40, (9), 975-80.

[112] Belyaev, N. D.; Kellett, K. A.; Beckett, C.; Makova, N. Z.; Revett, T. J.; Nalivaeva, N. N.; Hooper, N. M.; Turner, A. J., The transcriptionally active amyloid precursor protein (APP) intracellular domain is preferentially produced from the 695 isoform of APP in a β-secretase-dependent pathway. *J Biol Chem* 2010, 285, (53), 41443-54.
[113] Belayev, N. D.; Nalivaeva, N. N.; Makova, N. Z.; Turner, A. J., Neprilysin gene expression requires binding of the amyloid precursor protein intracellular domain to its promoter: implications for Alzheimer disease. *EMBO Rep* 2009, 10, (1), 94-100.
[114] Weinreb, O.; Mandel, S.; Amit, T.; Youdim, M.B., Neurological mechanisms of green tea polyphenols in Alzheimer's and Parkinson's diseases. *J Nutr Biochem* 2004, 15, (9), 506-16.
[115] Weinreb, O.; Amit, T.; Mandel, S.; Youdim, M.B., Neuroprotective molecular mechanisms of (-)-epigallocatechin-3-gallate: a reflective outcome of its antioxidant, iron chelating and neuritogenic properties. *Genes Nutr* 2009, 4, (4), 283–96.
[116] Melzig, M.F.; Janka, M., Enhancement of neutral endopeptidase activity in SK-N-SH cells by green tea extract. *Phytomedicine* 2003, 10, (6-7), 494-8.

In: Short-Term Memory: New Research
Editors: Garifallia Kalivas and Sappho F. Petralia
ISBN: 978-1-62100-860-6

Chapter 7

WORKING MEMORY AND LANGUAGE PROCESSING: EXTENDING AN INTERACTIVE MODEL TO CAPTURE SENTENCE-LEVEL DATA

Valantis Fyndanis
Aristotle University of Thessaloniki, Greece
Technological Educational Institute of Epirus, Greece

ABSTRACT

In the present chapter I propose an extension of the interactive model of short-term memory proposed by R. Martin and Lesch (1996), and R. Martin, Lesch, and Bartha (1999) – which was developed to capture word-level processing – so that it can capture, in addition, sentence-level information. I will illustrate the extended model's explanatory power with data from a Greek-speaking agrammatic patient on four previously reported tasks: sentence repetition task, sentence grammaticality judgment task, sentence-picture matching task, sentence completion task.

1. INTRODUCTION

Traditionally, short-term memory is considered to be a memory system which is responsible for maintenance of information for a short period of time (e.g., Atkinson and Shiffrin, 1968). An alternative term for *short-term memory*, by Baddeley and colleagues (Baddeley, 1986; Baddeley and Hitch, 1974), is the notion of a multi-component *working memory system*. They proposed that this system is responsible not only for short-term retention of different types of information (e.g., numbers, words), but also for their processing.

Many accounts of agrammatic Broca's aphasia involve the notions of *processing resources* (e.g., Fyndanis, Varlokosta, and Tsapkini, 2010; Swinney, Zurif, Prather, and Love, 1996; Zurif, Swinney, Prather, Solomon, and Bushell, 1993) or *working memory* (e.g., Kok, van Doorn, and Kolk, 2007). (It has been argued that the term *processing resources* is an equivalent concept for *working memory*; e.g., Caplan and Waters, 1999) In particular, it has repeatedly been suggested that the deficit in agrammatism is computational in nature, that is, agrammatic speakers have limited working memory capacity or reduced processing resources. However, these concepts are quite vague, since they do not make any claim about the specific locus of the deficit in agrammatic aphasia. If it is correct that working memory consists of a number of components (e.g., Baddeley, 1986, 2000; Baddeley and Hitch, 1974; Caplan and Waters, 1999; Martin and Lesch, 1996; Martin, Lesch, and Bartha, 1999), then the investigations in aphasia should aim at detecting the exact locus (component) of each patient's deficit. To do so, one needs an appropriate model as a framework, as well as the results from certain "complementary" tasks.

R. Martin and her colleagues (R. Martin and Lesch, 1996; R. Martin, Lesch, and Bartha, 1999) have proposed an interactive model of short-term memory, which links the (different) levels of long-term linguistic representations to the corresponding buffers in short-term memory where the linguistic representations are stored. However, while this model can perfectly be used as a framework for word-level deficits, it fails to capture sentence-level information, since it includes no component where syntactic and semantic processing could take place. In this study, an extension of R. Martin et al.'s (1996, 1999) model will be proposed to capture both word-level and sentence-level processing. Moreover, the extended model's explanatory power will be illustrated with results from a Greek-speaking agrammatic patient on four previously reported constraint tasks: sentence repetition task, sentence grammaticality judgment task, sentence-picture matching task, sentence completion task (Fyndanis, 2009, 2010; Fyndanis, Varlokosta, and Tsapkini, 2008, submitted, under review).

The chapter is organized as follows: In section 2 a brief outline of the original model of R. Martin and colleagues is given, whereas in section 3 the extension of the model is presented. In section 4 the results of the Greek-speaking agrammatic patient on the four above-mentioned tasks are presented and discussed within the framework of the extended model. Finally, the conclusions are reported in brief, in section 5.

2. A Brief Outline of R. Martin et al.' Model

Based on neuropsychological evidence, R. Martin and colleagues (e.g., Martin and Freedman, 2001; Martin and Lesch, 1996; Martin, Lesch, and Bartha, 1999) argued that linguistic information processing (at least at single-word level) and retention are not supported by the same capacity. (For a different approach, see N. Martin and Saffran, 1997). Instead, they argued that the output from word-level language processing is stored and maintained in limited-capacity buffers specific to each level of representation (e.g., lexical-semantic, phonological level) (see Figure 1) (R. Martin and Freedman, 2001). Furthermore, in contrast to other models of short-term memory/working memory (e.g., Baddeley, 2000; Baddeley and Hitch, 1974; N. Martin and Saffran, 1997), R. Martin and colleagues' model distinguishes between input and output phonological representations, while it also postulates two corresponding distinct buffers in the short-term memory system. Suggestions for such a separation have been made by other researchers as well (e.g., Allport, 1984; Shallice and Butterworth, 1977). Hence, as Figure 1 illustrates, R. Martin and colleagues have proposed an interactive model which integrates both the long-term linguistic representations – or in their words "long-term knowledge structure" – and the language-specific short-term memory system ("buffered representations"). The long-term knowledge structure comprises the phonological level (which includes input and output phonological sub-components), the lexical, and the semantic level. The short-term memory system includes input and output phonological buffers and a lexical-semantic buffer. This model postulates an interaction between the levels of the long-term knowledge structure, as well as links between its components and the corresponding buffers of the short-term memory system. In the long-term knowledge structure, there is a direct link between input and output phonological segments so that in order for the latter segments to be activated, prior transfer of activation to the lexical or semantic level is not necessary[1] The existence of such a link is reflected in the ability of unimpaired speakers to repeat non-words (R. Martin, Lesch, and Bartha, 1999).[2] Word comprehension and production occur in the long-term knowledge structure, whereas retention of the linguistic material occurs in the short-term buffers.

According to R. Martin, Lesch, and Bartha (1999), there is a direct relationship between the representations and processes involved in word comprehension and production and those involved in short-term memory.

Moreover, they argue that the representations (of each level) in the short-term memory system depend on the activation of the corresponding representations in the long-term knowledge structure, and, further, that the latter representations are activated at encoding, with this activation being maintained during retention, that is, as long as the representations are stored in the short-term buffers.

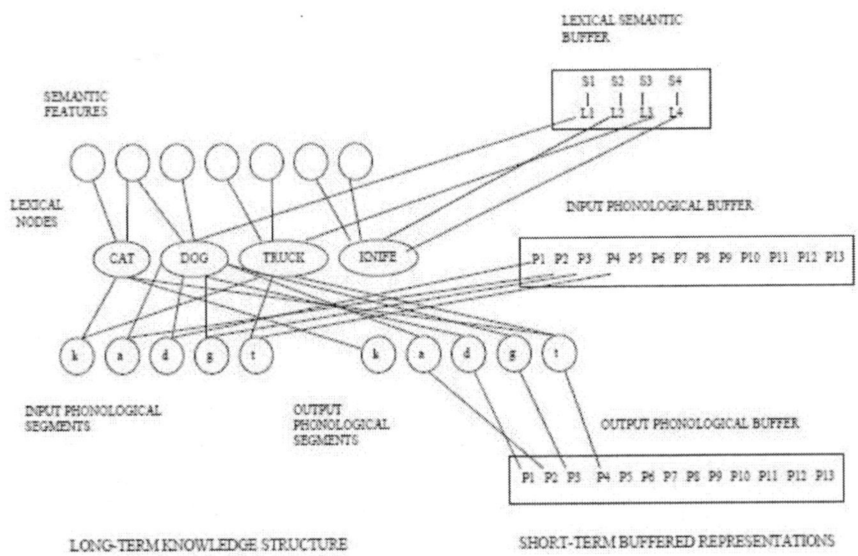

Figure 1. R. Martin et al.'s model of short-term memory (based on Martin, Lesch, and Bartha, 1999: 8) showing the different levels of processing and retention.

[1] We observe that this is not clear from Figure 1, as the links between input and output phonological segments are absent. Only the fact that these two types of segments appear at the same level suggests the above-mentioned possibility.

[2] This part of R. Martin et al.'s model corresponds to the sublexical route proposed (as one of the three possible routes) by Howard and Franklin's (1987, 1988: 20-22) model, which captures word repetition, among other things. This route allows the sublexical auditory-to-phonological conversion. The other two possible routes – according to Howard and Franklin's model – are the lexical and the semantic ones.

As far as the interactions between the components of the model are concerned, they are not "generalized", as only the components of the long-term knowledge structure interact with each other. Thus, in contrast to the buffers of short-term memory, which do not interact, the three-level representations in the long-term knowledge structure interact with each other after linguistic input has been perceived, so that there is feedforward and feedback of activation between the different levels. Since the activation in the levels of the long-term knowledge structure triggers the activation of the representations in the short-term memory buffers, it is suggested that the content of these buffers reflects the interactions that occur in the knowledge structure (R. Martin, Lesch and Bartha, 1999). Therefore, as per this model, if there is damage in the representations and processes involved in word perception and production, then the short-term memory system is expected to be affected as well, with predictable consequences depending on the specific representation or process being affected. Furthermore, it is possible that the ability to comprehend and produce a word is preserved, but short-term memory is impaired. That would might result in a clearly rapid decay of the representation at some level (op.cit).

3. Towards an Extension of R. Martin et al.'s Model

As mentioned in section 1, while R. Martin and colleagues' (R. Martin and Lesch, 1996; R. Martin, Lesch, and Bartha, 1999) model can capture word-level processing, it fails to capture sentence-level information, since it includes no component where syntactic and semantic processing could take place. Accordingly, an extension of the model will be proposed so that it can capture sentence-level data as well. It is worth mentioning, however, that the extension of the model proposed here is in a way tentative, as I will leave open issues pertaining to some of its aspects. Further research is needed to test the proposed model and shed light on the questions that still need to be addressed. The proposed extension mainly aims to offer a model that could be used to help researchers draw conclusions on the specific locus of the deficit of neurologically impaired speakers on the basis of constrained tasks, such as sentence repetition and grammaticality judgment tasks, and sentence-picture matching tasks, to name a few.

I suggest an extension of R. Martin and colleagues' (R. Martin and Lesch, 1996; R. Martin, Lesch, and Bartha, 1999) model by adding a sentence-level component. This new component would be responsible for syntactic parsing and semantic integration and would also have a storage capacity (see Figure 2).[3] As a result, it would be an additional component of the short-term memory system.[4] To be more accurate, since in this component computations/ operations such as syntactic parsing and semantic integration will take place (and not only storing), the extended model will be a model of working memory and not of short-term memory. In fact, this is how it will henceforth be referred to. Furthermore, we will refer to this new component as the *syntactic-semantic component*. This component would maintain links with the other three components of the working memory system (lexical-

[3] Thus, I assume that this component consists of two subcomponents, one for syntactic parsing and one for semantic integration. However, the question whether two separate components for syntactic parsing and semantic integration should be postulated is not addressed in the present study.

[4] It could be suggested that this component is similar to the work space for (syntactic) parsing argued for by Caplan and Hildebrandt (1988: 279-280).

semantic buffer, input phonological buffer, output phonological buffer). Certainly, these three buffers will maintain their links to the corresponding levels of the long-term knowledge structure. However, I propose the expansion of the function served by the output phonological buffer. Specifically, I suggest that the outputs of this buffer can be not only of word-level but of sentence-level as well. Such a possibility renders the model more economical, as otherwise the addition of another component should be proposed, namely of a sentence-level output phonological buffer. Nevertheless, since the language/cognitive system may not always opt for the most parsimonious solutions, future research needs to shed light on the question whether a single or two distinct (word-level and sentence-level) output phonological buffers should be postulated.

We could assume then, as proposed by the model, that sentence processing in repetition, for example, occurs in the following way: first, the phonological input representations are activated in the long-term knowledge structure upon the perception of the linguistic stimuli. This activation spreads to the higher levels of the knowledge structure, triggering the activation of the corresponding lexical-semantic representations. Subsequently, the latter representations are transferred (or just trigger the activation of the corresponding representations) to the lexical-semantic buffer of the working memory system and, thereafter, they are transferred to the syntactic-semantic component by feedforward spreading of activation. Furthermore, the syntactic-semantic component will be fed with syntactically relevant phonological cues or representations from the input phonological buffer. This seems reasonable since the syntactic-semantic component sometimes need phonological information – particularly, prosodic representations such as the intonational contóur of the sentence – in order to "extract" the underlying syntactic structure from the string of lexical-semantic representations (e.g., in the case of focused utterances).

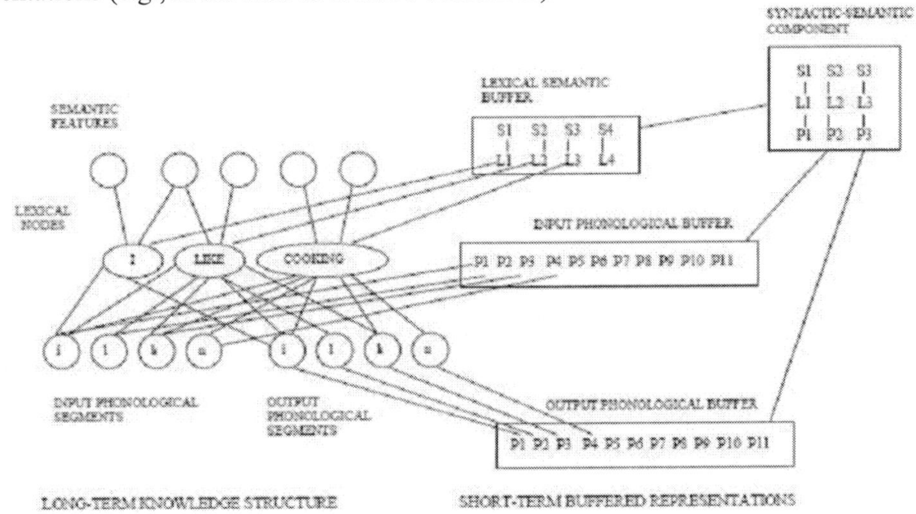

Figure 2. Extended version of R. Martin et al.'s (1999) model.

Consequently, the input for the syntactic-semantic component will be strings of "isolated" (not connected to each other at a "deep" level) lexical-semantic representations (including both lexical and grammatical elements), and possibly sententially-relevant phonological (prosodic) representations. Its output, on the other hand, will be processed (both syntactically and semantically) and "coherent" sequences, that is, sentences. Also, it is assumed that the syntactic-semantic component will transfer the syntactic-level phonological information (e.g., intonational contour) encoded in its output to the output phonological buffer, where the phonological representations of the words that make up the sentence will have already been activated (that is, prior to the above transfer). (Note that, as predicted by R. Martin et al.'s model, the activation of these representations in the output phonological buffer occurs by means of the interconnection of this component with the corresponding level of the long-term knowledge structure, that is, output phonological segments.) The sentence-level phonological information will combine with the single-word phonological representations (available in the output phonological buffer independently of the syntactic-semantic component) and this integration will yield the final, sentence-level output of the output phonological buffer.

4. Illustration of the Extended Model's Explanatory Power: Data from a Greek-Speaking Agrammatic Patient

In this section, an attempt will be made to illustrate the explanatory power of the proposed extended model by discussing the patterns of performance of a Greek-speaking agrammatic patient, GT, on four off-line constrained tasks within the framework offered by this model. First, I will briefly present GT's profile and results on a sentence repetition task, a sentence grammaticality judgment task, a sentence-picture matching task, and a sentence completion task. Subsequently, the results will be discussed within the present extended model with the aim of identifying the specific locus of his deficit.

4.1. GT's Profile

GT was a right-handed native speaker of Greek with nine years of education. He was 44 year-old at the time of testing. GT was diagnosed with non-fluent agrammatic aphasia following a single cerebrovascular accident (CVA) in the left hemisphere. The diagnosis was based on clinical consensus, the Greek standardized version of the Boston Diagnostic Aphasia Examination (BDAE) (Goodglass and Kaplan, 1983; Greek version by Papathanasiou, Papadimitriou, Gavrilou, and Mihou, 2008), and samples of spontaneous speech (picture description and conversation), analysed following the coding procedures described in Thompson, Shapiro, Tait, Jacobs, Schneider, and Ballard (1995). His speech rate was remarkably slower compared to that of his control participant. GT is an atypical non-fluent aphasic individual, since, although he presents a mean length of utterance of 5.58 words, his output is characterized by flat intonation and unclear articulation; moreover, he produces grammatical sentences only in 52% of the cases. The combination of the relatively reduced mean length of his utterances and the high proportions of ungrammatical sentences he produces is taken as evidence for agrammatism (following Faroqi-Shah and Thompson, 2004). Finally, the imaging data revealed that the lesions of GT involved mainly the basal ganglia of the left hemisphere. GT's testing took place 4.5 months post-onset. GT's detailed language testing data are reported in Fyndanis, Varlokosta, and Tsapkini (under review).

4.2. GT's Results on Four off-Line Tasks

GT participated in a number of off-line tasks aiming to test his ability to handle certain functional categories in Greek (subject-verb Agreement, Tense, Aspect, Complementizer Phrase, Negation). His results from these tasks have already been reported in other studies (Fyndanis, 2009, 2010; Fyndanis, Tsapkini, Varlokosta, Petropoulou, and Papathanasiou, 2006; Fyndanis, Varlokosta, and Tsapkini, 2010, submitted, under review). For the purposes of the present study, I will only discuss the results from a sentence repetition task, a sentence grammaticality judgment task, a sentence-picture matching task, and a sentence completion task (Tables 1, 2, 3, and 4, respectively). The sentence repetition, grammaticality judgment, and completion tasks were developed to test GT's ability to repeat, comprehend/judge and produce, respectively, subject-verb Agreement, Tense, and Aspect sentences.[5] In all three tasks, each condition included 56 items. The sentence-picture matching task, consisted of 18 items, was administered to test GT's ability to comprehend Tense only.[6] Although the results from these tasks have already been reported in other studies, they have not been discussed within the framework offered by the extended model of working memory and language processing proposed here. These data will be discussed in light of this model for two reasons: first, the above-mentioned tasks – as will be shown later on – are complementary; second, in all these tasks the stimuli used to test Agreement, Tense and Aspect differed in length. The Aspect sentences were longer than the Tense sentences, and the Tense sentences were longer than the Agreement sentences. Specifically, in the sentence repetition, grammaticality judgment, and completion tasks, the mean length for Agreement, Tense, and Aspect sentences were 4.39, 6.04 and 9.36 words, respectively. (The Tense sentences included in the sentence-picture matching task had 5.11 words on average). Length is considered to be one of the factors that contribute to the computational load of a sentence, especially when it is processed only in the auditory modality (e.g., Cheimariou, Varlokosta, Economou, Kakavoulia, and Protopapas, 2010; Fyndanis, Varlokosta, and Tsapkini, 2010), as is the case with these experiments. Indeed, we observed that in the sentence repetition, grammaticality judgment and completion tasks, the longer the sentences (Aspect > Tense > Agreement) the worse GT performed on them. Thus, to explore the functional locus of GT's deficit, in the following section the results from the four tasks will be discussed within the framework of the proposed extended model.

---

[5] As Comrie (1976) states "Tense relates the time of the situation referred to to some other time, usually to the moment of speaking. The commonest tenses found in languages [...] are present, past, and future: a situation described in the present tense is located temporally as simultaneous with the moment of speaking [...]; one described in the past is located prior to the moment of speaking [...]; one described in the future is located subsequent to the moment of speaking [...]" (pp. 1-2). Aspect, on the other hand, refers to "different ways of viewing the internal temporal constituency of a situation. [...] Aspect is not concerned with relating the time of the situation to any other time-point, but rather with the internal temporal constituency of the one situation" (Comrie, 1976: 3). The most important aspectual distinction is between *perfectivity* and *imperfectivity*: the former indicates the view of a situation as a whole, without distinction of the various separate phases making up that situation, whereas the latter pays attention to the internal structure of the situation (op. cit.: 16). Thus, the difference in the way the action of reading a book is seen in the sentences *John read a book yesterday* and *John was reading a book when I entered* is an aspectual difference which reflects the *perfectivity* vs. *imperfectivity* distinction, respectively.

[6] For an extensive presentation of the design of the sentence completion task, see Fyndanis, Varlokosta, and Tsapkini, under review; the sentence grammaticality judgment task and the sentence-picture matching task are reported in detail by Fyndanis, Varlokosta, and Tsapkini (submitted); an extensive presentation of the design of all four tasks is given in Fyndanis (2009).

Table 1. Distribution of GT's response types in the sentence repetition task (raw data and %)

	short sentences (Agreement)	medium sentences (Tense)	long sentences (Aspect)
Verbatim sentence repetitions	55 (98%)	51 (91%)	23 (41%)
Acceptable non verbatim repetitions	0 (0%)	5 (9%)	31 (55%)
Incorrect repetitions	1 (2%)	0 (0%)	2 (4%)

Table 2. Raw scores (incorrect) for GT, percentage of errors and comparisons (Fisher's exact test for count data) in the sentence grammaticality judgment task

Agreement (short)	Tense (medium)	Aspect (long)	Total	Agr vs. T	T vs. Asp	Agr vs. Asp
17/56 (30%)	21/56 (38%)	33/56 (59%)	71/168 (42%)	$p = .550$	$p = .037$	$p = .004$

Table 3. Raw scores (incorrect) and percentage of GT's errors in the sentence-picture matching task

Comprehension of Tense (medium sent.)
9/18 (50%)

Table 4. Raw scores (incorrect) for GT, percentage of errors and comparisons (Fisher's exact test for count data) in the sentence completion task

Agreement (short)	Tense (medium)	Aspect (long)	Total	T vs. Agr	T vs. Asp	Agr vs. Asp
3/56 (5%)	32/56 (57%)	46/56 (82%)	81/168 (48%)	$p = .000$	$p = .007$	$p = .000$

4.3. Discussion

4.3.1. Representational or Computational Deficit?

First of all, given the present framework, the question whether GT's deficit is representational or computational in nature should be addressed. In the sentence grammaticality judgment and completion tasks, we observe that the longer the sentences were (Aspect > Tense > Agreement), the lower the accuracy of GT' performance was. This can be taken as evidence that GT had reduced processing resources, resulting in his difficulty successfully processing long sentences (at least in the auditory modality, as is the case with the experiments discussed here). Also, in the sentence repetition task, the longer the sentences (Aspect and Tense sentences), the less often GT repeated them verbatim. This finding as well indicates that GT had reduced processing resources. As has been argued by Fyndanis and colleagues (Fyndanis, 2009; Fyndanis, Varlokosta, and Tsapkini, 2010, under review), sentence length is not the only factor that contributes to the (increased) computational load of Aspect and Tense sentences; another factor that increases the load of these sentences is the fact that both Aspect and Tense, unlike Agreement, carry interpretable features (Chomsky, 1995, 2000, 2001; Nanousi, Masterson, Druks, and Atkinson, 2006; Varlokosta, Valeonti, Kakavoulia, Lazaridou, Economou, and Protopapas, 2006). It has been suggested that "interpretable categories", such as Aspect and Tense, require processing and integration of both grammatical and extralinguistic/conceptual information, whereas processing of only grammatical information is sufficient for "uninterpretable categories", such as Agreement (Fyndanis, 2009; Fyndanis, Varlokosta, and Tsapkini, 2010, under review; Kok, van Doorn, and Kolk, 2007). As a consequence, Aspect and Tense are computationally "heavier" than Agreement. Another source of evidence that GT had a computational deficit comes from his pattern of performance on a constituent ordering task (Fyndanis et al., 2006) which included less and more demanding syntactic structures. GT performed lower on more demanding conditions (affirmative sentences in present perfect) than on less demanding conditions (affirmative sentences in present tense).

4.3.2. Focusing on GT's Working Memory

Having argued for the processing/computational nature of GT's deficit, we now have to focus on the working memory system of the proposed extended model, since its left part (long-term knowledge structure) would be of interest only in the case of a representational or single-word processing deficit.

An interesting finding is that, although GT performed almost at ceiling (96% correct) on the long sentences in the repetition task (despite the omissions he made), he performed at chance on the same sentence type in the grammaticality judgment task (41% correct). This contrast means that the difficulty GT had with the verbatim repetition of the long sentences cannot be attributed – at least exclusively – to a deficit in the output phonological buffer, since clearly this component is not involved in sentence grammaticality judgment. Of course, a deficit in this buffer could not be ruled out; however, the finding above constitutes independent evidence that GT's deficit undoubtedly involves some other component or components of his working memory system as well (lexical-semantic buffer, syntactic-semantic component, input phonological buffer) or some of their links.

To find out which part/component of GT's working memory is affected, let's focus on his pattern of performance on the sentence repetition task. Since GT incorrectly repeats only three sentences overall, one might argue that his working memory is not severely impaired. Nevertheless, while GT performs at ceiling on the short sentences, repeating them verbatim 98% of the time, he repeats verbatim 91% and only 41% of the medium and long sentences, respectively. Thus, as afore-mentioned, the longer the sentences (Aspect and Tense sentences), the less often GT repeated them verbatim,[7] which indicates that his working memory is affected to some extent. Interestingly, however, despite some omissions, almost always GT avoids the incorrect repetitions of the long and medium stimulus sentences. It has been argued that when the "to-be-repeated" sentence exceeds the capacity of the short-term

[7] A similar pattern of performance was exhibited by an English-speaking aphasic patient reported by Saffran and Marin (1975).

memory, its processing is required before its repetition (e.g., Bastiaanse, 1995).[8] Thus, it could be argued that GT processes at least the long sentences (9.36 words). Besides, the fact that GT repeats 5 of the 56 medium sentences correctly but not verbatim suggests that – at least occasionally – he processes these sentences as well. In particular, GT makes selective omissions, as he tends to omit (from both long and medium sentences) only the optional elements of the sentences, such as adjuncts (e.g., *ávrio* "tomorrow", *epí δéka leptá* "for ten minutes") and pronominal subjects (e.g., *esí* "you-sg", *emís* "we"). (Note that Greek is a null-subject language, thus omitting pronominal subjects is "legal".) This indicates that GT had successfully processed and comprehended at least the important part (verb and arguments) of the stimulus sentences, before he made omissions during their repetition. This, however, suggests that, even in the long-sentence condition, most of the time GT had available all the sentence material in the syntactic-semantic component. This seems to be reasonable, since to selectively omit some sentential elements, the position of which varies across sentences (in the repetition task reported here, the adjuncts were usually sentence-initial, whereas the pronominal subjects in the middle of the aspectual or tense sentences), one has to have all the sentential material available in the syntactic-semantic component. This, in turn, implies that all the sentence material was available in the lexical-semantic and input phonological buffers as well, and that, in addition, the links between the latter components and the syntactic-semantic component were intact. If the deficit involved the lexical-semantic buffer or/and the input phonological buffer, then not all the linguistic input (of at least the long sentences) could be stored in them, which would in turn result in the deficient storage of the stimulus sentence in the syntactic-semantic component. In this case, not all the "important" parts of the long sentences could always be stored in the syntactic-semantic component. That would inevitably result in ungrammatical sentence repetitions. Hence, since the lexical-semantic buffer and the input phonological buffer do not seem to be affected, it appears that we could not assume impaired links of these buffers with the syntactic-semantic component. These links must function smoothly, because otherwise the transfer and storing of all the linguistic material into the syntactic-semantic component, where the selective sentence production is planned, would be impossible.

Therefore, if the line of reasoning above is correct, it seems that GT's deficit lies in the syntactic-semantic component. As has become evident from his performance on the sentence grammaticality judgment and sentence-picture matching tasks as well, not always is GT able to successfully process the aspectual and tense adverbials, and semantically integrate them with the verbal morphology, which marks Aspect and Tense. As a result, he often fails to establish a single, integrated sentence representation. For this reason, in the repetition task, he chooses to phonologically encode and produce only the part of the lexical-semantic representations that he had previously processed and integrated successfully. Consequently, GT's ability for sentence comprehension is only partially preserved – in the sense that his comprehension system *intermittently* works smoothly –, which often does not allow him to acceptably paraphrase the whole stimulus sentence.

As mentioned earlier, although GT's results can be accounted for by assuming that in some demanding conditions (long sentences and, secondarily, medium sentences) he faces problems in the syntactic-semantic component, the possibility of a co-existing impairment in

[8] Certainly, this does not mean that sentence processing never occurs when all the sentential material is stored in short-term memory. However, in this case the phonological (sublexical) sentence repetition is possible as well.

the output phonological buffer should not be ruled out. Therefore, apart from his inability to successfully integrate aspectual or tense adverbials with verbal morphology, it is not unlikely that GT is not able to phonologically produce sentences exceeding a certain length. In this case, it might be argued that GT chooses to produce only a part of the linguistic material available in the syntactic-semantic component, specifically only the part which is successfully integrated (being, thus, sufficient for a grammatical repetition of the sentence), and which, at the same time, does not exceed the length limit imposed by the output phonological buffer. Certainly, in order to argue for such a possibility, we should assume that the output phonological buffer provides feedback to the syntactic-semantic component with respect to the maximum amount of linguistic material than can phonologically be encoded. Such an assumption is not incompatible with the extended version of R. Martin et al.'s model proposed here, since this postulates the interconnection between the syntactic-semantic component and the buffers of the short-term memory system. Nevertheless, this possibility would imply that the maximum amount of linguistic material that the output phonological buffer could accommodate would coincide with the maximum amount of linguistic material that GT would be able to syntactically process and semantically integrate. This coincidence appears to weaken the possibility of an impaired output phonological buffer.

4.3.3. A Comment on R. Martin and Freedman (2001)

Finally, I will comment on an issue raised by R. Martin and Freedman (2001), which seems to be in contrast to the proposed extended model. They claim that the apparently memory-related comprehension patterns of patients with a short-term memory deficit might be attributed to some sentence processing deficit, which is exacerbated by their short-term memory deficit. Therefore, R. Martin and Friedmann do not consider sentence processing to occur within a component of the working memory system, such as that postulated in the present study. Or, to put it in a different way, by referring to a short-term memory deficit they only imply an impaired storage capacity. However, for the syntactic-semantic component proposed here to work effectively, both an unimpaired storage capacity and sufficient processing resources (to allow for normal (not slowed) sentence processing) are required. Thus, a broader definition of the short-term memory system could accommodate sentence processing as well, which would lead to its transformation into a working memory system. If we take the performance on sentence repetition tasks on the one hand and the performance on sentence grammaticality judgment tasks and sentence-picture matching tasks on the other hand to better reflect the state of the short-term/working memory system and the sentence processing mechanism, respectively, which agrees with R. Martin and Freedman's (2001) line of reasoning, then we can make the following observation: *Prima facie*, indeed, GT's short-term/working memory deficit seems to be independent of his comprehension deficit. For instance, he repeats verbatim the medium (Tense) sentences 91% of the time, which indicates that his short-term/working memory capacity is sufficient to handle sentences of this length, whereas with the same sentences he scores correct only 50% and 62% of the time in the sentence-picture matching task and in the sentence grammaticality judgment task, respectively. However, this dissociation between repetition and judgment/comprehension tasks does not necessarily reveal different degrees of comprehension and short-term/working memory impairments. Since GT often fails to process and semantically integrate the medium/Tense sentences, which is clear from his performance on the two judgment/comprehension tasks, in the repetition task most of the time he resorts to sublexical repetition of these sentences. This seems plausible, since the Tense sentences consisted of around six words on average. Therefore, in the repetition task, GT manages to circumvent his inability to integrate temporal adverbials with verbal morphology by following the sublexical route. Instead, in the sentence-picture matching and sentence grammaticality judgment tasks, in both of which such an integration is indispensable, there is no way to circumvent this deficit. As a result, GT's performance on the Tense sentences is significantly lower in the latter two tasks than in the sentence repetition task. However, if indeed semantic integration occurs in the syntactic-semantic component, as proposed here, then the function of this component, which is one of the working memory components, is critical for comprehension.

5. Conclusion

In this chapter an extension of R. Martin and colleagues' (R. Martin and Lesch, 1996; R. Martin, Lesch, and Bartha, 1999) interactive model of short-term memory and language was proposed, so that it can capture sentence-level processing. Its usefulness was illustrated by discussing the data of a Greek-speaking agrammatic patient on four constrained tasks. It was demonstrated that the proposed extended model can fruitfully be used as a framework in the endeavor to detect the functional locus of the underlying breakdown of neurologically impaired patients with (morpho)syntactic deficits. In particular, the proposed model ideally could be employed as a framework to discuss data on sentence repetition tasks. However, as demonstrated here, the functional locus of a neurologically impaired speaker could best be detected when results from sentence repetition tasks combine with results from other "complementary" tasks, such as sentence grammaticality judgment tasks and/or sentence-picture matching tasks.

Acknowledgments

I thank Kyrana Tsapkini and Spyridoula Varlokosta for their contribution to the design of the tasks discussed in this chapter. I also express my gratitude to Gary Dell, Randy Martin and Tim Shallice for discussing with me issues on working memory. Furthermore I thank Christina Manouilidou, Ryan Taylor, Aikaterini Klepousniotou, and Fabiana Galiussi for their editorial help. Finally, I am grateful to Maria Kambanaros for reviewing this chapter and providing useful comments.

References

Allport, D. A. (1984). Auditory verbal short-term memory and conduction aphasia. In Bouma, H. and Bouwhuis, D. G. (Eds.), *Attention and performance X: Control and language processes* (pp. 351-364). Hillsdale, NJ: Erlbaum.

Atkinson, R. C. and Shiffrin, R. M. (1968). Human memory: A proposed system and its control processes. In Spence, K. W. and Spence, J. T. (Eds.), *The psychology of learning and memory: Advances in research and theory, Vol. 2* (pp. 89-195). New York: Academic Press.

Baddeley, A. (1986). *Working memory*. Oxford: Clarendon Press.

Baddeley, A. (2000). The episodic buffer: A new component of working memory? *Trends in Cognitive Sciences*, *4*, 417-423.

Baddeley, A. D. and Hitch, G. (1974). Working memory. In Bower, G. A. (Ed.), *The Psychology of Learning and Motivation* (pp. 47-89). New York: Academic Press.

Bastiaanse, R. (1995). Broca's aphasia: A syntactic and/or a morphological disorder? A case study. *Brain and Language*, *48*, 1-32.

Caplan, D. and Hildebrandt, N. (1988). *Disorders of syntactic comprehension*. Cambridge, MA: MIT Press.

Caplan, D. and Waters, G. (1999). Verbal working memory and sentence comprehension. *Behavioral and Brain Sciences*, *22*, 77-126.

Cheimariou, S., Varlokosta, S., Economou, A., Kakavoulia, M., and Protopapas, A. (2010). Error patterns of Greek aphasic speakers in sentence completion and grammaticality judgment. *Procedia – Social and Behavioral Sciences*, *6*, 181-182.

Chomsky, N. (1995). *The minimalist program*. Cambridge, MA: MIT Press.

Chomsky, N. (2000). Minimalist inquiries: The framework. In Martin, R., Michaels, D., and Uriagereka, J. (Eds.), *Step by Step* (pp. 89-155). Cambridge, MA: MIT Press.

Chomsky, N. (2001). Derivation by phase. In Kenstowicz, M. (Ed.), *Ken Hale: A life in language* (pp. 1-52). Cambridge, MA: MIT Press.

Comrie, B. (1976). *Aspect*. Cambridge, New York: Cambridge University Press.

Faroqi-Shah, Y. and Thompson, C. K. (2004). Semantic, lexical, and phonological influences on the production of verb inflections in agrammatic aphasia. *Brain and Language*, *89*, 484-498.

Fyndanis, V. (2009). *Functional categories in Greek agrammatism* (in Greek). Unpublished PhD thesis. Aristotle University of Thessaloniki, Greece.

Fyndanis, V. (2010). Short-term memory and language processing: Extending an interactive model to capture sentence-level data. *Procedia-Social and Behavioral Sciences*, *6*, 70-71.

Fyndanis, V., Tsapkini, K., Varlokosta, S., Petropoulou, K., and Papathanasiou., I. (2006). Negation in agrammatism: Evidence from Greek. *Brain and Language, 99*, 162-163.

Fyndanis, V., Varlokosta, S., and Tsapkini, K. (2008). The functional categories of the verbal complex in Greek agrammatism. Poster presentation at the 46th Annual Meeting of the Academy of Aphasia.

Fyndanis, V., Varlokosta, S., and Tsapkini, K. (2010). Exploring *wh*-questions in agrammatism: Evidence from Greek. *Journal of Neurolinguistics*, *23*, 644-662.

Fyndanis, V., Varlokosta, S., and Tsapkini, K. (under review). Agrammatic production: Interpretable features and selective impairment in verb inflection. *Lingua.*

Fyndanis, V., Varlokosta, S., and Tsapkini, K. (submitted*)*. Comprehension and judgment in agrammatic aphasia: Evidence from Greek.

Goodglass, H. and Kaplan, E. (1983). *Boston Diagnostic Aphasia Examination*. Malvern: Lea and Febinger.

Howard, D. and Franklin, S. (1987). Three ways for understanding written words and their use in two contrasting cases of surface dyslexia. In Allport, D. A., MacKay, D., Prinz, W., and Scheerer, E. (Eds.), *Language perception and production: Relationships between listening, speaking, reading and writing* (pp. 340-366). London: Academic Press.

Howard, D. and Franklin, S. (1988). *Missing the meaning? A cognitive neuropsychological study of processing words by an aphasic patient*. Cambridge, MA: MIT Press.

Kok, P., van Doorn, A., and Kolk, H. (2007). Inflection and computational load in agrammatic speech. *Brain and Language*, *102*, 273-283.

Martin, N. (2001). Repetition disorders in aphasia: Theoretical and clinical implications. In Berndt, R. S. (Ed.), *Handbook of Neuropsychology* (2nd ed., 3rd vol., pp. 137-155). Amsterdam: Elsevier Science B.V.

Martin, N. and Saffran, E. M. (1997). Language and auditoty-verbal short-term memory impairments: Evidence for common underlying processes. *Cognitive Neuropsychology*, *14*, 641-682.

Martin, R. C. and Freedman, M. L. (2001). Relations between language and memory deficits. In Berndt, R. S. (Ed.), *Handbook of Neuropsychology* (2nd ed., 3rd vol., pp. 239-256). Amsterdam: Elsevier Science B.V.

Martin, R. C. and Lesch, M. F. (1996). Associations and dissociations between language impairment and list recall: Implications for models of STM. In Gathercole, S. E. (Ed.), *Models of short-term memory* (pp. 149-178). East Sussex, UK: Psychology Press.

Martin, R. C., Lesch, M. F., and Bartha, M. C. (1999). Independence of input and output phonology in word processing and short-term memory. *Journal of Memory and Language*, *41*, 3-29.

Nanousi, V., Masterson, J., Druks, J., and Atkinson, M. (2006). Interpretable vs. uninterpretable features: Evidence from six Greek-speaking agrammatic patients. *Journal of Neurolinguistics*, *19*, 209-238.

Papathanasiou, I., Papadimitriou, D., Gavrilou, V., and Mihou, A. (2008). Psychometric properties of BDAE in normal adult population: The effect of age and gender (in Greek). *Psychology* (Greek edition), *15*, 398-410.

Saffran, E. M. and Marin, O. S. M. (1975). Immediate memory for word lists and sentences in a patient with deficient auditory short-term memory. *Brain and Language*, *2*, 420-433.

Shallice, T. and Butterworth, B. (1977). Short-term memory impairment and spontaneous speech. *Neuropsychologia*, *15*, 729-735.

Swinney, D., Zurif, E., Prather, P., and Love, T. (1996). Neurological distribution of processing resources underlying language comprehension. *Journal of Cognitive Neuroscience*, *8*, 174-184.

Thompson, C. K., Shapiro, L. P., Tait, M. E., Jacobs, B. J., Schneider, S. L., and Ballard, K. J. (1995). A system for the linguistic analysis of agrammatic language production. *Brain and Language*, *51*, 124-127.

Varlokosta, S., Valeonti, N., Kakavoulia, M., Lazaridou, M., Economou, A., and Protopapas, A. (2006). The breakdown of functional categories in Greek aphasia: Evidence from agreement, tense, and aspect. *Aphasiology*, *20*, 723-743.

Zurif, E., Swinney, D., Prather, P., Solomon, J., and Bushell, C. (1993). An on-line analysis of syntactic processing in Broca's and Wernicke's aphasia. *Brain and Language*, *45*, 448-464.

Reviewed by Dr. Maria Kambanaros

In: Short-Term Memory: New Research
Editors: Garifallia Kalivas and Sappho F. Petralia
ISBN: 978-1-62100-860-6

Chapter 8

THE UNIQUE CONTRIBUTION OF WORKING MEMORY TO READING ACQUISITION IN ARABIC

Raphiq Ibrahim
The Edmond J. Safra Brain Research Center for the Study of Learning Disabilities, Learning Disabilities Department, University of Haifa, Israel

ABSTRACT

Previous research has shown that the process of reading acquisition in Arabic by beginning readers is more challenging and might be slower than in other languages (Saiegh-Haddad, 2003). Furthermore, recent study showed that reading in Arabic is slower than reading in other languages, even among skilled native Arabic speakers (Azzam, 1984; Eviatar & Ibrahim, 2004; Abu-Rabia, 2001). This chapter summerize the role of short-term memory, represented by Working Memory (WM) measures in developmental reading problems, considering: 1) The unique contribution of WM to reading in language that has a unique and complex structure, Arabic; 2) Domain-general or -specific explanations of decoding and reading difficulties. Specifically, the chapter tries to explain whether a supra-lexical factor (working memory), affects meta-lingual performance, which is critical for the development of reading skill in Arabic language readers; and whether this effect differs with age, from 1st through 12th grade of school. Based on recent published studies (Ibrahim, 2011; Abu-Ahamad, Ibrahim & Share, 2011), short-term memory was found to be involved in and affect phonemic manipulations at all grade levels: the longer the manipulated stimulus, the poorer the performance. The implications of these findings in addition to other aspects of the related issue are discussed.

1. THEORETICAL BACKGROUND

Working memory means the ability to hold several facts or thoughts in memory temporarily while solving a problem or performing a task. These cognitive processes that maintain information in the mind during active processing of information were coined by Baddeley and Hitch (1974) as working memory. This capacity enables the coding, processing and recording of information during cognitive activity. Baddeley (1986) replaced the unitary short-term store with a working memory system consisting of three components: an attention-like central executive, a phonological loop holding speech-based information, and a visuo-spatial sketchpad specialised for spatial and visual coding. This working memory system is of relevance to non-memory activities such as comprehension and verbal reasoning. The phonological loop and visuo- spatial sketchpad have both been sub-divided into two-component systems, one component for storage and one for processing. The central executive fulfils several functions, but many of its characteristics remain unclear. In the context of language processing, the information stores of long-term memory are also of importance in learning through reading and reading comprehension. Thus, memory and reading are in close interaction with each other. Insufficient working memory capacity or poorly organized long-term memory can cause difficulties with reading or reading comprehension. The term *phonological memory* has been used to denote the idea that reading measures (decoding, reading comprehension, and reading time) are mediated by two working memory (WM) systems: the phonological loop memory component, and the visuospatial sketchpad component that performs a similar function for visual information (Baddeley & Hitch, 1974). These two subsystems provide active storage that is capable of combining information from sensory input and the central executive. The executive is now assumed to be a purely attentional system whose role extends beyond memory function (Baddeley, 2000, 2003; Baddeley & Wilson, 2002), but there is no consensus regarding the terms for the different components of memory. The distinction between short-term memory (STM) and WM is less clear: STM is typically used to describe situations in which small amounts of material are held passively (such as in digit or word span tasks) and then reproduced in an untransformed fashion; WM is considered a processing resource of limited capacity involved in the preservation of information while simultaneously processing the same or other information (Swanson & Ashbaker, 2000; Swanson & Siegel, 2001). Note that the model assumes that a short-term memory does support working memory performance (Cowan, 1999). We focus upon Cowan's (1999) Embedded Process model since it explicitly incorporates a role for Long-term Memory (LTM) which Baddeley's model does not. Baddeley coined the term "articulatory loop" (so called "Phonological working memory") for the process of rapid verbal repetition of the to-be-remembered information, which greatly helps maintain it in memory. Phonological working memory has a crucial role in connecting speech sounds and recognizing speech and letter correspondence. This activity is central at the first stages of acquiring reading skills. Thus, phonological working memory also plays a key part in this stage. Difficulties with learning to read can be connected with either unclearness of phonological working memory representations (insufficient ability to distinguish phonological differences) or with a fast filling up of the phonological working memory.

1.1. Language, Learning, and Working Memory

It is well agreed that working memory is required to understand spoken language; to comprehend what is read; to write sentences, and perform some math operations. For example, comprehension of sentences that are complex in structure, relies heavily on adequate working memory. Research on children with language delays, that is children who develop language much later than the norm but who have normal nonverbal intelligence, shows that they have working memory problems. They are referred to as having specific language impairment (SLI) and are at risk for having reading disabilities. Children between the ages of 4 and 6 with SLI showed in general limited working memory capacity and delays in vocabulary development. The syntactic development of children also is affected by working memory. Generally, people use working memory when preservation of word order (syntax) is important to correctly understand a sentence. Working memory allow the listener to hold verbal information in mind long enough to make sense of the sequence of words, process them for long-term storage, and to perform verbal problem-solving tasks.

As the working memory plays a central role in language learning (spoken and written), if it is weak, learning can be considerably improved by selecting material that places less burden on the working memory. Plain language is one of the most expedient tools that reduce the burden on the linguistic working memory. Clear, well parsed and structurally short language facilitates the functioning of the working memory. It reduces the burden of the new information (short sentences and familiar vocabulary) and makes it easier for a person to link new information into old (logicality and clearness of text references). Activation of processing during reading (i.e. deep processing) is also a good means to improve reading comprehension and the organization of new information in a manner optimal to reading.

Numerous studies found that good readers are more successful in STM tasks than weak readers, who find it difficult in the short term to retain verbal material presented either aurally or visually. The reduced range of memory in the weak readers appears in a variety of verbal material such as numbers, letters, phrases, and sentences. The performance of these tasks depends on the efficient storage of information in a phonological code, which lessens the burden on the WM so that it can be freely occupied in the process of higher understanding. Thus, in addition to deficient phonological awareness, weak readers also have weaker short-term verbal memory, although it is still not clear which of the various processing components is responsible for this. Many authors attribute it to the ability to store unfamiliar phonological forms (Share & Stanovich, 1995). In addition, the defective function of the short-term phonological memory is liable to affect access to the auditory channel lexicon (Breznitz, 2006). Tallal (1980) claimed that a functional lack of auditory temporal processing may cause a specific deficit in the organization of phonological information in the mind (Tallal, 1980). According to this theory even the difficulty in rapid manipulation – slowness in carrying out tasks of rapid manipulation, say retrieving the names of objects, colors, numbers and letters – is due to phonological deficiency, and does not indicate additional defects as claimed by theories that attribute this to difficulties in automatization (Bowers & Swanson, 1991). With repeated and extensive practice at processing information some tasks require less effort and become more automatic. Namely, when such skills become automatic, the brain is relieved of having to process individual units of information. This allows the brain to perform more complex processing and problem solving tasks. It also improves the efficiency of the working memory system. The question that I try to answer in this chapter is "to what extent the characteristics of a language like Arabic, requires different functioning of memory so that the long-term memory can function actively, while its contents should support comprehension during reading a text".

2. WORKING MEMORY AND READING ARABIC

Several studies made the connection between efficiency of basic linguistic mechanisms (phonology, orthography) and efficiency of cognitive processes of reading, such as memory and working memory (WM) (Share & Stanovich, 1995; Vellutino, Fletcher & Snowling, 2004). These studies, which compared ordinary and dyslexic children, concluded that the dyslexics' problems in deciphering and organizing phonological information are likely to cause difficulties in the storage and retrieval of words in short and long memory. These difficulties may in turn impair the effectiveness with which the individual makes connections between the auditory and graphical components of written words, and the development of orthographic patterns. As a result, the processing of written words will be inefficient and impose a burden on the working memory. Following research on reading acquisition of Arabic showed that it is slower than of Hebrew (Abu-Rabia, 1997; Saiegh-Haddad, 2003), and our earlier study on the contribution of diglossia and graphemic complexity to the inhibition and slowness of reading acquisition (Ibrahim, Eviatar & Aharon-Peretz, 2007), this chapter try to determine how such factors affect cognitive abilities, like memory components.

2.1. Memory and Diglossia in Arabic

The spoken form of Arabic, *ammia*, the local dialect, is used by speakers of the language in a specific geographic area for daily verbal communication, and is the native language of virtually all Arabic speakers. It differs from the literary form, , known as 'written Arabic' or 'Modern Standard Arabic' (MSA), which is the language that all speakers of Arabic the world over read and write. Spoken Arabic (SA) appears entirely in colloquial dialect and has no written form. Thus, from the ecological point of view, SA and MSA can be considered an example of *diglossia*: a social environment in which a community uses two forms of the same language concomitantly (Ferguson, 1959). From a linguistic point of view, literate Arabic speakers could be considered, de facto, bilinguals, fueling the controversy over whether the two forms of Arabic represent different languages (Eid, 1990). According to Maamouri (1998), the gap between the language of orality (spoken dialect at home) and the language of literacy (literary Arabic, LA) seems to be a major cause of low learning achievement in school and low adult literacy levels everywhere in the Arab world. Maamouri added that there are phonological, morphological, lexical and syntactical "distances" between the two forms. These studies attempted to determine whether there is a diglossia effect on phonological awareness such that phonological manipulations are more difficult to perform in the literary language. Saiegh-Haddad (2003) hypothesized that this difficulty slows reading acquisition in Arabic compared to other languages.

In an earlier study Ibrahim and colleagues found that *diglossia* and the phonological distance between the two varieties of Arabic are related to the native decoding ability of young Arab children (Ibrahim & Aharon-Peretz, 2005; Ibrahim, 2009). When the relationship between the two forms of Arabic was compared to that between Hebrew and SA, using the priming technique, the representation of LA is that of L2, similar to Hebrew, while that of SA and LA have the status of two separate languages in the cognitive systems of Arab adults.

The effect of phonological distance on phonological awareness has been studied, but not its contribution to specific components, including lexical distance, stimulus type (words versus non-words) and tasks involving working memory (target phoneme location in tasks and stimulus length on phonological awareness). Furthermore, these effects have not been studied beyond childhood. The present research may help clarify whether and how early literary lexical information should be acquired in order to consolidate quality lexicon (Perfetti, 2008) and to enable faster acquisition of the written language.

2.2. Researces in Arabic

Over the past several decades a large body of research has focused on the preschool foundations of reading development. Much of this work has been motivated by the need for early identification and intervention aimed at preventing later literacy difficulties (Snow, Burns, & Griffin, 1998). It is important to keep in mind, however, that reading is a not a single unitary construct, but includes at least two distinct components. The first is the identification of printed words (word recognition), and the second the comprehension of the text. It is often unclear whether the findings of studies aimed at elucidating the factors that place the pre-school child at risk for later reading difficulties apply to word recognition, reading comprehension, or both. Studies examining reading comprehension have demonstrated that this skill is partly dependent on efficient word recognition such that good comprehenders are typically good decoders (Perfetti ,1985 ,1999; Shankweiler, Lundquist, Katz, Stuebing, & Fletcher, 1999; Stanovich, 1982, 1991). But this literature has pointed to the role of higher-order cognitive abilities in reading comprehension. Cain, Oakhill, and Bryant (2004), for example, showed in a longitudinal study that measures of vocabulary, working memory, inference making and comprehension monitoring, all contributed to reading comprehension skills in 8-11 year olds. It appears that reading comprehension relies on a wide range of abilities including "lower-level" skills such as word recognition, as well as higher-order "supra-lexical" abilities such as vocabulary and syntax and high-level cognitive skills.

In a recent study on reading acquisition of Arabic among native Arabic speakers, we explored whether underlying processes that predict word identification vary according to the complexity or depth of the script (Abu-Ahamad, Ibrahim & Share, 2011). Although early reading acquisition in Arabic takes place within the orthographic context of fully vowelized script, which is generally considered a highly transparent orthography, this script has numerous complexities that are likely to pose a challenge to the novice reader. We focused on the extent to which intra-lexical and extra-lexical (or supra-lexical) factors, assessed in kindergarten, predict individual differences in later word recognition. Specifically, to what extent can word identification in Arabic be characterized as "modular"? In the final months of kindergarten, native Arabic speakers were administered a battery of tests assessing a variety of intra-lexical factors (phonemic awareness, phonological processing, visual-orthographic processing, pre-school print concepts and morphological awareness) and supra-lexical factors (nonverbal ability, receptive vocabulary, syntactic awareness and working memory). Word identification and reading comprehension were assessed at the beginning of 2nd grade The results revealed that decoding skill in Arabic at the beginning of 2nd grade is relatively poor compared to English and Hebrew. Word identification skill depended mainly on sub-lexical and lexical abilities, which together explained 33% of the variance in 2nd grade. The strongest predictors were phonemic awareness and phonological processing, followed by early print concepts, morphology and visual-orthographic processing. Alongside these intra-lexical abilities, supra-lexical abilities accounted for 11% of the variance in word recognition, consistent with the multiple complexities of the script. Reading comprehension skill was found to rely heavily on decoding skill as well as higher-order linguistic and cognitive abilities.

In my recent study (Ibrahim, 2011) that examined the influence of the diglossia of the Arabic language on the development of phonological ability, the WM skills were assessed at the end of each of the first through the last school years (1st grade through 12th grade). This enabled us to determine the effect of the WM components (phonological versus visual) – singularly and in combination – on the reading abilities within a language. Specifically, the study examined to what extent the visual STM and phonological STM are involved in and affect phonemic manipulations by assessing meta-lingual performance in written language compared to spoken language that has no visual memory. In addition, this work examined whether various aspects of diglossia — lexical distance, stimulus type (words versus non-words), target phoneme location in tasks, and stimulus length — affect phonological awareness among Arabic language readers, and whether this effect is different along a continuum of grades, beginning from childhood when reading is acquired, until adulthood when the reading level has matured. Other researchers reported a dissociation on successful intervention in reading between early and later grades (Foorman, Francis, Shaywitz, Shaywitz & Fletcher, 1997). Hence, a comparison of reading skills at different grades in school is crucial. It was hypothesized that the lexical distance will affect the ability to carry out the tasks of phonemic analysis and deletion; and that the participants would perform the tasks better with spoken words, to which they are more frequently exposed, than literary words; and that this influence will lessen with age, especially since the rate index was not examined. The results showed that performance was better when the deletion was at the beginning than at the end of the word. In addition, it was found a main effect for the type of task indicating a clear difference in performance between deletion of the initial sound and deletion of the final sound of the components. A main effect of grade was also found supporting the clear differences between the grades regardless of the type of task with a clear interaction between the task and grade. The analysis of deletion location revealed that the percentage of the components of literary words was much larger than the percentage of spoken words. The significant differences in performance between initial deletion and final deletion occurred only in grades 1 and 3, partly confirming the assumption that the influence of the location of the deletion from words would influence the performance of the phoneme deletion task.

The influence of stimulus length on the performance of the phonemic deletion and phonemic analysis tasks was examined. Components were divided into 3 categories: short components (3 sounds), medium-length components (5 sounds), and long components (6-7 sounds). Performance on the shorter words was much better than on the medium-length and long words in both tasks; performance on the medium-length words was better than on long words only on the task of phonemic analysis. Like with phonemic analysis, there was a clear advantage to executing spoken words over literary words, and an advantage was even found in the performance of non-words over both spoken and literary words. This was so even when the phonological structures were identical among the groups. This finding demonstrates that performance of the spoken language reflects more knowledge, experience, control, and maturity, and consolidation of the linguistic and meta-lingual mechanisms of the spoken language, compared to the performance of the literary language. The better performance of spoken words than literary words, which concurs with the findings of Saiegh-Haddad (2003), might reflect stronger and more consolidated semantic connections in the spoken language, and stronger control over the phonemes and phonological and syllabic structures belonging to the spoken language.

The whole findings on the involvement of memory in meta-lingual performances indicate that STM is involved in and affects phonemic manipulations: the longer the manipulated stimulus, the poorer the performance. These results were obtained for all age groups, supporting the involvement of memory in general and the active memory in particular in phonological processing. The findings also lend support to the view that the source of difficulty in STM is phonological memory, which is considered to be one of the important components of phonological processing. The phonemic deletion task, which also examined phonological awareness, yielded the opposite trend: performance was better in the literary language than in the spoken one. This contradicts both our assumptions and Saiegh-Haddad's findings (2003) that phonological awareness abilities are better in spoken Arabic than literary Arabic. Moreover, while there was a moderate correlation between the tasks we devised to assess the phonological awareness of the participants, they actually tapped two different processes of phonological processing. This dissociation is explained in part by research showing that the phonemic deletion task depends in part on the visual modes, namely the orthographical structures stored in the orthographical lexicon; and the report that phonemic analysis is more dependent on auditory modes (Ibrahim, 2008). The relationship between mode of stimulus presentation and better performance on the literary language than the spoken language in the phonemic analysis task is strengthened by the finding of better performance on the phonemic analysis of a non-word than the analysis of both literary and spoken words. Even in the research by Saiegh Haddad (2004), kindergarten and 1st grade children showed a low level of performance on phonemic identification of literary words in comparison to both spoken and non-words (Saiegh-Haddad, 2004). The researcher explained her findings by saying that "the phonological representation of the literary language was blurred, which caused the automatic activation of the dominant representations of the spoken language for literary structures" (pp. 506). The findings in the Ibrahim's research can be explained by the connection with auditory modes, especially since performance in the spoken language (with dominant structures) was poorer than the performance of non-words.

This better performance of non-words over spoken words and literary words might be due to higher investment and lack of automation in responses, especially when the words are not known to the children. Non-words require more resources of auditory attention and immediate word analysis based only upon auditory-phonological modes, without the use of orthographic and/or semantic lexicons. Direct analysis by means of auditory modes lessens the chance of distortions in other mechanisms, and is likely to reduce errors in performance.

The low level of meta-lingual performance (word analysis) in the literary language seen in all our grades has far-reaching implications. It makes reading acquisition in the lower grades difficult, especially when the process is carried out in the literary language over which the children have less control, as well as over its meta-lingual components (Elbro, 1996). In the higher grades, the low level of meta-lingual ability may impact on the higher processes in reading comprehension and written expression, which are dependent, in part, on language knowledge and a rich vocabulary. This means that the efficiency of the reading processes, whether basic or high level, may be affected by the poor control over linguistic and meta-lingual mechanisms in the literary language (Abu-Rabia, 2000; Vellutino et al., 2004).

It can be assumed that the reduction in phonemic analysis ability, which is a basic ability in reading and writing, slows reading acquisition in the Arabic language, as found in previous studies (Ibrahim et al. 2007); and that it constitutes a risk for the development of higher functions such as reading comprehension and expression in writing which depends, partly, on the intactness of basic reading processes. The prominent role of phonemic awareness in Arabic decoding and the low levels of decoding accuracy suggest that Arabic must be regarded as a low-transparency script. The finding by Ibrahim et al. (2007) that supra-lexical factors were modest but not "marginal" predictors of word identification is in accordance with the "transparency-by-modularity" interaction proposed by Share (2008), and suggests that Arabic is "semi-modular" in contrast to the highly modular nature of Hebrew. Their results showed that word identification constitute a major stumbling block for comprehending written Arabic in initial literacy learning. Finally, the substantial overlap observed between intra-lexical and supra-lexical abilities underscores the complexities of Arabic script and the challenges of diglossia.

The results of this study and our previous research led to two major conclusions: 1) sensitivity to *diglossia* is driven by the language of the test: lexical distance that exists between literary and spoken Arabic, and its influence on the ability to carry out phonemic manipulation, is different in the beginning Arabic speaker and the more experienced one. 2) Memory involvement in meta-lingual performances is driven by the mode of stimuli presentation: the longer the manipulated stimulus, the poorer the performance. These findings were obtained for all age groups, and strengthen the view of the involvement of memory in general and of the active memory in particular in phonological processing.

3. Conclusion

Working memory accounted for a few percentage points of the variance in word recognition. This finding converged with studies that showed an association between deficits in working memory and deficits in word recognition (e.g., Siegel & Ryan, 1989; Swanson & Alexander, 1997). However it important to note that working memory no longer continued to contribute to word recognition once general ability was controlled. As already mentioned in the results section, Saiegh-Haddad (2005) showed that Arabic pseudoword reading fluency in first grade was primarily predicted by letter recoding speed (a composite measure of accuracy and speed), followed by working memory. Additionally, some studies have found that a deficit in working memory is also characteristic of poor readers of Arabic (Abu-Rabia, et al., 2003; Abu-Rabia & Siegel, 2002). In the current study, the contribution of working memory to word recognition was marginal, but this must be qualified by a methodological limitation: The present working memory task was very hard for the kindergarteners hence, future research will need to rectify this shortcoming.

A phonological memory measure composed of tasks involving storage and manipulation of verbal stimuli was found to affect decoding ability. Thus, such measures of WM combined with the more commonly used measures in kindergarten assessments may provide a better estimate of a child's future academic success. And, since the cognitive structure of WM is in place at early school age (Alloway, Gathercole, & Pickering, 2006), administering WM tests at a young age will pick up potential future reading difficulties.

The research also points to the importance of intentional exposure and promotion of the literary Arabic language at an early age. Exposing children to this form before they enter school should help prevent immaturity in meta-lingual mechanisms in the standard literary language, reduce the gap between the spoken and the standard language, and ultimately make the process of reading acquisition easier. The research also sheds light on the unique features of Arabic that contribute to the inhibition and slowness of the reading process, and argues strongly for the early identification of reading difficulties. Parents, kindergarten teachers, school teachers, and those in charge of developing curricula and intervention programs to apply recommendations must be made aware of these problems, especially in view of the data gathered in recent years documenting the low level of reading achievement among Arabic-speaking children in comparison with the speakers of other languages in Israel.

REFERENCES

Abu-Ahamad, H., Ibrahim, R., & Share. D.L. (In press). *Cognitive Predictors of Early Reading Ability in Arabic: A Longitudinal Study from Kindergarten to Grade 2.* In Elinor. S & Joshi. M. (Eds.), "Handbook of Arabic Literacy" - Springer.

Abu-Rabia, S. (1997). Reading in Arabic orthography: The effect of vowels and context on reading accuracy of poor and skilled native Arabic readers. *Reading and Writing: An Interdisciplinary Journal, 9,* 65-78.

Abu-Rabia, S. (2000). Effects of exposure to literary Arabic on reading comprehension in a diglossic situation. *Reading and Writing: An Interdisciplinary Journal, 13,* 147–157.

Abu-Rabia, S., & Siegel, L. (2002). Reading, writing and working memory skills among Arabic-English bilingual children. *Journal of Psycholinguistic Research, 31*, 661–678.

Alloway, T. P., Gathercole, S. E. & Pickering, S. J. (2006). Verbal and visuospatial short-term and working memory in children: are they separable? Child Development, 77, 1698-1716.

Baddeley, A. D. (1986). Working memory. London: Oxford University Press.

Baddeley, A. D., & Hitch, G. (1974). Working memory. In K.W. Spence and J. T. Spence (eds.) The Psychology of Learning and Motivation, vol 8. (pp. 67-89). New York: Academic Press.

Baddeley, A. (2000). The episodic buffer: a new component of working memory? Trends in Cognitive Sciences, 4(11), 417-423.

Baddeley, A. (2003). Working memory and language: an overview. Journal of Communication Disorders, 36, 189-208.

Baddeley, A.D. & Hitch, G.J. (1974). Working memory. In G.A. Bower (Ed.), Recent Advances in Learning and Motivation (Vol. 8, pp. 47–89). New York: Academic Press.

Baddeley, A. & Wilson, B. (2002). Prose recall and amnesia: implications for the structure of working memory. *Neuropsychologia*, 40, 1737-1743.

Bowers, P. G. & Swanson, L.Y.(1991). Naming Speed Deficits in Reading Disability: Multiple Measures of a Singular Process. *Journal of Experimental Child Psychology*. 51, 195-219.

Breznitz, Z. (2006). Fluency in reading, synchronization of processing. Lawrence elbaum associated publishers.Mahwah.New Jersey Ch.1-6.

Cowan, N. (1999). An embedded-process model of working memory. In A. Miyake and P. Shah (Eds.) Models of Working Memory: Mechanisms of active maintenance and executive control. (pp. 102-134). New York: Cambridge University Press.

Cain, K., Oakhill, J., & Bryant, P. E. (2004). Children's reading comprehension ability: Concurrent prediction by working memory, verbal ability, and component skills. *Journal of Educational Psychology*, 96, 31–42.

Eid, M. (1990). Arabic linguistrics: The current scene. In M. Eid (Ed) Perspectives on Arabic linguistics I. (pp 3 37). Amsterdam: John Benjamins Publishing Company.

Elbro, C. (1996). Early linguistic abilities and reading development: A review and a hypothesis. *Reading and Writing: An Interdisciplinary Journal*, 8, 453-485.

Eviatar, Z. & Ibrahim, R. (2004). Morphological and orthographic effects on hemispheric Processing of nonwords: A Cross-linguistic comparison. *Reading and Writing,*17, 691-705.

Ferguson, C. A. (1959). Diglossia. *Word, 14*, 47–56.

Foorman, B, R., Francis, D. J., Shaywitz, S. E., Shaywitz, B. A., & Fletcher, J. M. (1997). The case for early reading intervention, In A. B. Blachman (Ed.). Foundations of reading acquisition and dyslexia: Implications for early intervention (pp. 243-264). Mahwah: Laurence Erlbaum.

Ibrahim, R. (2008). Does visual and auditory word identification have a language-selective input?: Evidence from word processing in Semitic languages. *The Linguistics Journal,* 3(2), 82-102.

Ibrahim, R. (2009). The cognitive basis of diglossia in Arabic: Evidence from a repetition priming study within and between languages. *Psychology Research and Behavior Management.* 12, 95-105.

Ibrahim, R. (2011). Literacy problems in Arabic: Sensitivity to diglossia in tasks involved working memory. *Journal of Neurolinguistics.*

Ibrahim, R., & Aharon-Peretz, J (2005). Is literary Arabic a second language for native Arab speakers?: Evidence from a semantic priming study. *The Journal of Psycholinguistic Research, 34*(1), 51–70.

Ibrahim, R., Eviatar, Z., & Aharon-Peretz, J. (2007). Metalinguisitic awareness and reading performance: A cross-language comparison. *Journal of Psycholinguistic Research*, 36, 297-317.

Maamouri, M. (1998). *Language education and human development: Arabic diglossia and its impact on the quality of education in the Arab region.* Discussion paper prepared for The World Bank, The Mediterranean Development Forum.

Perfetti, C. A. (1985). *Reading ability.* New York: Oxford University Press.

Perfetti. C. A. (1999). Comprehending written language: A blueprint of the reader. In A. D. Frederici (Ed.). *Language comprehension: A biological perspective* (pp. 167-208). Berlin: Springer-Verlag.

Perfetti, C. (2008). Reading Ability: Lexical Quality to Comprehension. *Scientific Studies of Reading,* 11, 357-383.

Saiegh-Haddad, E. (2003). Linguistic distance and initial reading Acquisition: The case of Arabic diglossia. *Applied Psycholinguistics, 24*, 431-451

Saiegh-Haddad, E. (2004). The impact of phonemic and lexical distance on the phonological analysis of words and pseudowords in a diglossic context. *Applied Psycholinguistics, 25*, 495-512.

Shankweiler, D., Lundquist, E., Katz, L., Stuebing, K. K., Fletcher, J. M., Brady, S., et al. (1999). Comprehension and decoding: Patterns of association in children with reading difficulties. *Scientific Studies of Reading, 3*, 69-94.

Share, D. L., & Stanovich, K. E. (1995). Accommodating individual differences in critiques: Replies to our commentators. *Issues in Education: Contributions from Educational Psychology*, *1*, 105-121.

Share, D. L. (2008). On the Anglocentricities of current reading research and practice: The perils of over-reliance on an "outlier" orthography, *Psychological Bulletin*, 134, 584-615.

Siegel, L. S., & Ryan, E. B. (1989). The development of working memory in normally achieving and subtypes of learning disabled. *Child Development*, *60*, 973-980.

Snow, C. E., Burns, M. S., & Griffin, P. (1998). *Preventing reading difficulties in young children*. Washington, DC: National Academy Press.

Stanovich, K. E. (1982). Individual differences in cognitive processes of reading, Part 1: Word decoding. *Journal of Learning Disabilities ,15,* 485-493.

Stanovich, K. E. (1991). Discrepancy definition of reading disability: Has intelligence led us astray? *Reading Research Quaterly*, *26*, 7-29.

Swanson, H. L. & Ashbaker, M. H. (2000). Working memory, short-term memory, speech rate, word identification and reading comprehension in learning disabled readers: Does the executive system have a role? *Intelligence,* 28 (1), 1-30.

Swanson, H. L. & Siegel, L. (2001). Learning disabilities as a working memory deficit. *Issues in education,* 7 (1), 1-48.

Tallal, P. (1980). Auditory temporal perception, phonics, and reading disabilities in children. *Brain and Language*, 9, 182-198.

Vellutino, F.R., Fletcher, J.M. & Snowling, M.J. (2004). Specific reading disability (dyslexia):What have we learned in the past four decades? *Journal of Child Psychology and Psychiatry*, 45, 2-40.

In: Short-Term Memory: New Research
Editors: Garifallia Kalivas and Sappho F. Petralia
ISBN: 978-1-62100-860-6

Chapter 9

AN *IN VITRO* MODEL FOR ANALYZING THE CONVERSION OF SHORT-TERM TO LONG-TERM MEMORY

Keiko Tominaga-Yoshino* and Akihiko Ogura
Laboratory of Synaptic Plasticity
Osaka University Graduate School of Frontier Biosciences
Suita, Osaka, Japan

ABSTRACT

Short-term memory is instantaneously established by modifying the synaptic transmission efficiency of existing synapses.

Long-Term Potentiation (LTP) of the rodent hippocampus is a cellular model most often used to investigate this instantaneous synaptic modification, as it has been shown that intense activity in an input pathway leads to an immediate enhancement in synaptic transmission efficiency.

Although such instantaneous synaptic modification is assumed to lead to structural changes that ensure life-long memory, how this conversion occurs is poorly understood. While morphological changes observed in the late phase of LTP are expected to offer some insight on the matter, the longevity of these changes is unknown. Using stable cultures of rodent hippocampal slices, we recently found that repeated, but not single, inductions of LTP lead to a distinct, slow developing and long lasting enhancement of synaptic strength coupled with the formation of new synapses, a phenomenon we name RISE (Repetitive LTP-Induced Synaptic Enhancement).

In this article, we describe fundamental properties of this novel synaptic plasticity phenomenon and propose an *in vitro* model for analyzing its cellular mechanisms that underlie the conversion of short- to long-term memory.

* E-mail address: tomyk[at]fbs.osaka-u.ac.jp

INTRODUCTION

In a widely-read neurobiology textbook "From Neuron To Brain" by J. Nicholls and colleagues [1], the boundary between short-term and long-term memories is placed between PTP (Post-Tetanic Potentiation) and LTP (Long-Term Potentiation).

In the Figure 12.1 of the book (fourth edition), the former is a minute-order phenomenon and the latter is an hour-order one. Presumably this classification is based on the difference in the cellular mechanisms underlying PTP (primarily presynaptic) and LTP (primarily postsynaptic).

In a similarly renowned neurobiology textbook "Neuroscience: Exploring the Brain" by M. Bear and colleagues [2], the boundary is placed between the hour-order event and the day-order one (Chapter 24 of the third edition). Presumably this classification is based on psychological phenomenology. The memory retention curve of Ebbinghaus [3] consists of two decay phases, the fast (exponential) and the slow (asymptotic), with no discussion on the mechanisms that cause them. Overall, distinction between short-term and long-term memories has been subjective.

So we re-define in this chapter the short-term memory as that originates from instantaneous modulation at the precedently existing synapses through post-translational modification processes and the long-term memory as that results from non-instantaneous modulation of neural circuits including structural changes such as formation of new synapses through transcriptional modification processes. And we assume that part of the former is converted to the latter. By this re-definition, mechanisms underlying this conversion should become treatable.

In this chapter, we describe our original in vitro model system that may help analyzing the cellular mechanisms underlying this transformation.

1. STRUCTURAL PLASTICITY

While sustained memory most probably requires some sort of structural changes [4], it is not true that any structural changes themselves be permanent. For example, neurotransmitter release is accompanied by a structural change including the fusion of a synaptic vesicle to a membrane. Although the membrane surface area transiently increases with the added vesicle, it returns to its original size immediately after [5]. The postsynaptic membrane should be the same. Receptor externalization must be coupled with membrane addition which should expand the surface of postsynaptic area, but the state of surface increment would not necessarily persist long.

Another example is the formation of new presynaptic boutons and postsynaptic spines, which must be accompanied by cytoskeletal reorganization. Yet again, however, cytoskeletal changes can be brief, as seen in developing neural circuits where axon's growth cones extend by actin polymerization, but often shorten immediately after by actin depolymerization [6].

LTP in the hippocampus is an instantaneous modification of synaptic transmission, which is followed by structural modifications [7]. However, the duration of these structural modifications are unknown. In a historic monograph "The Understanding of the Brain" [8], Sir John Eccles predicted that new synapse is formed through hypertrophy and branching of pre- or postsynaptic structure (Figure 5-18 of the first edition). While hypertrophy of the postsynaptic structure (dendritic spine) does appear to occur in LTP, whether branching follows or not is unclear.

2. Necessity for *In Vitro* Model System that Allows Long-Term Examination

Whether LTP proceeds to persistent synaptic enhancement supported by the formation of new synapses should be examined in the specimen that allows observation over a period of days. The acute slice preparation isolated from the adult rodent hippocampus, the specimen often used in the LTP studies, can be maintained in some conditions only for several hours.

LTP was first discovered in the brain *in vivo* [9]. And this LTP is shown to persist long [10]. Then, is the brain *in vivo* appropriate for examining the fate of LTP? Since living animals behave "at the animals' disposal" beyond the control of experimenter, the animals may voluntarily recall the "nightmare experience" repeatedly, as LTP-inducing stimuli cause epileptic convulsions. In other words, the experimenter cannot regard *a priori* that the LTP evoked by him/her persists by itself.

The specimen we propose as appropriate is the stable culture of hippocampal slice [11]. The hippocampi are taken from a newborn (within a week after birth) rodent pup, which are cut into slices of ~400 μm thickness and maintained *in vitro* aseptically. During the first two weeks of maintenance, the slices construct intrinsic synaptic connections according to their own genetic program and then stabilized [12]. The circuits formed within the cultures are equivalent to those in the acute slices prepared from an adult animal. LTP can be evoked by the protocols identical to those used in the acute slice. Yet, the cellular phenomena that occur in consequence of stimulation can be pursued by physiological, morphological, biochemical and genetic means over weeks (even months) under the full control of the experimenter.

3. RISE, a Novel Persistent Synaptic Plasticity Phenomenon

We have successfully induced LTP in such stable cultures of rat hippocampal slice. For fear of bacterial contamination, we applied chemical means (100 μM glutamate applied for 3 minutes) to induce LTP in the synapses between CA3 and CA1 pyramidal cells (Schaffer-CA1 synapses). The state of enhanced synaptic strength (*i.e.* LTP) lasted for 2-4 hours but disappeared in 24 hours. Structural change (increase in the number of synaptophysin-immunoreactive spot) coupled with LTP induction was also observed immediately after the stimulation, but became insignificant after 24 hours.

However, when LTP induction was repeated three times at 24-hour intervals, the situation changed [13]. Although the all three LTP also disappeared, synaptic enhancement began to develop gradually after the disappearance of the third, with the synaptic strength reaching a significantly enhanced level at day 7 (the day of first induction of LTP was defined as day 0). This enhanced state lasted for at least three weeks (it should last even longer, since there was no signature of diminishment) [Figure 1].

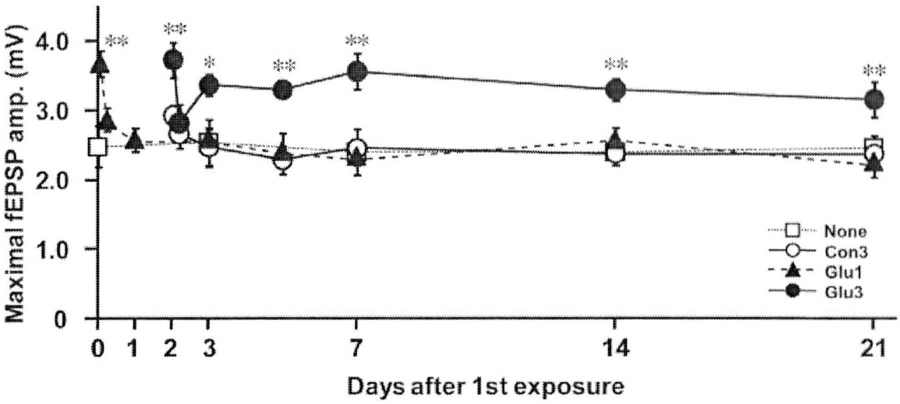

Figure 1. Increases and decreases in synaptic strength after single or repeated inductions of LTP in stable rat hippocampal cultures. LTP was evoked by pharmacological means (100 μM glutamate for 3 minutes in a milieu containing 3 mM Ca^{2+}/0 mM Mg^{2+}). The index for synaptic strength shown here is the maximal field EPSP (fEPSP) amplitude recorded at the CA1 pyramidal cell layer, which is the response to supramaximal electric pulse stimulation given at the CA3 pyramidal cell layer. The maximal fEPSP is shown as mean values of the values recorded from a large number of cultures. Morphological indices were also measured (not shown here) and found to behave in parallel with the electrical index shown here. Data shown are from ref. 13.

Immunohistochemical studies using the antibodies synaptophysin (a marker protein for presynaptic sites) and drebrin (a marker protein for postsynaptic compartments) showed this delayed synaptic enhancement was accompanied by an increase in the number (density) of synapses. Electron-microscopy confirmed the increase in excitatory synapses by observing the number of synaptic vesicle-containing presynaptic boutons that opposed postsynaptic spines equipped with PSD (PostSynaptic Density). We named this novel synaptic plasticity phenomenon RISE (Repetitive-LTP-Induced Synaptic Enhancement) to distinguish it from the canonical single-evoked LTP.

LTP that triggers the development of RISE is L-LTP (Late-phase LTP), which is known to be dependent on PKA (Protein Kinase A) activation. Lowering the dose of applied glutamate enables us to selectively induce E-LTP (Early-phase LTP). However, repetitive inductions of E-LTP do not trigger RISE. In contrast, applying forskolin, an activator of adenylyl cyclase that leads to the activation of PKA, three times in 24-hour intervals triggers RISE, but not if it is applied only once or twice [14].

4. Meaning of Repetition in the Formation of Memory

Three inductions of L-LTP are necessary and sufficient for triggering RISE. As judged from the synaptic strength measured three weeks after the repeated LTP induction, two times is ineffective, whereas four or five times is no more effective than [13] [Figure 2]. This then begs the question, what does the necessity of three times mean?

In "Conditioned Reflexes: An Investigation of the Physiological Activity of the Cerebral Cortex [15]" by I. P. Pavlov, the Old Testament in memory research, the necessity of repetition in the establishment of conditional reflex appears to be regarded as obvious. There is no mentioning on what is progressing during the repetition of training.

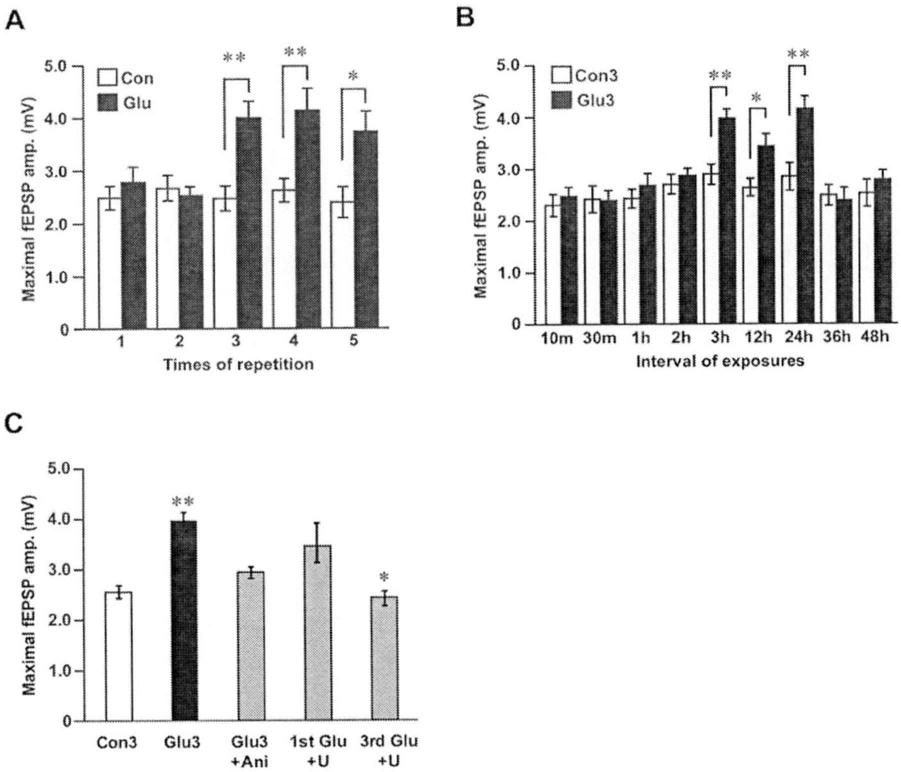

Figure 2. Pharmacological effects on RISE establishment Electrical index shown here is the same as that in Figure 1. LTP inductions using glutamate were done at days 0, 1 and 2; the synaptic strength was assayed at day 7-8. (A) Dependency on times of repetition. (B) Dependency on interval of repetition. (C) Dependency on protein synthesis and MAPK kinase activity. Anisomycin (30 μM) was applied for 2 hours beginning 30 minutes before each glutamate application. U0126 (20 μM) was applied for 2 hours beginning 30 minutes before the first or third glutamate application. Data shown are extracted from ref. 13 and supplemented by unpublished results from the authors.

In "The organization of behavior [16]", the New Testament in memory research, D. O. Hebb defined the "cell assembly" as a population of neurons that are activated by a sensory input and assumed that the connections between any two of them are strengthened by simultaneous activity. These neurons are either previously assembled or just incidentally activated by the input stimulus and thereby assembled at that time. By this assumption, both formation of memory and its recollection are explained. What real process did Hebb suppose by strengthening? In the Chapter 4 of the book above, a picture is shown in which the presynaptic boutons increase in number by simultaneous activity, suggesting that the boutons increase in number stepwise upon every repetition.

In the same chapter Hebb mentions the possibility that an activated axon could support the growth of contiguous cells and thus the cell assembly would grow in size.

The ideas are insightful. In this scheme, however, the effect of every repetition is assumed to be identical. Is that obvious? In other words, is it not possible that the effect of the second or the third experience would differ from the effect of the first experience?

We therefore applied U0126, an inhibitor of MAPK (Mitogen-Activated Protein Kinase) kinase, U0126 at the dose of 20 μM, but it does suppress the development of RISE when administered at the third LTP induction. Yet it had no effect when applied at the first LTP induction (Tominaga-Yoshino, unpublished observation), suggesting that the first and third LTP have distinct significcance in the development of RISE [Figure 2A].

Separately, cDNA-array analysis revealed many genes that are specifically up-regulated or down-regulated specifically after the second LTP or third LTP [17]. This result suggests that an orderly expression of distinct genes with each LTP induction leads to the formation of new synapses. In other words, the repeated LTP-induction may not result in a simple accumulation of the same effects.

5. Proper Intervals Should be Placed between LTP Inductions to Produce RISE

There is a remarkable property in the repeated LTP inductions for triggering RISE. That is a dependency on the interval of repetition. The LTP induction must be spaced 3-24 hours. Repetition with intervals of $\leq$ 2 hours or $\geq$ 36 hours are ineffective [13] [Figure 2B].

What cellular process does this 3-24 hours' interval reflect? The most straightforward interpretation might be the effective lifetime of some protein(s). The first LTP leads to the production of a protein X whose lifetime spans 3-24 hours, a typical for proteins. If the second LTP is induced during the lifetime of X, a protein Y is produced by using X. If the third LTP is induced during the lifetime of Y, a protein Z is produced by using Y. Z then initiates the process of synaptogenesis.

This is plausible since RISE depends on protein synthesis. Anisomycin, a translation inhibitor, abolishes RISE development [Figure 2C]. Still, this fact does not necessarily support the above interpretation, since L-LTP itself is dependent on protein synthesis. The above hypothesis can only be confirmed if X, Y and Z are identified, although there is already evidence suggesting Z includes a glutamate receptor subunit and cytoskeleton-regulatory proteins (described later).

6. RISE is Equipped with Input-Pathway-Specificity

To maintain aseptic conditions for many weeks, we usually induced LTP by chemical means to trigger RISE. However, this protocol induced LTP in the entire slice so that we could not discuss about the input-pathway specificity of RISE. Input-pathway specificity, the nature that plastic change occurs limitedly in the activated pathway, is one of the most fundamental requirements for a model phenomenon in a memory study.

To test the input-pathway specificity of RISE, we adopted a protocol in which the third L-LTP is induced by electric means in one of the input pathways after physically dividing the Schaffer collateral pathway by a knife-cut [18]. Utilizing the fact that RISE required three times of LTP induction, the first and second LTP was induced chemically, which was a compromise to the minimization of bacterial contamination. The result was that RISE was produced in the stimulated pathway selectively in fact. This result provides a further support to RISE as a useful model in memory study.

7. Morphological Consequences of Synapse Formation

LTP is accompanied by structural changes in the dendritic spines, the postsynaptic compartment of excitatory synapses in the hippocampus. Among those changes is a perforation, where the PSD transforms from its usual disc shape to a doughnut or horseshoe shape. Some investigators assume that this perforation is a preliminary step for the synapse's division and thus multiplication [19].

In our cultures as well, electron microscopy (EM) reveled an increase in perforated spines after LTP induction [20]. Then, if spine perforation would be followed by the spine's multiplication, the occurrence of perforated spines should decrease when the spines increase in number and newly-born small spines appear. However, our EM study did not observe this. After the spine number increased by the establishment of RISE, the perforated spines remained high in frequency. Even when small spines grew in size and the mean spine size returned to a pre-stimulation level, the perforated spines remained still frequently observed. These results suggest that the perforation might not be transitory form toward division but rather might reflect elevated activity of the synapse. In other words, new spines might form independently of perforation.

For example, we recently examined RISE effects by time-lapse chasing of single CA1 pyramidal neurons, finding that new spines sprouted from dendritic stems rather than existing spines divided into two (Oe *et al.* unpublished observation). This resembles behavior in the developing brains [21], suggesting a mechanistic similarity for synaptogenesis between fetal and adult brains.

8. RISE and Protein Synthesis

As described above, protein synthesis is required for the development of RISE. Thus proteomic differential screenings of proteins expressed after the second and the third LTP induction may help identify which proteins are responsible for triggering the RISE (*i.e.* protein(s) Z referred to in section 6).

A cDNA microarray analysis was carried out [17], which resulted in identification of >700 up-regulated genes specifically increased after the third LTP induction (taking a significance level of >20% increase as compared with the second LTP). In addition, >500 genes were down-regulated specifically after the third LTP induction(>20% decrease as compared with the second LTP).

Since RISE is a slow and large-scale remodeling of neural circuit, those up- and down-regulated genes (proteins) should include not only the ones related to the *cause* of RISE but also the ones related to the *result* of RISE. We are interested in the former genes (proteins), but it is practically impossible to check experimentally the functions of those >1200 species one by one, and in their combinations.

Meanwhile, one gene and one class of genes and their corresponding proteins attracted our attention. The one gene is *gria1* (gene of GluR1), which expresses a subunit of the AMPA-type glutamate receptor. When GluR1 makes a homomeric tetramer, a juvenile form of AMPA receptor that is Ca^{2+}-permeable is resulted [22].

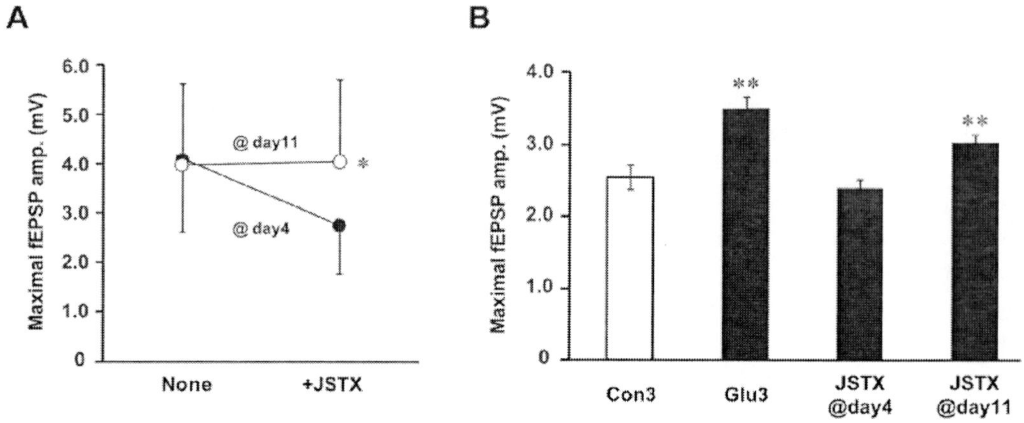

Figure 3. The Ca^{2+}-permeable AMPA receptor is both a cause and effect of RISE development. (A) Mazimal fEPSP amplitude before and after application of JSTX (0.5 μ¥M). Note that the JSTX-sensitive component was present at day 4 after the repeated glutamate application, but then became absent at day 11 (the day of the first glutamate application is referred to as day 0). (B) Blockage of RISE by JSTX (0.5 μM) applied for 1 day beginning at day 4 after repeated glutamate applications. Electrical index of synaptic strength was monitored at day 14. Data shown are unpublished results from the authors.

On the other hand, when GluR1 forms a heteromeric tetramer with a GluR2 subunit, a mature form of AMPA receptor impermeable to Ca^{2+} is resulted. According to the cDNA analysis, after the third LTP induction, GluR1 was significantly up-regulated, whereas GluR2 expression remained unchanged, suggesting that Ca^{2+}-permeable AMPA receptor (CP-AMPAR) is formed in newly-born synapses.

Electrophysiological examination revealed that EPSP (Excitatory Post Synaptic Potential) recorded during the developing phase of RISE significantly contained a component sensitive to JSTX (Joro-Spider ToXin), a toxin known as a specific blocker of CP-AMPAR [23]. What is more important is that the application of JSTX during that phase inhibited the occurrence of RISE as monitored 2 weeks later (Tominaga-Yoshino, unpublished observation; published in a preliminary form by Tominaga-Yoshino *et al.* ref. 24) [Figure 3]. This means that CP-AMPAR formation would be not only a *result* of RISE but also a *cause* of RISE. Ca^{2+} influx through CP-AMPAR may control cytoskeletal rearrangement, since Ca^{2+} is known to regulate polymerization and depolymerization of actin [25].

The class of genes of interest is actin-associated proteins. Cofilin plays a pivotal role in cytoskeletal rearrangement, since phosphorylated cofilin accelerates the polymerization of actin, whereas dephosphorylated cofilin accelerates actin depolymerization. The expression level of cofflin protein rose after the second LTP, and the phosphorylation level of cofilin rose after the third LTP.

These results suggest a scheme that actin-based cytoskeleton tends to depolymerize after the second LTP and tends to polymerize after the third LTP. The elevated phosphorylation of cofilin should be the encouraged expression of cofilin-regulating factors including *ssh1*, *limk1* and *pak4*, which occurred in fact [17].

9. LOSS, LTD-Repetition-Operated Synaptic Suppression, a Mirror-Image of RISE

In acute hippocampal slices, a low-frequency electric stimulation or application of metabotropic glutamate receptor agonist can induce an activity-dependent weakening of synaptic transmission strength, a phenomenon known as LTD (Long-Term Depression) in CA3-CA1 synapses [26]. This is robustly reproducible in the cultured slices [27]. The LTD in the cultured slice lasted less than 24 hours. However, when LTD was induced three times, the situation greatly changed. After the third LTD had disappeared, another synaptic weakening developed slowly, lowering the state of synaptic transmission for more than three weeks.

When we examined the culture undergoing synaptic weakening by immunohistochemistry using pre- and postsynaptic marker proteins or by electron microscopy, the number of synapses had decreased. We named this phenomenon LOSS (LTD-repetition-Operated Synaptic Suppression) to discriminate it from the conventional single LTD. Like RISE, three LTD inductions were necessary and sufficient to produce LOSS. Including the time-courses of development, RISE and LOSS are apparently symmetric long-lasting synaptic plasticity phenomena. This opposing nature may in turn gave a clue on their underlying cellular mechanisms [28].

In dissociated hippocampal cell culture, three repetitive activations of PKA at stimulations equivalent to three repetitive inductions of L-LTP, but not a single activation, leads to an increase in synapse density that quite resembles RISE [29]. This is probably mediated by the production and release of endogenous BDNF (Brain-Derived Neurotrophic Factor), since the application of a BDNF scavenging protein (a chimeric protein between BDNF-receptor and immunoglobulin G's Fc fragment) during repeated PKA activations abolishes this increase. Conversely, exogenously applied BDNF promotes this increase [30].

Recently, a precursor form of BDNF (proBDNF) was found to counter BDNF effects including apoptosis prevention and neurite extension [31]. Knowing this, we applied a proBDNF scavenger (anti-proBDNF/BDNF antibody) during the repeated LTD inductions, confirming the inhibition of LOSS development. Furthermore, masking the putative proBDNF receptor ($p75^{NTF}$) inhibited the development of LOSS [32]. These results concomitantly strengthen the theories that RISE is BDNF-mediated and LOSS is proBDNF-mediated.

10. Can RISE be an *In Vitro* Model for Conversion of Short-Term Memory to Long-Term Memory?

Behavioral examinations have shown that memory is not stored in the hippocampus but rather is transferred to and consolidated in the cerebral cortex [33]. Therefore, it is of critical interest to determine if RISE or RISE-equivalent phenomenon occurs in the cerebral cortex too. The canonical viewpoint that LTP itself represents the long-term memory is endorsed by the fact LTP occurs not only in the hippocampus but in the cortex as well (ref. 34 in the visual cortex, ref. 35 in the cingulate cortex).

To address this question, we established a culture that included the hippocampus and its target entorhinal cortex. In this expanded culture we confirmed that RISE-like synaptic strengthening coupled with synapse formation occurred in the cortex (Iijima, unpublished observation; reported in a preliminary form by Iijima et al., 2008; ref. 36). Currently, we are analyzing the time course and cellular processes involved in information transfer from the hippocampus to the cortex.

A more fundamental issue regarding RISE is whether it really relates to memory expressed in animal behavior. Such studies require examining memory-related animal behaviors by enhancing or suppressing genes related to RISE development. Genes for BDNF and its receptor TrkB are obvious targets, but their genetic manipulations have potentially global and profound effects in the brain development, as it has already been shown [37] compromising any conclusions about RISE. Furthermore, while RISE is distinct from LTP, it is not independent of LTP. Consequently, drug applications that inhibit RISE are not informative if they also inhibit LTP. Thus, the identification of RISE-specific genes and RISE-specific drugs independent of LTP are needed to strengthen any conclusions about RISE in behavioral memory.

As described here, at least in the system of cultured brain slices, single LTP brings about a synaptic modification that is durable for less than 24 hours, whereas three repeated LTP inductions lead to the synaptic modification RISE that is maintained for over three weeks and is supported by structural changes including synapse formation. Further analysis of the molecular and cellular processes during the LTP repetition should help reveal the underlying mechanisms for the two effects, providing important insight on the conversion from short-term memory to long-term memory.

This study was funded by Kaken-hi of the Japanese MEXT (Ministry of Education, Culture, Sports, Science and Technology) to A. O. and K.T., and also was supported by the Global COE program of MEXT at Osaka University.

CONCLUSION

1. We established a novel in vitro model system for analyzing the cellular mechanisms that underlie the transformation from short-term memory (instantaneous modulation in existing synapses) to long-term memory (long-lasting structural modification including synapse formation and elimination).
2. In organotypic slice cultures of the rat hippocampus, repetitive inductions, but not a single induction, of LTP leads to a slowly-developing long-lasting enhancement of synaptic transmission coupled with new synapse formation, the development of which depends on the times and intervals of repetition. We name this synaptic plasticity as RISE (Repetitive-LTP-Induced Synaptic Enhancement).
3. Proteins for cytoskeletal rearrangement are recruited after the third LTP induction, suggesting that the repetition that is usually required for memory consolidation is not a simple accumulation of the same effects.
4. A mirror-image synaptic weakening phenomenon coupled with synapse elimination is brought about after repeated inductions, but not a single induction, of LTD. We name this synaptic plasticity as LOSS (LTD-repetition-Operated Synaptic Suppression). The symmetric nature of RISE and LOSS suggests symmetric

opposing mechanisms for their development, such as effects of BDNF and its precursor protein (proBDNF).

REFERENCES

[1] Nicholls JG, Martin AR, Wallace BG, Fuchs PA (2001) From Neuron to Brain (4th edition). Sinauer, Sunderland.

[2] Bear MF, Connors BW, Paradiso MA (2007) Neuroscience: Exploring the Brain (3rd edition). Lippincott Williams and Wilkins, Baltimore.

[3] Ebbinghaus H (1885) Über das Gedächtnis. English translation "Memory: A Contribution to Experimental Psychology (1913)". Teachers College, Columbia University, New York.

[4] Rampon C, Tsien JZ (2000) Genetic analysis of learning behavior-induced structural plasticity. Hippocampus 10:605-609.

[5] Miller TM, Heuser JE (1984) Endocytosis of synaptic vesicle membrane at the frog neuromuscular junction. *J. Cell Biol.* 98:685-698.

[6] Smith SJ (1988) Neuronal cytomechanics: The actin-based motility of growth cones. *Science* 242:708-715.

[7] Matsuzaki M, Honkura N, Ellis-Davies GC, Kasai H (2004) Structural basis of ong-term potentiation in single dendritic spines. *Nature* 429:761-766.

[8] Eccles JC (1973) The Understanding of the Brain. McGraw-Hill, New York.

[9] Bliss TVP, Lømo T (1973) Long-lasting potentiation of synaptic transmission in the dentate area of the anaesthetized rabbit following stimulation of the perforant path. *J. Physiol.* 232:331-356.

[10] Bliss TVP, Gardner-Medwin AR (1973) Long-lasting potentiation of synaptic transmission in the dentate area of the unanaesthetized rabbit following stimulation of the perforant path. *J. Physiol.* 232:357-374.

[11] Gähwiler BH, Capogna M, Debanne D, MaKinney RA, Thompson SM (1997) Organitypic slice cultures: A technique has come of age. *Trends Neurosci.* 20:471-477.

[12] Muller D, Buchs PA, Stoppini L (1993) Time course of synaptic development in hippocampal organitypic cultures. *Dev. Brain Res.* 71:93-100.

[13] Tominaga-Yoshino K, Urakubo T, Okada M, Matsuda H, Ogura A (2008) Repetitive induction of late-phase LTP produces long-lasting synaptic enhancement accompanied by synaptogenesis in cultured hippocampal slices. *Hippocampus* 18:281-293.

[14] Tominaga-Yoshino K, Kondo S, Tamotsu S, Ogura A (2002) Repetitive activation of protein kinase A induces slow and persistent synaptogenesis in cultured hippocampus. *Neurosci. Res.* 44:357-367.

[15] Pavlov PI (1927) Lektsii o Rabote Bolyshih Polusharij Golovnogo Mozga. English translation "Conditioned Reflexes: An Investigation of the Physiological Activity of the Cerebral Cortex (1927)". Oxford University Press, London.

[16] Hebb DO (1949) The Organization of Behavior: A Neuropsychological Theory. J Wiley and Sons, Hoboken.

[17] Kawaai K, Tominaga-Yoshino K, Urakubo T, Taniguchi N, Kondoh Y, Tashiro H, Ogura A, Tashiro T (2010) Analysis of gene expression changes associated with long-

lasting synaptic enhancement in hippocampal slice cultures after repetitive exposures to glutamate. *J. Neurosci. Res.* 88:2911-2922.
[18] Oe Y, Tominaga-Yoshino K, Ogura A (2011) Local establishment of repetitive-LTP-induced synaptic enhancement in cultured hippocampal slices with divided input pathways. *J. Neurosci. Res.* (in the press).
[19] Toni N, Buchs PA, Nikonenko I, Bron CR, Muller D (1999) LTP promotes formation of multiple spine synapses between sigle axon terminal and a dendrite. *Nature* 402:421-425.
[20] Urakubo T, Ogura A, Tominaga-Yoshino K (2006) Ultrastructural features of hippocampal CA1 synapses with respect to synaptic enhancement following repeated PKA activation. *Neurosci. Lett.* 407:1-6.
[21] Kwon HB, Sabatini BL (2011) Glutamate induces de novo growth of functional spines in developing cortex. *Nature* 474:100-104.
[22] Ogura A, Nakazawa M, Kudo Y (1992) Further evidence for the calcium permeability of non-NMDA receptor channels in cultured hippocampal neurons. *Neurosci. Res.* 12:606-616.
[23] Tsubokawa H, Oguro K, Masuzawa T, Nakaima T, Kawai N. (1995) Effects of a spider toxin and its analogue on glutamate-activated currents in the hippocampal CA1 neuron after ischemia. J. Neurophysiol. 74:218-225.
[24] Tominaga-Yoshino K, et al. (2007) Involvement of Ca^{2+}-permeable AMPAR in the production of repetitive-LTP induced synaptic enhancement (RISE). Program No.147.3.2007 Neuroscience Meeting Planner. San Diego, CA:.Society for Neuroscience. Online.
[25] Stossel TP et al. (1985) Nonmuscle actin-binding proteins. Annu. Rev. Cell Biol. 1:353-402.
[26] Bear MF, Abraham WC (1996) Long-term depression in hippocampus. *Annu. Rev. Neurosci.* 19:437-462.
[27] Kamikubo Y, Egashira Y, Tanaka T, Shinoda Y, Tominaga-Yoshino K, Ogura A (2006) Long-lasting synaptic loss after repeated induction of LTD: Independence to the means of LTD induction. *Eur. J. Neurosci.* 24:1606-1616.
[28] Shinoda Y, Kamikubo Y, Egashira Y, Tominaga-Yoshino K, Ogura A (2005) Repetitive induction of mGluR-dependent LTD causes slowly developing persitent reduction in synaptic strength accompanied by synapse elimination. *Brain Res.* 1042:99-107.
[29] Yamamoto M, Urakubo T, Tominaga-Yoshino K, Ogura A (2005) Long-lasting synapse formation in cultured rat hippocampal neurons after repeated PKA activation. *Brain Res.* 1042:6-16.
[30] Koshimizu H, Kiyosue K, Hara T, Hazama S, Suzuki S, Uegaki K, Nagappan G, Zaitsev E, Hirokawa T, Tatsu Y, Ogura A, Lu B, Kojima M (2009) Multiple functions of precursor BDNF to CNS neurons: negative regulation of neurite growth, spine formation and cell survival. *Molecular Brain* 2, e27.
[31] Lu B, Pan PT, Woo NH (2005) The yin and yang of neurotrophin action. *Nat. Rev. Neurosci.* 6:603-614.
[32] Egashira Y, Tanaka T, Soni P, Sakuragi S, Tominaga-Yoshino K, Ogura A (2010) Involvement of the $p75^{NTR}$ signaling pathway in persistent synaptic suppression

coupled with synapse elimination following repeated LTD induction. *J. Neurosci. Res.* 88:3433-3446.

[33] Kesner RP (2000) Behavioral analysis of the contribution of the hippocampus and parietal cortex to the processing of information: interactions and dissociation. Hippocampus 10:483-490.

[34] Artola A, Singer W (1987) Long-term potentiation and NMDA receptors in rat visual cortex. Nature 330:649-652.

[35] Chapman PF, Kairiss EW, Keenan CL, Brown TH (1990) Long-term synaptic potentiation in the amygdala. Synapse 6:271-278.

[36] Iijima K, Oe Y, Tominaga-Yoshino K, Ogura A (2009) Is memory transfer reproducible in vitro? A long-lasting synaptic enhancement after repeated LTP induction in cultured brain slice. *IUPS Abstract* P1AM6-3.

[37] Lipsky RH, Marini AM. (2007) Brain-derived neurotrophic factor in neuronal survival and behavior-related plasticity. Ann. NY Acad. Sci. 122:130-143.

In: Short-Term Memory: New Research
Editors: Garifallia Kalivas and Sappho F. Petralia
ISBN: 978-1-62100-860-6

Chapter 10

CAV2.1-MEDIATED NMDA RECEPTOR SIGNALING IN SHORT-TERM MEMORY

Eiki Takahashi*

Research Resources Center, RIKEN Brain Science Institute, Japan

ABSTRACT

The Cav2.1 channel is highly expressed in the nervous system and regulates the presynaptic modulation of the glutamate release machinery. N-methyl-D-aspartate (NMDA)-receptor signaling mediates short-term memory. Because Cav2.1 and NMDA receptors are present at a variety of synapses, the use of systemic injections makes it difficult to evaluate the behavioral performance. In this regard, studies using microinfusions into specific neural regions are a useful tool to understand the relevant neuronal circuits. The antiepileptic drug levetiracetam has been reported to inhibit presynaptic Cav2.1 functions, reducing glutamate release. Rolling Nagoya mice carrying a mutation in the α1 subunit of the Cav2.1 (Cav2.1α1) demonstrate severe ataxia from about 2 weeks of age. Heterozygous rolling Nagoya (rol/+) mice show normal spontaneous alternations in behavior in the Y-maze test, a measure of short-term spatial memory. In this study, we have shown that a dose of levetiracetam injected into the hippocampus did not affect the controls but decreased the spontaneous alternation in rol/+ mice. The results suggest that the Cav2.1α1 mutation, through a decrease in the Ca^{2+} influx, lowers the threshold for learning impairment and that Cav2.1-mediated NMDA receptor signaling in the hippocampus is involved in short-term spatial memory. The combination of the sub-threshold pharmacological and genetic approach presented here is easily performed and can be used to study functional signaling pathways in neuronal circuits.

Keywords: Cav2.1 channel; levetiracetam; N-methyl-D-aspartate (NMDA) receptor; Rolling Nagoya mice; short-term spatial memory; signaling pathway

---

* Corresponding author: Eiki Takahashi, DVM, PhD, DJCLAM. Research Resources Center, RIKEN Brain Science Institute, Hirosawa 2-1, Wako, Saitama, Japan, 351-0198; E-mail: etakahashi@brain; Telephone: 81-48-467-5871; Facsimile: 81-48-467-9692.

INTRODUCTION

Voltage-gated Ca^{2+} (Cav) channels play an important role in regulating diverse neuronal functions attributed to elevated intracellular Ca^{2+} concentrations [1, 2, 19]. Two major Cav2 channel types, Cav2.1 (P/Q type) and Cav2.2 (N type), critically function at the presynaptic terminals [2, 37]. Cav2.1 is a molecular complex consisting of several subunits: α1, α2-δ, β, and γ [4]. The α1 subunit is essential for channel functioning and determines fundamental channel properties [4]. It has been reported that the glutamatergic system is one of the neurotransmitter systems regulated by Cav2.1 [17] and that N-methyl-D-aspartate (NMDA)-dependent processes are likely to be involved in the mechanisms of short-term memory [33].

Rolling Nagoya mice carrying a mutation in the α1 subunit of the Cav2.1 channel (Cav2.1α1) demonstrate severe ataxia from about 2 weeks of age [25, 27]. Although we found differences between 22-month-old rol/+ and +/+ mice, 2-month-old rol/+ mice showed no apparent decrease in short-term memory compared with 2-month-old +/+ mice using the Y-maze test [31]. However, the precise physiological role of Cav2.1 in regulating short-term memory has not been elucidated.

Cognitive impairment is observed in epilepsy and appears most frequently in patients with complex partial seizures [15, 36]. These perturbations may result from abnormalities in the neuronal circuits important for normal processing of cognitive processes, as well as from epileptiform activity in the brain [22]. Furthermore, antiepileptic medication may lead to a deterioration in normal cognitive processes [8]. Levetiracetam [(S)-alpha-ethyl-2-oxo-1-pyrrolidine acetamide] is an antiepileptic drug used to treat patients with partial and generalized seizures [5, 14, 23]. Levetiracetam inhibits presynaptic Cav2.1 functions, reducing glutamate release [18]. Our previous studies have shown that the systemic administration of a lower dose of levetiracetam to 2-month-old rol/+ mice results in spontaneous alternative dysfunction in the Y-maze test [33]. These results indicate that Cav2.1-mediated NMDA receptor signaling is critical in spatial short-term memory. However, because Cav2.1 and the NMDA receptor are present at a variety of synapses, the use of systemic injections makes it difficult to evaluate behavioral performance. In this regard, studies using microinfusions into specific neural regions are a useful tool to specifically understand the relevant neuronal circuits. Glutamatergic transmission within the nucleus accumbens and hippocampus is thought to play a central role during cognitive activity. We have shown that the local intra-accumbens or -hippocampal injection of NMDA antagonists impair the spontaneous alternation of mice in the Y-maze test [34, 35]. These results suggest that the NMDA receptor signaling within the nucleus accumbens and the hippocampus is involved in short-term memory. We have also shown that intra-accumbens injection of levetiracetam decreased spatial short-term memory [35]. This is likely to be due to the regulation of glutamate release by Cav2.1 in the nucleus accumbens. However, the precise physiological role of Cav2.1-regulated short-term memory in the hippocampus has not been determined.

In the present study, the relationship between short-term memory and Cav2.1-mediated glutamatergic transmission within the hippocampus was investigated using 2-month-old rol/+ mice treated with levetiracetam and observed in the Y-maze test.

MATERIALS AND METHODS

Animals

All animal procedures were approved by the Animal Experiments Committee of RIKEN and were handled in accordance with the Institutional Guidelines for Experiments using Animals. The rolling Nagoya mice were provided by the RIKEN BioResource Center with the support of the National BioResource Project of the Ministry of Education, Culture, Sports, Science and Technology in Japan. Male +/+ and rol/+ F1 progeny were derived from a cross between rol/+ mice and genotyped by PCR using tail DNA [31]. The mice were given free access to water and food pellets (CRF-1; Oriental Yeast Co., Ltd., Tokyo, Japan) and were housed under a 12/12-h light/dark cycle (lights on from 08:00 to 20:00) at 23 ± 1°C and 55 ± 5% humidity.

Drugs and Surgery

For the local infusion studies, NMDA (Sigma-Aldrich, St. Louis, MO, USA) (2.0 or 4.0 μg/μL) and levetiracetam (Sigma-Aldrich) (0.2 or 2.0 μg/μL) were dissolved in saline (vehicle). Under anesthesia and using standard stereotaxic procedures, stainless-steel guide cannulae (22-gauge) were implanted into the dorsal hippocampus (anterior to bregma, -2.0 mm; lateral to midline, ± 2.0 mm; ventral from the dura, -2.0 mm). Mice were allowed to recover for at least 1 week following surgery.

Behavioral Test

Y-maze testing was conducted between 10:00 and 16:00 by a trained experimenter who was blinded with regard to the mouse strains. Separate groups of male 2-month-old +/+ and rol/+ mice were used in the behavioral test. The light intensity in the testing room was 35 lux. The mice were moved into the behavioral testing room at least 2 h prior to testing. In our previous studies, we found that there is no significant difference between the strains in the number of arm entries and spontaneous alterations after this habituation time [33, 34]. The mice were injected in the testing room immediately after habituation. The mice were briefly (approximately 1 min) anesthetized with 2% isoflurane to facilitate insertion of the injection cannula on testing days. Infusions into the hippocumpus (0.5 μL) were made at a rate of 0.2 μL/min approximately 32 min prior to the behavioral testing. The injection cannula (26-gauge) was left in place for 2 min following the infusion. The mice that were not treated with levetiracetam received an equivalent volume of vehicle. The Y-maze test was conducted using a previously reported procedure [26]. The mice were placed in the one of the compartments and allowed to move freely for 10 min. The percentage of spontaneous alterations was calculated as: (actual alteration/maximum alteration) × 100. At the completion of the experiments, frozen brain sections were examined under a light microscope. The mice with injection needle placements outside the boundaries of targeted areas were excluded from behavioral analysis. To examine the effects of an intra-hippocampal drug injection on spatial short-term memory in the Y-maze, the following groups of mice were used; vehicle-injected mice (+/+, rol/+), 1.0 μg/side NMDA-injected mice (+/+, rol/+), 2.0 μg/side NMDA-injected mice (+/+, rol/+), 0.1 μg/side levetiracetam-injected mice (+/+, rol/+), 1.0 μg/side levetiracetam-injected mice (+/+, rol/+). Each group contained 12 mice.

Data are presented as mean ± standard error of the mean (SEM). Statistical analyses for the behavioral tests were conducted using Excel Statistics 2006 (SSRI, Tokyo, Japan). Data were analyzed using repeated-measures ANOVA with Tukey's test.

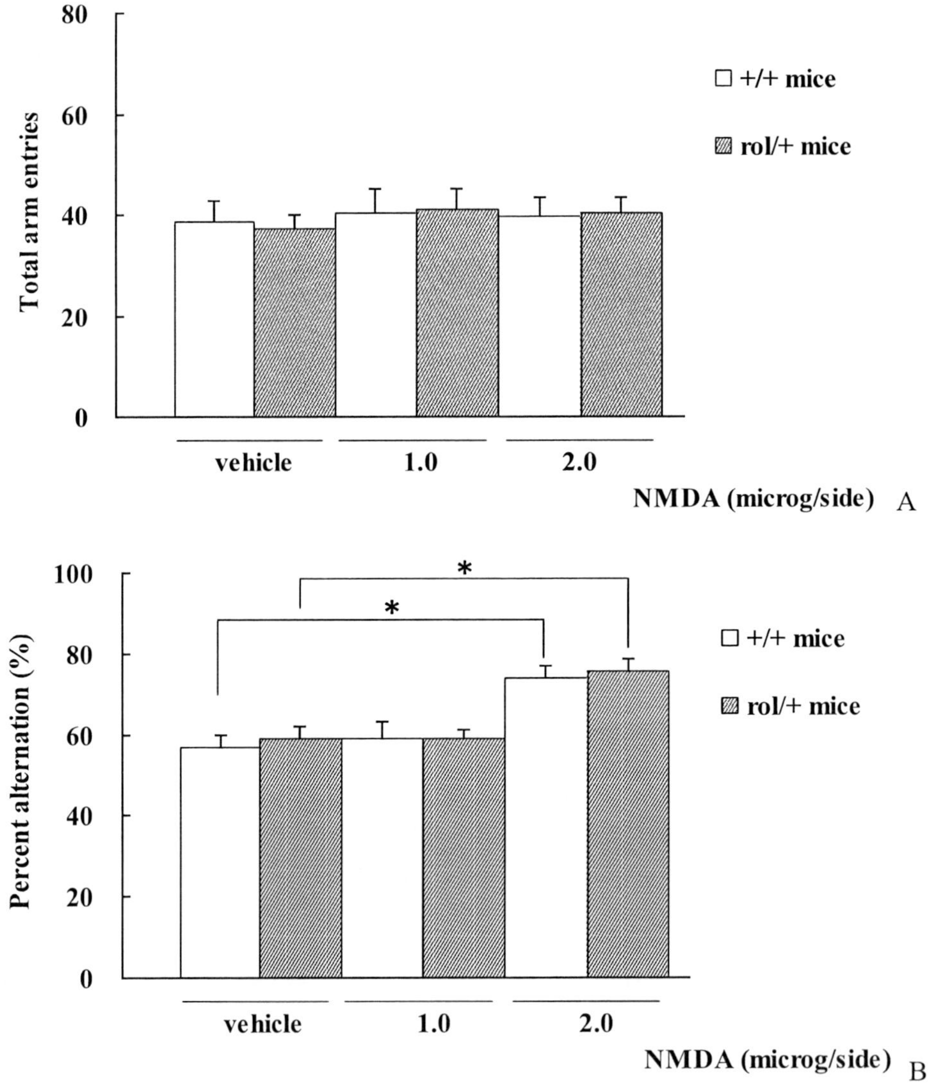

Figure 1. Effects of intra-hippocampus injections of NMDA on the number of total arm entries (A) and spontaneous alteration (B) in the Y-maze test. The following mice were used in the test: vehicle-injected +/+ (n = 12), vehicle-injected rol/+ (n = 12), 1.0 μg/side NMDA-injected +/+ (n = 12), 1.0 μg/side NMDA-injected rol/+ (n = 12), 2.0 μg/side NMDA-injected +/+ (n = 12), and 2.0 μg/side NMDA-injected rol/+ mice (n = 12). The data are presented as the mean ± standard error of the mean (SEM). * $P < 0.05$, compared with the appropriate control (Tukey's test).

RESULTS

Effect of Intra-hippocampal NMDA Injection on Short-term Memory

Regarding the number of arm entries following intra-hippocampal NMDA injections (Figure 1A), there was no significant effect of genotype ($F(1,66) = 0.285$, $p > 0.05$), dose ($F(2,66) = 0.034$, $p > 0.05$), or genotype × dose interaction ($F(2,66) = 0.121$, $p > 0.05$). Regarding spontaneous alterations (Figure 1B), there was no significant effect of genotype ($F(1,66) = 0.191$, $p > 0.05$) or genotype × dose interaction ($F(2,66) = 0.954$, $p > 0.05$), but there was a significant effect of dose ($F(2,66) = 7.911$, $p < 0.01$). Post-hoc analyses showed that the spontaneous alterations in the 2.0-μg/side NMDA-injected +/+ mice were higher than in the vehicle-injected +/+ mice ($p < 0.05$, Tukey). The spontaneous alterations in the 2.0 μg/side NMDA-injected rol/+ mice were also higher than in the vehicle-injected rol/+ mice ($p < 0.05$, Tukey).

Effect of Intra-hippocampal Levetiracetam Injection on Short-term Memory

Regarding the number of arm entries following an intra-accumbens injection of levetiracetam (Figure 2A), there was no significant effect of genotype ($F(1,66) = 0.271$, $p > 0.05$), dose ($F(2,66) = 1.811$, $p > 0.05$), or genotype × dose interaction ($F(2,66) = 0.222$, $p > 0.05$). Regarding the spontaneous alterations (Figure 2B), there were significant effects of genotype ($F(1,66) = 4.911$, $p < 0.05$), dose ($F(2,66) = 12.311$, $p < 0.01$), and genotype × dose interaction ($F(2,66) = 3.512$, $p < 0.05$). Post-hoc analysis showed significant differences between the 0.1-μg/side levetiracetam-injected +/+ and rol/+ mice ($p < 0.01$, Tukey). There were fewer spontaneous alterations in the 0.1-μg/side levetiracetam-injected rol/+ mice compared with the vehicle-injected rol/+ mice ($p < 0.01$, Tukey). There were fewer spontaneous alterations in the 1.0-μg/side levetiracetam-injected +/+ mice than in the vehicle-injected +/+ mice ($p < 0.01$, Tukey). There were also fewer spontaneous alterations in the 1.0-μg/side levetiracetam-injected rol/+ mice than in the vehicle-injected rol/+ mice ($p < 0.01$, Tukey).

DISCUSSION

In the present study, we used a behavioral method without reinforcers to evaluate whether hippocampal-dependent Cav2.1-regulated glutamatergic signaling has an important role in spatial short-term memory. To examine memory formation in rodents, various kinds of behavioral stimuli may be used, such as food for an eight-arm radial maze test, water immersion for a water maze test, or electrical stimulation for a fear-conditioning test [7]. Although animals learn rules through positive or negative reinforcement during the training phase, human cognitive performance is not usually tested with reinforcers such as intense hunger. Thus, cognitive tests without reinforcers would be more appropriate for studying the relationship between Cav2.1 functioning and memory formation. Spontaneous alternation is used as a measure of exploratory behavior and spatial short-term memory, which are related to hippocampal-dependent functions [6]. The Y-maze test is based on the spontaneous tendency of rodents to enter a novel arm more often than the other arms due to the innate tendency of mice to explore novelty [13].

The intra-hippocampal NMDA infusion had similar dose effects, enhancing the spatial short-term memory in +/+ and rol/+ mice, suggesting that the postsynaptic NMDA receptor signaling in the hippocampus does not impair rol/+ mice. The Ca^{2+} current amplitude exhibited a 40% reduction in the homozygous rolling Nagoya mice compared with wild-type controls [25]. This result suggests that the Cav2.1 mutation in rol/+ mice may result in a decreased Ca^{2+} influx and lower the threshold for glutamate release, thereby playing a role in cognitive impairment. This possibility was confirmed using systemic injections of a combination of sub-threshold doses of levetiracetam in the Y-maze test, which triggers a short-term memory deficit in rol/+ mice, but not in wild-type controls [33]. In the present study, intra-hippocampal injections of levetiracetam (1.0 μg/side) decreased spatial cognition in the wild-type control and rol/+ mice. However, intra-hippocampal injections of levetiracetam (0.1 μg/side) had no effect on spatial cognition in the wild-type controls, but it impaired spontaneous alternation behavior in rol/+ mice. A previous study showed that a combination of intra-accumbens sub-threshold doses of levetiracetam induced a short-term memory deficit in the rol/+ mice, but not in wild-type controls [35]. Systemic injections of a combination of sub-threshold doses of the NMDA receptor antagonist MK-801 in the Y-maze test triggered a short-term memory deficit in the rol/+ mice but not in the wild-type controls [31]. Intra-hippocampal and -accumbens injection of a combination of sub-threshold doses of MK-801 did not affect the controls but decreased spatial cognition in rol/+ mice [34, 35]. These results indicated that the hippocampus and nucleus accumbens are important regions in spatial short-term memory formation and that spatial short-term memory information within both regions is processed by Cav2.1-regulated glutamatergic transmission.

Levetiracetam specifically binds to SV2A, a protein abundant on synaptic vesicles [16, 21], and reduces glutamate release [18]. We have shown that a dose of levetiracetam that was ineffective in wild-type controls blocked spatial short-term memory in rol/+ mice. Therefore, the interaction between Cav2.1 and SV2A is important in glutamate release, and the combination of sub-threshold doses for a decrease in Ca^{2+} influx and synaptic vesicle function on the presynapse lowers the threshold for glutamate release and spatial short-term memory impairment. Because SV2A interacts with synaptotagmin 1 to enhance the release of neurotransmitters, different sub-threshold doses or different drugs might have different effects on signaling, leading to various phenotypes [16, 21].

It has been reported that glutamatergic afferents from the hippocampus provide the main source of information to the nucleus accumbens during several types of cognitive activity [11, 12, 29, 30]. Ca^{2+} influx via the channels triggers neurotransmitter production and release in a cooperative process with other components of neurotransmitter-biosynthesizing enzyme activation and vesicle fusion machineries [2, 3, 24]. Given the pivotal role of Ca^{2+} channels in controlling neurotransmitter production and release, defects in the expression, localization, structure, or modulation of presynaptic Ca^{2+} channels may result in aberrant glutamatergic signaling, leading to various patterns of neural network dysfunction. We have shown that Cav2.1-regulated glutamatergic signaling in the hippocampus and nucleus accumbens is important in short-term spatial learning. An interesting question is whether there are differences in the effects observed after manipulation of the hippocampus and nucleus accumbens.

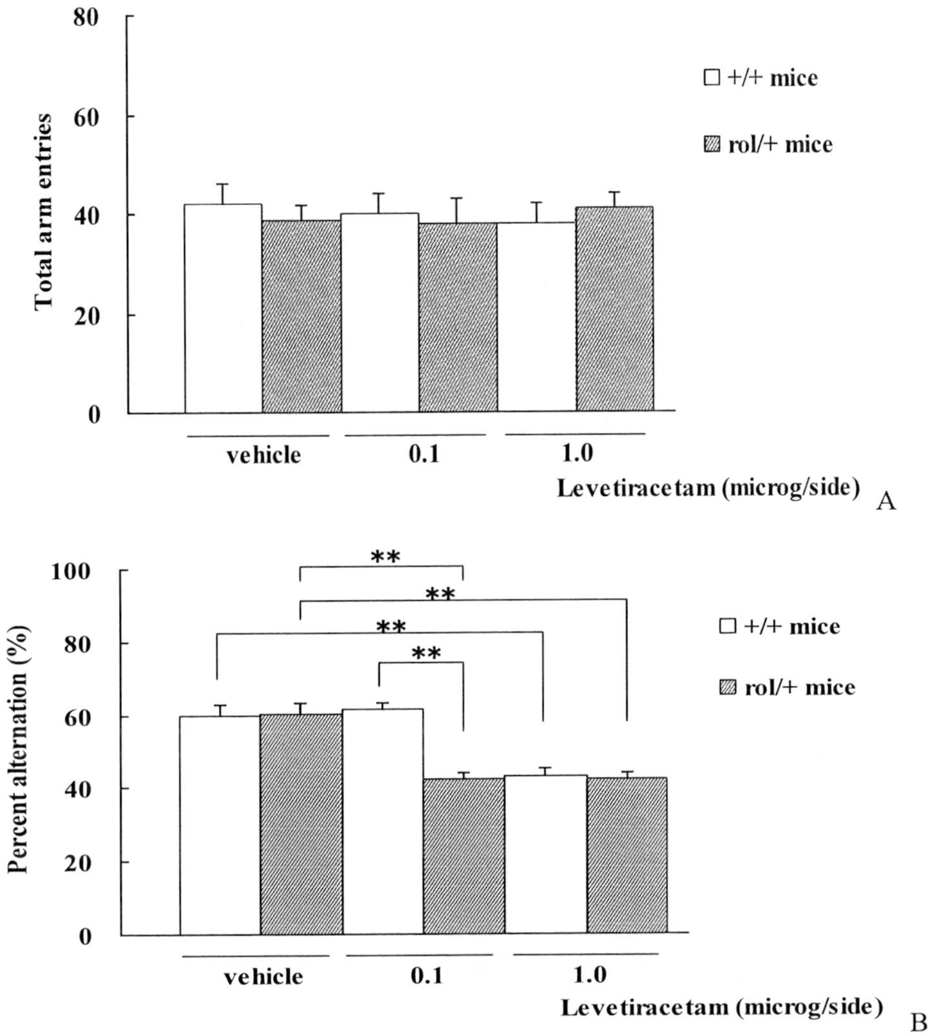

Figure 2. The effects of intra-hippocampus injections of levetiracetam on the number of total arm entries (A) and spontaneous alteration (B) in the Y-maze test. The following mice were used in the test: vehicle-injected +/+ (n = 12), vehicle-injected rol/+ (n = 12), 0.1 μg/side levetiracetam-injected +/+ (n = 12), 0.1 μg/side levetiracetam-injected rol/+ (n = 12), 1.0 μg/side levetiracetam-injected +/+ (n = 12), and 1.0 μg/side levetiracetam-injected rol/+ mice (n = 12). The data are presented as the mean ± standard error of the mean (SEM). ** $P < 0.01$, compared with the appropriate control (Tukey's test).

The hippocampus is involved in object-location memory, a measure of short-term spatial memory [9]. Sub-threshold doses of levetiracetam and NMDA receptor antagonist CPP, which are effective when administered separately at threshold doses, have a combined effect on memory in the object-location test [33], indicating that Cav2.1-mediated NMDA-receptor signaling is likely to be important in the hippocampus-dependent short-term memory. Therefore, the use of sub-threshold doses of pharmacological agents in combination is also useful in analyzing functional signaling pathways in neuronal circuits. Reported mutations of the Cav2.1α1 gene in mice include leaner and tottering, as well as rolling [28]; leaner has a mutation in a splice donor consensus sequence, which results in altered C-terminal sequences [10], and tottering has a mutation in the S4–S5 linker of domain II [10]. The P-type Ca^{2+} current amplitude in homozygous tottering and leaner mice was reduced by 25% and 75%, respectively, compared with that in wild-type controls [20, 25]. The severity of ataxia differs in the order leaner mice > tottering mice > rolling mice [10]. Whereas homozygous leaner and tottering mice exhibit seizures similar to human epilepsy, rolling mice do not [10]. Nevertheless, none of the heterozygous leaner, tottering, or rolling mice exhibited apparent behavioral abnormalities. These results indicate that the threshold dose for phenotypes differ in different mutants. In a previous study, 22-month-old rol/+ mice demonstrated decreased spatial short-term memory in the Y maze test compared with 22-month-old +/+ mice, although we found no difference between 2-month-old +/+ and rol/+ mice [31]. Expression analyses showed that the mutant-type Cav2.1α1 mRNA was expressed at a higher level in the 22-month-old than in the 2-month-old rol/+ mice [32]. One of the factors contributing to a deficit in memory formation in the 22-month-old rol/+ mice would be an age-related increase in mutant-type Cav2.1α1 expression, resulting in a decline in the depolarization-induced Ca^{2+} influx through Cav2.1 channels and a deficit in memory formation. These results indicate that the mutant-type Cav2.1α1 expression dosage in the 2-month-old rol/+ mice is a sub-threshold dose. Consequently, a detailed comparison of combinations of allelic variants, pharmacological concentrations, local infusion regions, and gene expression dosages may be helpful in understanding the relationships among the many different biophysical, structural, and synaptic signaling abnormalities and observed behavioral deficits.

In the present study, intra-hippocampal injections of levetiracetam (0.1 μg/side) were ineffective in wild-type controls but disrupted spatial short-term memory in rol/+ mice. These findings, using local infusions, demonstrate that alterations in genetic structure combined with sub-threshold doses of pharmacological agents can be useful for inducing the effects of phenotypes in silent mutants and for identifying functional signaling pathways. In particular, rol/+ mice given microinfusions with selective glutamatergic compounds in specific regions, such as the hippocampus, may be a useful model for delineating changes in memory associated with Cav2.1-mediated signal transduction.

Conclusion

Neuronal voltage-dependent Cav2.1 channel mediates the presynaptic machinery for vesicular release of neurotransmitters. Rolling Nagoya mice carrying Cav2.1α1 gene mutation show ataxia, whereas rol/+ mice do not show abnormal behavior in the Y-maze test, which is a measure of spatial short-term memory. NMDA-dependent processes are involved in the mechanisms of short-term memory. Levetiracetam inhibits presynaptic Cav2.1 functions, reducing glutamate release. In the present study, to examine the relationship between hippocampal-dependent Cav2.1-mediated synaptic transmission and short-term memory, we conducted the Y-maze test using rol/+ mice treated with NMDA or levetiracetam. Similar spontaneous alternation patterns were noted in wild-type and rol/+ mice after intra-hippocampal injection with NMDA (0–2.0 μg/side). Intra-hippocampal injections of levetiracetam (0.1 μg/side), which had no effect in wild-type controls, decreased spatial cognition in rol/+ mice. Intra-hippocampal injections of levetiracetam (1.0 μg/side) decreased spatial cognition in both genotypes. The study presented here demonstrates the importance of hippocampal Cav2.1/NMDAR signaling in spatial short-term memory. These results also indicate that Cav2.1α1 mutations lowers the threshold for short-term memory impairment, probably through the decrease in Ca^{2+} influx, and that the combination sub-threshold pharmacological and genetic approach is useful to study functional pathways in neuronal circuits.

REFERENCES

[1] Berridge MJ, Lipp P, Bootman MD. The versatility and universality of calcium signalling. *Nat Rev Mol Cell Biol.* 2000. 1:11-21.

[2] Catterall WA. Structure and function of neuronal Ca^{2+} channels and their role in neurotransmitter release. *Cell Calcium.* 1998. 24:307-323.

[3] Catterall WA. Interactions of presynaptic Ca^{2+} channels and snare proteins in neurotransmitter release. *Ann NY Acad Sci.* 1999. 868:144-159.

[4] Catterall WA and Few AP. Ca2+ channel regulation and presynaptic plasticity. *Neuron.* 2008. 59:882-901.

[5] Cereghino JJ, Biton V, Abou-Khalil B, Dreifuss F, Gauer LJ, Leppik I. Levetiracetam for partial seizures: results of a double-blind, randomized clinical trial. *Neurology.* 2000. 55:236-442.

[6] Conrad, CD, Grote KA, Hobbs RJ, Ferayorni A. Sex differences in spatial and nonspatial Y-maze performance after chronic stress. *Neurobiol Learn Mem.* 2003. 79:32-40.

[7] Crawley JN. Learning and Memory. In: Crawley JN, editor. What's wrong with my mouse? Behavioral phenotyping of transgenic and knockout mice. New York. *Wiley-Liss.* 1992. 83-130.

[8] Devinsky O. Cognitive and behavioral effects of antiepileptic drugs. *Epilepsia.* 1995. 36:S46-S65.

[9] Ennaceur A, Neave N, Aggleton JP. Spontaneous object recognition and object location memory in rats: the effects of lesions in the cingulate cortices, the medial prefrontal cortex, the cingulum bundle and the fornix. *Exp. Brain Res.* 1997. 113:509-519.

[10] Fletcher CF, Lutz CM, O'Sullivan TN, Shaughnessy JDJ, Hawkes R, Frankel WN, Copeland NG, Jenkins NA. Absence epilepsy in tottering mutant mice is associated with calcium channel defects. *Cell.* 1996. 87:607-617.

[11] Floresco SB, Seamans JK, Phillips AG. Differential effects of lidocaine infusions into the ventral CA1/subiculum or the nucleus accumbens on the acquisition and retention of spatial information. *Behav Brain Res.* 1996. 81:163-171.

[12] Friedman DP, Aggleton JP, Saunders RC. Comparison of hippocampal, amygdala, and perirhinal projections to the nucleus accumbens: combined anterograde and retrograde tracing study in the Macaque brain. *J Comp Neurol.* 2002. 450:345-365.

[13] Granon S, Save E, Buhot MC, Poucet B. Effortful information processing in a spontaneous spatial situation by rats with medial prefrontal lesions. *Behav Brain Res.* 1996. 78:147-154.

[14] Grant R., Shorvon SD. Efficacy and tolerability of 1000-4000mg per day of Levetiracetam as add-on therapy in patients with refractory epilepsy. *Epilepsy Res.* 2000. 42:89-95.

[15] Hermann B, Wyler A, Somes G, Berry A, Dohan F. Pathological status of the mesial temporal lobe predicts memory outcome from left anterior lobectomy. *Neurosurgery.* 1992. 31:652-657.

[16] Janz R, Goda Y, Geppert M, Missler M, Sudhof TC. SV2A and SV2B function as redundant calcium regulators in neurotransmitter release. *Neuron.* 1992. 24:1003-1016.

[17] Jarvis SE, Zamponi GW. Trafficking and regulation of neuronal voltage-gated calcium channels. *Curr Opin Cell Biol.* 2007. 19:474-482.

[18] Lee CY, Chen CC, Liou HH. Levetiracetam inhibits glutamate transmission through presynaptic P/Q-type calcium channels on the granule cells of the dentate gyrus. *Br J Pharmacol.* 2009. 158:1753-1762.

[19] Liu L, Zwingman TA, Fletcher CF. In vivo analysis of voltage-dependent calcium channels. *J Bioenerg Biomembr.* 2003. 35:671-865.

[20] Lorenzon NM, Lutz CM, Frankel WN, Beam KG. Altered calcium channel currents in Purkinje cells of the neurological mutant mouse leaner. *J Neurosci.* 1998. 18:4482-4489.

[21] Lynch BA, Lambeng N, Nocka K, Kensel-Hammes P, Bajjalieh SM, Matagne A, Fuks B. 2004. The synaptic vesicle protein SV2A is the binding site for the antiepileptic drug levetiracetam. *Proc Natl Acad Sci* USA. 2004. 101:9861-9866.

[22] Lynch MW, Rutecki PA, Sutula TP. The effects of seizures on the brain. *Curr Opin Neurol.* 1996. 9:97-102.

[23] Mazza M, Martini A, Scoppetta M, Mazza S. Effect of levetiracetam on depression and anxiety in adult epileptic patients. *Prog Neuropsychopharmacol Biol Psychiat.* 2008. 32:539-543.

[24] Mendoza IE, Schmachtenberg O, Tonk E, Fuentealba J, Díaz-Raya P, Lagos VL, García AG, Cárdenas AM. Depolarization-induced ERK phosphorylation depends on the cytosolic Ca^{2+} level rather than on the Ca^{2+} channel subtype of chromaffin cells. *J Neurochem.* 2003. 86:1477-1486.

[25] Mori Y, Wakamori M, Oda S, Fletcher CF, Sekiguchi N, Mori E, Copeland NG, Jenkins NA, Matsushita K, Matsuyama Z, Imoto K. Reduced voltage sensitivity of activation of P/Q-type calcium channels is associated with the ataxic mouse mutation rolling Nagoya (tg(rol)). *J Neurosci.* 2000. 20:5654-5662.

[26] Niimi K, Takahashi E, Itakura C. Improved short-term memory and increased expression of NR2B observed in senescence-accelerated mouse (SAM)P6. *Exp Gerontol.* 2008. 43:847-852.

[27] Oda S. The observation of rolling mouse Nagoya (rol), a new neurological mutant, and its maintenance. *Jikken Dobutsu.* 1973. 22:281-288.

[28] Pietrobon D. Calcium channels and channelopathies of the central nervous system. *Mol Neurobiol.* 2002. 25:31-50.

[29] Sargolini F, Roullet P, Oliverio A, Mele A. Effects of lesions to the glutamatergic afferents to the nucleus accumbens in the modulation of reactivity to spatial and non-spatial novelty in mice. *Neuroscience.* 1999. 93:855-867.

[30] Sargolini F, Roullet P, Oliverio A, Mele A. Effects of intra-accumbens focal administrations of glutamate antagonists on object recognition memory in mice. *Behav Brain Res.* 2003. 138:153-163.

[31] Takahashi E and Niimi K. Spatial learning deficit in aged heterozygous Cav2.1 channel mutant mice, rolling mouse Nagoya. *Exp Gerontol.* 2009. 44:274-279.

[32] Takahashi E, Niimi K, Itakura C. Age-related spatial and nonspatial short-term memory in Cav2.1α1 mutat mice, rolling mouse Nagoya. *Behav Brain Res.* 2009. 204:241-245.

[33] Takahashi E, Niimi K, Itakura C. Subthreshold pharmacological and genetic approaches to analyzing Cav2.1-mediated NMDA receptor signaling in short-term memory. *Eur J Pharmacol.* 2010. 645:113-118.

[34] Takahashi E, Niimi K, Itakura C. Impairment of spatial short-term memory following acute administration of the NMDA receptor antagonists in the heterozygous rolling Nagoya mice carrying Cav2.1α1 mutation. *Behav Brain Res.* 2010. 213:121-125.

[35] Takahashi E, Niimi K, Itakura C. Role of Cav2.1-mediated NMDA receptor signaling in the nucleus accumbens in spatial short-term memory. *Behav Brain Res.* 2011. 218:353-356.

[36] Thompson PJ and Corcoran R. Everyday memory failures in people with epilepsy. *Epilepsia.* 1992. 33:S18-S20.

[37] Yokoyama CT, Myers SJ, Fu J, Mockus SM, Scheuer T, Catterall WA. Mechanism of SNARE protein binding and regulation of Cav2 channels by phosphorylation of the synaptic protein interaction site. *Mol Cell Neurosci.* 2005. 28:1-17.

INDEX

A

B

C

D

E

F

G

H

I

J

K

L

M

N

O

P

Q

R

S

T

U

V

W

Y